# Palliative Care: Explorations and Challenges

*Edited by*

Judith M. Parker and Sanchia Aranda
University of Melbourne

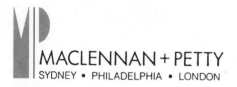

MACLENNAN + PETTY
SYDNEY • PHILADELPHIA • LONDON

*First published 1998*
*Reprinted 2000*

MacLennan & Petty Pty Limited
PO Box 145, Rosebery, Sydney NSW 1445, Australia

National Library of Australia
Cataloguing-in-Publication data:

Palliative care: explorations and challenges

Bibliography
Includes index

ISBN 0 86433 120 7

1. Palliative treatment. 2. Terminal care. 3. Nursing.
I. Parker, J. M. (Judith Milburn), 1936– .
II. Aranda, Sanchia.
610.7361

Printed and bound in Australia

# Contents

## Part I   Exploring Palliative Care

## Part II   Death and Caring for the Dying

## Part III Challenges in Context

# Foreword

*Palliative Care: Explorations and Challenges* is not a timid book. Rather, it is a book that challenges traditional ideas about terminal illness and care of the dying. The authors examine difficult questions about palliative care that are currently being discussed and debated in many countries. Questions about improved accessibility to palliative care, alternative models of palliative care, and cost effective delivery of palliative care services are posed.

Dr Parker frames the book thoughtfully in the first chapter, providing a helpful historical context within which to place current debates about palliative care. The notion of the human body as a de-spiritualised commodity cared for within a healthcare system governed increasingly by marketplace forces, provides the reader with a cogent analysis of the context within which debates about provision of palliative care are occurring. Underpinning these debates are a number of pressures: the need for more integrated and accessible palliative care services, increasing expectations that economic factors associated with healthcare delivery be documented and controlled, a need for palliative care research to guide practice and verify care outcomes, a recognition of current limits in palliative care knowledge, and a steady commitment to a palliative care model that honours existential and spiritual concerns as well as symptom management and illness-specific needs. These issues are considered from the perspectives of the individual practitioner, educator, researcher, and healthcare administrator. Implications for clinical practice, healthcare policy, palliative care education, and palliative care research are offered.

An underpinning theme that emerges from the text is a question about the complexity of palliative care services and the multiplicity of care needs to be considered. For example, to what extent does the palliative care system address the needs of individuals with different illnesses (e.g., Alzheimer's disease, AIDS). In many parts of the world (e.g., Canada), the fastest growing group of individuals affected by AIDS is young heterosexual women and their children. How well will our models of palliative care respond to the suffering of these individuals who have needs for highly technical, often expensive, long-term care? To what degree are palliative care providers responding to the care needs of individuals and families at different stages of the life cycle? In many parts of the world, the palliative care needs of children have been sorely under-met and under-studied. What efforts must be undertaken to redress this gap in the palliative care system? And as the demographic profile of our population changes toward one with an increasing number of older individuals, how will the current palliative care network and broader healthcare system adapt to accommodate diminishing resources of ageing family carers? Parker and Aranda's book calls us to consider innovative and responsive ways of providing palliative care to a broader and more complex community of patients and families.

This book also raises questions about the extent to which a 'generic' model of palliative care can serve individuals and families of different cultural backgrounds. Will questions about cultural differences related to care of the terminally ill reveal helpful practice information? Or, will we find that when it comes to death and dying, comfort and suffering, pain and hope, we are more alike than different? And if differences in palliative care delivery are indicated, how might such changes be sensitively and practically incorporated?

In addressing controversies regarding specialised versus integrated palliative care services, the book asks us to consider seriously the extent to which palliative care services are reserved for 'end of life' phases of care. Although the World Health Organization has proposed a definition of palliative care compatible with care aimed at treatment, current practice usually involves a 'lane change' from treatment aimed at cure to a palliative care referral when all else has 'failed'. This book challenges practitioners, educators, researchers and policy-markers to consider more effective ways of providing individuals with access to palliative care at various phases of an illness trajectory.

And finally, ethical issues associated with practice and research are discussed by a number of authors. Difficult ethical issues that arise in the clinical moment are described and the reader is reminded of the various ways individuals approach their dying. Issues such as euthanasia are also discussed, calling for informed and sensitive community debate about the relationship between palliative care and requests for death.

The authors are to be congratulated for an ambitious and timely book that makes a substantial contribution to palliative care knowledge. According to Carper (1978), care is informed by four types of knowledge: experiential knowledge of expert practitioners, aesthetic knowledge gained through sensitivity to artistic and poetic expressions of the death and dying experience, ethical knowledge developed through consensus and moral reasoning, and scientific knowledge generated from systematic examination of astute clinical research questions. A fifth source of knowledge, sociopolitical knowledge, has been added to this taxonomy by White (1995). Without an understanding of how change occurs at an organisational and societal level, health practitioners cannot shape the context within which palliative care is provided. *Palliative Care: Explorations and Challenges* draws from all five of these sources of knowledge and offers valuable analyses about how to respond to the diverse needs of those who require palliative care.

**Linda J. Kristjanson** RN PhD
*Professor, School of Nursing*
*Edith Cowan University*
*Perth*
*Western Australia*

# References

Carper, B. (1978). Fundamental ways of knowing. *Adv Nurse Sci, 1* (1), 13–23.
White, J. (1995). Patterns of knowing: Review, critique, and update. *Adv Nurs Sci, 17* (4), 73–86.

# Acknowledgments

The idea for this book came out of the many discussions we had at the School of Nursing at La Trobe University in the context of setting up and conducting a postgraduate program in cancer nursing and palliative care. We are very grateful for the support and encouragement we received, particularly from the members of the Cancer Nursing Course Committee and from Associate Professor June Buckenham, Head of School. We would also like to thank Professor G.J.A. Clunie, Dean of the Faculty of Medicine, Dentistry and Health Sciences at the University of Melbourne whose support has provided us with the time necessary to bring the book to fruition. An edited work is always a team effort and we appreciate the efforts and co-operation of the many contributors to this volume. They have all provided significant threads which interweave to form a rich and varied tapestry of palliative care. We are grateful to Jenny Curtis for believing in us and encouraging us to do the book. Our final and most heartfelt thanks goes to Carla Taines and to Anna Ingham, without whose editorial skills, patience, determination and sheer hanging in there with us, this work would never have seen the light of day.

# Contributors

**Jennifer Abbey** (RN, PhD, FRCNA) has been involved in aged care as a practitioner and educator for over two decades. She was until recently Assistant Dean, Research, in the School of Nursing, Flinders University, South Australia. Her PhD research focused on the culture of residential aged care, particularly as that culture impinges on palliative care and the treatment of people with dementia. She has been an invited speaker at national and international conferences on this subject. She sees the need for advanced specialist practice for gerontic nurses and is shortly returning to the clinical arena.

**Sanchia Aranda** (RN, MN, BAppSc(AdvNurs), MRCNA) has had extensive experience in cancer nursing and palliative care practice and education. As a senior lecturer in the School of Nursing at La Trobe University Sanchia developed a very successful Cancer and Palliative Care Nursing major within the Graduate Diploma in Advanced Nursing. She is currently the Associate Professor of Palliative Care (Nursing) in the University of Melbourne School of Postgraduate Nursing and the Centre for Palliative Care. Sanchia is a board member of the International Society of Nurses in Cancer Care and is a past chairperson of the Clinical Oncological Society of Australia's nursing group.

**Michael Ashby** (MBBS, MRCP, FRCR, FRACP, MRACMA) is Professor of Palliative Care, Department of Medicine, Monash University, based at McCulloch House, Monash Medical Centre, Clayton, Victoria. He trained in medicine and radiotherapy and oncology in the United Kingdom and in 1989 was appointed as the first director of Palliative Care at Royal Adelaide Hospital and Mary Potter Hospice. He was appointed to his present position in 1995, which involves clinical, teaching and research responsibilities based in a new purpose-built in-patient unit. His special interests include medical education, ethics and clinical pharmacology as it applies to care at the end of life.

**Helen Austin** (MBBS GradDipHSM) held a variety of positions for 14 years at Bethlehem Hospital including terms as medical officer to the Neurological Unit, the Hospice Unit and as medical director. During this time she gained experience in the care of people with chronic progressive neurological disorders such as motor neurone disease and multiple sclerosis as well as in-patient hospice care. In 1996 she joined the staff of the Centre for Palliative Care at the University of Melbourne and took up clinical positions at Caritas Christi Hospice, Peter MacCallum Cancer Institute and the Caritas Christi Order of Malta Hospice Home Care Service. Her particular interests include quality activities and the ethical dilemmas associated with the end of life.

**Katrina Breaden** (RN, MN, BAppSc, MRCNA) is a lecturer in nursing at the Tasmanian School of Nursing and teaches in both the undergraduate and postgraduate nursing programs. Her professional and research interests lie in the areas of hospice and palliative care, and she is currently completing an English National Board qualification in Pain Management.

**Rosemary Calder** (BA(Hons)) has been manager of Aged Services Redevelopment in the Department of Human Services, Victoria, since 1995 and has been responsible for policy and strategic development of state-funded residential, specialist acute, rehabilitation and other health services for older people since 1990. The funding and development of statewide palliative care services has also been a major responsibility. Rosemary has a background in sociology and has worked in health services and aged care policy research and service development for more than 15 years. Prior to joining the department, she was senior policy and research officer for the Australian Council on the Ageing for nine years.

**Ysanne B. Chapman** (RN, BNursEd, MSc(Hons), DipNursEd) has more than 30 years in nursing, with over ten years in the academy. She has worked in many aspects of nursing practice, favouring end of life care as her career progressed. Presently enrolled as a full-time PhD student with the Department of Clinical Nursing at the University of Adelaide, Ysanne is researching sadness as experienced by community nurses in their work with palliative clients. Ysanne's most recent academic appointment was as a senior lecturer with the Tasmanian School of Nursing at the University of Tasmania.

**Graham English** (BA, MA, DipRelEd) teaches in the School of Education at the Australian Catholic University, Sydney. His books include *I go in hope, Someone keeps sending me flowers* and, with Barry Dwyer, *Catholics in Australia: Our story*, and *Faith of our fathers and mothers*. His cartoons and illustrations have appeared in a number of books and magazines, particularly in *Women–church* magazine, a journal dedicated to a feminist critique of religion. He teaches a course in spirituality for palliative care nurses in the School of Nursing at ACU.

**Rosalie Hudson's** (RN, GradDipGer, BAppSc, BTheol, TheolM, FRCNA) nursing experience includes hospice/palliative care in both community and in-patient settings, aged care and administration, and she is currently director of nursing/manager of Melbourne Citymission Nursing Home. Rosalie has tertiary degrees in both nursing and theology and has published widely on issues of death and dying. In 1994 she co-authored *Unique and ordinary: Living and dying in a nursing home.* She is a PhD candidate, exploring the issue of death, personhood and community within the nursing home context.

**Roger Hunt's** (BM, BS, GradDipPH) views have been formed through caring for dying patients for over thirteen years. He is former chairperson of the South Australian Association for Hospice and Palliative Care and is currently, a senior consultant and clinical lecturer. His interests include epidemiology, clinical research, ethics, art and song.

**Olga Kanitsaki** (AM, RN, RM, GradDipWardManag&HospNsg, BAppSc, MEdStud, FRCNA) is the Head of the Centre for Environmental and Social Health Nursing, La Trobe University and teaches in undergraduate and postgraduate courses. Olga is also heavily involved with cross-cultural research, has served on many committees and was the founder of the Transcultural Health Care Council. Her services in nursing, particularly in the area of multicultural health, were recognised in 1995 when she was made a Member of the Order of Australia (AM). She is completing a PhD at La Trobe University School of Sociology, Anthropology and Politics.

**Susan Lee** (RN, DipAppSci, BAppSci, MBioeth, MRCNA) is a lecturer at the School of Nursing, Monash University and since 1990 has taught in the area of palliative care. In 1993, she developed a successful and well-recognised Post Graduate Diploma in Palliative Care. Since 1992, Susan has served on the Committee of Management of the Peninsula Hospice Service and is currently the chair; she is also on the board of directors of the Victorian Association for Hospice and Palliative Care. Susan has spoken widely on palliative care issues at palliative care, oncology and ethics forums. As a guest of the Japanese Society of Hospice and Homecare in 1996, she spoke at their National Conference on Community Based Palliative Care and visited palliative care services in Japan.

**Elizabeth Manias** (RN, CritCareCert, BPharm, MPharm, MNursStud, MRCNA) is a lecturer in the Faculty of Nursing at the Royal Melbourne Institute of Technology and a doctoral candidate in the School of Nursing at La Trobe University. Elizabeth obtained her general nursing registration at the Alfred Hospital, Melbourne, and later worked as a clinical nurse specialist in the intensive care unit of St Vincent's Hospital. As part of her Master of Nursing Studies degree, she investigated nurses' experiences and perceptions of 'Not For Resuscitation' (NFR) practices in metropolitan teaching hospitals. Her doctoral research involves a critical ethnographic study of the discursive practices of nurse–nurse and nurse–doctor relationships in intensive care. Elizabeth continues to work on a part-time basis in the intensive care unit of St Vincent's Hospital.

**Marguerite Menon** (RN, RM, DipNEd, GradDipHealthEd, BEd, MEd) graduated at Royal Prince Alfred Hospital in 1962. Following wide clinical experiences in medical, theatre, midwifery and nursing education, she lived in Spain and on return to Australia researched cross-cultural issues for migrant nurses (1987). Marguerite has more than 20 years experience in education, administration and public health. In 1995, she was appointed manager to establish the Palliative Care Education Resource Centre at Caritas Christi Hospice in Melbourne. Her doctoral studies are investigating the palliative care system in Australia.

**Margaret Noone** (IBVM) is a member of the Loreto Order of Religious Sisters. With a background in education, she spent many years researching the needs of families who have a child with a progressive life-threatening illness, in Australia and overseas. She worked at the Child in Need Institute in villages around Calcutta, studied theology at Berkeley, California and worked at the Centre for Attitudinal Healing in California as a family counsellor. After returning to Australia in 1985, she became the first co-ordinator of Very Special Kids and is now Director. While on a Churchill Fellowship in 1989, Margaret carried out research on families with sick children in England, Scotland, Canada and the USA. Margaret Noone has written and published a number of articles and is a regular speaker at conferences in Australia and overseas.

**Margaret O'Connor** (RN, BTheol, MN) commenced her nursing career in 1972 at Mercy Private Hospital in Melbourne and then worked in the community settings. Margaret's first position in palliative care was at Melbourne Citymission Hospice Service in 1985, where she worked as a community nurse before moving to Mid-Eastern Palliative Care Association in Nunawading (Melbourne) and eventually taking up the position of nursing co-ordinator. She is currently the director of Caritas Christi and Order of Malta Hospice Home Care Service at Kew. Margaret is currently enrolled as a Doctor of Nursing student. During 1996 Margaret became chairperson of the Victorian Association for Hospice and Palliative Care.

**Yvonne Panek-Hudson** (RN, DipHealthSci(Nurs), GradDipCancerNurs) is a clinical nurse specialist in Oncology/Bone Marrow Transplantation at the Royal Melbourne Hospital. Yvonne's major interest both clinically and academically is the provision of palliative care for the bone marrow transplant patient. This topic will be the focus of her MA thesis. Yvonne is also a sessional lecturer in cancer nursing at the Victoria University of Technology and assists in the co-ordination of the Bone Marrow Transplantation Module at La Trobe University.

**Judith Parker** (RN, PhD) took up the position of foundation Professor and Head of School of Postgraduate Nursing at the University of Melbourne in 1996, where she is charged with developing collaborative research, practice and scholarly endeavours between the university and the clinical practice domain. She was previously Professor of Nursing in the School of Nursing, La Trobe University where she developed, implemented and taught in postgraduate nursing programs and surpervised a number of PhD candidates. Judith has published in the fields of her major clinical research interests of cancer nursing and palliative care, and has established and is foundation editor of the very successful and highly regarded international refereed journal *Nursing Inquiry*.

**Claire Parsons** (RN, RM, MSocSc, PhD) was, at the time of writing this chapter, director of research in the Centre for Research in Public Health & Nursing and director of the National Centre in HIV Social Research: People with HIV/AIDS and Their Carers. Her background is in nursing, medicine and social sciences and she has published in the fields of public health and nursing, including works on women's health, cross-cultural issues in health care, and HIV/AIDS. She has taught mainly in medical social science, public health and research methods.

**Ruth Redpath** (FRCS, FRCR) is a Melbourne-born and educated medical graduate who went on to train in surgery and radiation oncology. For 14 years she worked within the British National Health Service, her last appointment being as Consultant Radiation Oncologist at St Bartholomew's Hospital and the Hospital for Sick Children, Great Ormond Street, London. In 1982, she became involved in the development of community palliative care services at Dandenong and in setting up hospital palliative care consultancy services. She was also responsible for establishing the academic unit at Monash Medical Centre with a particular commitment to teaching undergraduate medical students and recently qualified doctors. She has also contributed to government advisory bodies and has been president of the Victorian Association for Hospice and Palliative Care and the Australian Association for Hospice and Palliative Care.

**Jennifer Richmond** (RN, RM, GradCertGer) is a nurse and writer who became interested in palliative care after hearing Dame Cicely Saunders speak in Perth in 1977. Almost a decade later, via community and in-patient rural health nursing, Jennifer found her way to Melbourne Citymission where she nursed in both in-patient and domiciliary hospice services, as well as spending several years as a bereavement counsellor. In the past 10 years, Jennifer has written, co-written and edited a number of nursing publications, including *Bereavement: A survivor's guide* (for Melbourne Citymission) and, with Rosalie Hudson, *Unique and ordinary: Reflections on living and dying in a nursing home.*

**Bruce Rumbold** (MSc, MA, PhD, BD (Hons), PhD) is Professor of Pastoral Studies, Whitley College, University of Melbourne. Bruce Rumbold spent his twenties first as a graduate student in solid state physics in Melbourne, then in practical theology in Manchester. In England his research brought him in contact with the hospice movement. Returning to Melbourne he spent his thirties as a parish minister, and his forties developing a pastoral studies program in the theological school at Whitley College. During this time he maintained an involvement with the hospice and palliative care movement in Australia, and recently did further graduate work in health sociology. Now entering his fifties, he continues to teach at Whitley and develop his research interests in the nature and practice of care.

**Susan Sherson** (RN, CertCritCare) is currently a Nurse Educator in Staff Development and Equal Employment Opportunity Co-ordinator at the Royal Melbourne Hospital, where she had previously been a student, staff and charge nurse, and nursing careers advisor. She has also worked in Vietnam, New Guinea and the United Kingdom where she pursued critical care nursing. Her book, *House of love*, tells of her nursing and personal experiences as a member of the first Australian Surgical Team sent to the Mekong Delta during the war in South Vietnam. Other publications include *100 years of nursing education at 'The Melbourne' Hospital— A vignette of history* and *Always your voice will call*, a brief history of MacRobertson Girls' High School. Her main teaching interests are in the area of ethics as related to clinical practice. In 1993 she was awarded the Jane Bell Fellowship and travelled to the United States, the Netherlands and United Kingdom to study these issues further.

**Annette Street** (BEd(Hons), PhD) is currently Associate Professor and Postgraduate Co-ordinator in the School of Nursing at La Trobe University, Melbourne. Annette has conducted research and consultancies throughout Australia, New Zealand, Thailand and in the USA. Her current research projects are centred in palliative care, specifically around issues for nurses dealing with the changes to the structure of palliative care services and also for GPs caring for terminally ill people in the community. Her books *Inside nursing* and *Nursing replay*, along with her other published monographs, are used in graduate programs in nursing and education in a number of English-speaking countries.

**Anne Turley** (MBus) has been Director and General Manager of Melbourne Citymission Hospice Services since 1988. She is a past president of the Victorian Association for Hospice and Palliative Care, and past secretary of the Australian Association for Hospice and Palliative Care. She was a member of the Victorian Health Minister's Taskforce on Palliative Care and is currently a member of the Ministers Palliative Care Implementation Committee. In 1994 she completed an extensive research project on facilitating Continuity of Care for clients across service providers. Since 1988 she has been a part-time lecturer in pastoral care with the Evangelical Theological Union. She is co-editor of the book *The creative option of palliative care*. Ordained in New Zealand in 1977, she has a background in church ministry, chaplaincy and counselling.

**Kate White** (MN) established the first palliative care nurse consultant position at St Vincent's Hospital, Sydney and worked in this role for ten years. Kate was the first overseas student accepted in the ENB Course at St Christopher's Hospice, London, successfully completing this in 1988. Kate played a pivotal role in the development of the Graduate Diploma in Palliative Care Nursing at the Australian Catholic University, and she now works as lecturer and clinical research fellow at the Australian Catholic University and St Vincent's Campus (Sydney). Currently she is undertaking doctoral studies in the area of quality of life. She is also co-leader of the Designated Research Group in Oncology and Palliative Care Nursing at the University of Western Sydney, president of the Association of Palliative Care Nurses, and serves on several international editorial boards.

**Lesley Wilkes** (RN, CM, RnalCert, BSc(Hons), GradDipEd(Nurs), MHPEd, MCN, PhD, FRCNA) is Professor of Nursing, Wentworth Area Health Service/University of Western Sydney, Nepean. She has over 25 years experience as a nurse, nurse academic/researcher and nurse educator manager. She played an integral role in the development and implementation of the first university postgraduate program for palliative care nursing at the Australian Catholic University in 1987. She heads a funded research group of academics and clinicians at the University of Western Sydney Nepean focusing on palliative care and oncology nursing. Her publication record includes one book, chapters in books, refereed international journal articles and conference papers. She has managed some 15 research projects related to nursing education and nursing practice. Her research interests include caring, ethical issues for nurses, palliative care and oncology nursing.

**Patsy Yates** (MSocSci, RN) is a senior lecturer with the school of nursing at Queensland University of Technology and the Division of Oncology at Royal Brisbane Hospital. She has over ten years clinical and teaching experience in cancer nursing and palliative care, and currently co-ordinates the postgraduate programs in cancer nursing at QUT. Her research interests are in the area of psychosocial aspects of cancer and pain management.

# Introduction

## Judith Parker

This book explores some of the ideas that have guided and shaped palliative care principles and practices and that challenge some prevailing
notions underpinning the delivery of healthcare services to terminally ill
people. Today we are living in an era in which palliative care services
are being mainstreamed; that is to say, they are moving away from
hospice-oriented notions of care of dying people and coming under the
rubric of mainstream healthcare services with the emergence of a
new medical specialty, palliative medicine. Many chapters explore the
implications for practice of this shift.

*Palliative care: Explorations and challenges* is a book about many of the
complex, ambiguous, contradictory and personally threatening issues
surrounding terminal illness that confront policy-makers and healthcare
practitioners as we move into the new millennium. It is also a book that
provides important insights into aspects of healthcare delivery for those
seeking to understand health services in the context of terminal illness,
treatment and care. This is not a book, however, that attempts to provide
recipe answers to complex issues. Rather it seeks to demonstrate the
intricacies, the entanglements and the puzzlements that underlie our
sometimes simplistic and routinised practices in the provision of palliative care.

It is a book which, through its gaps, points to the need for much more
systematic research into the issues that distress dying people and their
families. The significance of the hospice movement has been not only the
emphasis it has given to the provision of more humane and holistic care
for dying people and their families. It has been one of the few contexts in
which research has been undertaken into pain management and symptom
control, particularly for cancer. As has been pointed out recently (Council
on Scientific Affairs. American Medical Association, 1996), hospice providers' experience shows that dying persons are far less likely to be
overwhelmed by existential anguish and spiritual concerns than they are
by fear of pain, loss of control, indignity and being a burden on their
families.

Yet there are serious shortcomings in literature on the management of cancer pain (Ad Hoc Committee, 1992); scant research has been undertaken on the management of the terrifying symptom of serious dyspnoea, and there is no systematic body of research literature on many of the very distressing symptoms that dying persons have to contend with, such as fatigue, hiccoughs, mouth sores, skin breakdown, constipation, incontinence, nausea and itching. There are ethical and pragmatic reasons for not undertaking research into these symptoms upon such vulnerable people, but, as a consequence, a systematic body of evidence-based literature which identifies best practice in palliative care has not evolved. This is an area that many of those working in palliative care are currently trying to address.

As is well known, the modern hospice movement has its origins in the work of Dame Cicely Saunders who opened St Christopher's Hospice in London in 1967. This was followed by a rapid expansion, with the hospice movement quickly spreading to North America and to Australia. The era that saw the emergence of the modern hospice was one in which there was a strong cultural avoidance of death and of intimations of mortality in western society. A number of factors contributed to this including changing demographics, advances in medical technology, the bureaucratic structure of health services and the cold war obsessions with nuclear annihilation.

Today we are confronted with more subtle forms of death avoidance as the demographic trends apparent in the 1960s intensify and we have ever more sophisticated medical diagnostic and treatment technologies available to us. We find ourselves in an increasingly market-driven and commodified healthcare environment in which commercial interests appear to be driving many of the decisions made about health care. We live in a world characterised less by political divisions between the left and the right and more by pluralisation and proliferation of multiple lifestyles in a global context of advanced information and communication technologies.

In this chapter I want to draw first upon the work of Philippe Ariès (1974) to show how our orientations to death are linked to wider cultural factors and to indicate how, by the middle of this century, death had come to be thought of as fundamentally alien. I then want to link this to the ways in which notions of the body have evolved over this time within western culture resulting, also by the middle of the century, in a medicalised understanding of both the body and of death. It was thus in a context of death avoidance in a medicalised culture that the hospice movement evolved. I also draw on more recent literature to suggest how, in postmodernity, death has been pushed even further away and the body has come to be thought of as a commodity. I then suggest that current health services are being structured in ways which reinforce and sustain these ideas of death and of the body, and that the main-streaming of palliative care services needs to be understood in this context. This raises questions about how the key values that led to the emergence of the hospice movement are to be retained or constituted anew in a very different societal formation. Finally this chapter points to how some of the issues raised in this chapter are addressed by the various contributors.

## Orientations to death and cultural change

The French historian Philippe Ariès (1974) points out that as cultures change, so do orientations to death. He identifies a quasi-static, orienta-tion to death that prevailed traditionally in the early middle ages in Europe, in which people were familiar with death. While sudden deaths of course occurred, people normally had time to realise they were going to die. One awaited death, lying down, facing heaven and ritually prepared for it, 'with neither fear nor dispair, half way between passive resignation and mystical trust'. Dying in this period was also a public ceremony in which family, friends and neighbours were present. Ariès describes this as a 'sort of vulgate of death'; it was ordinary, it implied a collective notion of destiny in which people accepted death as part of the order of nature. It is summarised by the phrase *et moriemur*, and we shall all die. It implies a notion of the person as part of a collectivity with no distinction drawn between nature and culture.

Ariès notes that while this attitude has never been totally abandoned, and indeed continues today among some communities, it became subtly modified among the literati in the upper classes, somewhere in the late middle ages around the twelfth century. It was at this time that writers and thinkers were rediscovering the concept of the individual in the writings of the ancient Greeks. Introduced into the old idea of collective destiny there arose a concern for the individuality of each person and with this, death gradually became personal and dramatic. There emerged more personal, more inner feelings about death, and a passion for being and anxiety about not living fully enough. As Ariès notes, '[d]eath became the occasion when man [*sic*] was most able to reach an awareness of himself'. He describes *la mort de soi*, one's own death, as revealing 'the importance given during the whole modern period to the self, to one's own existence' (1974, p. 55). He points out, however, that both of these orientations to death, the collective and the individual, demonstrated a familiarity with death. Whether death was understood as part of the order of nature or in relation to an individual biography it was known, comfortable, familiar; it was part of oneself.

Somewhere between the sixteenth and eighteenth centuries, he points out, a fundamental rupture occurred. Death was no longer a familiar aspect of one's being; it came to represent all that the individual was not. This break between the individual and death seems to be part of a wider division that was occurring in educated society at this time. Philosophers of the eighteenth century had absolute faith in the power of human reason and saw as their goal an enlightened humanity that would emerge through the development of human reason and culture. Everything not rational was cast into the realm of other and hence the strange mix and intermingling of death, eroticism, irrationality, beauty and a yearning for the other that characterised the romantic movement. Death was challenged and came to represent the erotic and the irrational, the violent and the beautiful. It came to be seen as other than self and linked to a new intolerance of separation and with this a passionate and romantic sorrow about the idea of death.

By the nineteenth century, the death of a loved one was accompanied by unprecedented and extremely ostentatious mourning, and importance was now given not so much to the death of the self as to *la mort de toi*, thy death. Ariès points out that while death had previously been a solemn event, it had also been 'an event as banal as seasonal holidays'. However, by the nineteenth century, death became omnipresent and was now accompanied by passionate and unique sorrow. Grieving people 'cried, fainted, languished and fasted' in an excess of hysterical mourning. He implies that this exaggerated pomp or ostentatious decor of death was a societal reaction to the weakening of the old familiarities people had once had with death. He argues further that by the twentieth century, there has been a flight from the idea of death. Death has become unnamable. In other words, the split between self and other (i.e. death) has been accelerated to the extent that there is a refusal to accept death; it has became shameful and forbidden. By the middle of the twentieth century, it had become, in the words of Gorer (1956), pornographic, so shameful and abhorrent that it could not be discussed or referred to openly.

One writer (Williams, 1966) undertook a survey of contributions to *Psychological abstracts* on the topic of death from 1931 to 1961 and reported that the evidence indicated that 'the universal fact of death remained a relatively taboo subject in Western culture and had, therefore, all the power of a repressed content seeking a channel of expression' (p. 420). In the 1960s and 1970s a vast literature on the topic of death avoidance emerged such that Kastenbaum reported in 1977 that 'every day it becomes more anachronistic to speak of death as the taboo topic it seemed to be only a decade or two ago' (p. 85). It was in this context that the death awareness movement developed in the United States fuelled particularly by the work of Kübler-Ross (1969). However, it is worth pointing out that Kastenbaum (1977) noted at the time that this movement was resulting in cosmetic rather than structural change and, as a consequence, more highly sophisticated forms of death denial and avoidance came into operation.

## The body and cultural change

While Ariès' work gives us insight into the ways in which death has been socially constructed over a millennium in western society, the work of historian and philosopher Ivan Illich (1986) gives similar insights into the historicity of the body. He points out that he had tended to think of his body as a natural fact, as outside the historian's domain, until, in a study of the twelfth century, he came to realise that 'each historical moment is incarnated with an epoch-specific body'. Bodies exist only in the context of a historical epoch, forming the felt equivalent of an era, to the extent that a specific group can experience the age. He says:

> In most periods, women seem to have different kinds of bodies than men, serfs different from those of lords. The first repairmen of the new windmills which appeared in the 13th century, itinerant mechanics, were shunned by city and country folk alike because of their feel. (1986:7)

A major influence upon how bodies have come to be understood and experienced in western society has been that of medical science. Since the rise of natural science in the seventeenth century, the body has come to be conceived of as an object like other objects in nature which are amenable to the investigations of natural science. The social context that saw the rupture between self and death has seen a similar rupture between the mind and the body. In modernity, the rational mind came to be regarded as the site of agency, as autonomous, free and independent. The body on the other hand was understood as passive and determinate; it was re-garded as separate, as an object to be managed and controlled by medical science. Philosopher and physician Drew Leder (1990) claims that medi-cine has been profoundly Cartesian in spirit, insofar as it is fundamentally concerned with gaining mastery over the threat of death posed by the mortal body. The body reminds us of our mortality and hence of death. My body may be mine, but it is not me; it is something else. In modernity, the body, like death, became other.

Ivan Illich suggested in 1975 that much of western society had become medicalised as a consequence of advanced technology and industrial expansionism in the field of medical care. In this context death too had become medicalised and separated from everyday life, surrounded by the trappings of medical technologies such as life-support systems. In revisiting his work a decade later, Illich (1986) points out that he wrote the book to highlight the institutional, social and cultural effects of the medi-cal system which he described as iatrogenic, but that he failed to recognise the extent to which the 'body-percept itself had become iatrogenic'. He 'overlooked the degree to which at mid-century, the experience of "Our bodies *and* Our Selves" had become the result of medical concepts and cares'.

In reflecting on the impact that medicine has made upon western society, he suggests that around the middle of this century, the medical establishment reached an unprecedented influence over the social construction of bodies. By the 1960s medicine had achieved paramount importance in determining what the body is and how it ought to feel. However, he argues that by the 1970s this hegemonic power of medicine had begun to wane. Medicine began to share its power to objectify people with other agents. More importantly, by the 1980s he claims, 'a new model has sprung up that engenders people who objectify themselves: who conceive of themselves as "producers" of their bodies. It is now but part of a new epistemological matrix in the process of being formed'. Interestingly, he muses on the fact that the post-Cartesian ownership of the body in everyday speech (my body, the body I have) is now being superseded in some quarters particularly among young people who 'identify' with their body and speak of the body 'I am'. What Illich was identifying in 1986 are some significant cultural shifts that we now refer to as the commodification of the body in postmodernity.

The epistemological matrix Illich refers to can also be thought of as the social formation of postmodernity, which shares many aspects of the social formation of modernity; but is also very different in a number of key areas. Postmodernity has a logic tied very closely to current socio-economic forms, changing technologies and the globalisation of culture. In the context of the ready availability of television, increased international travel and trade, and improved communication systems, many traditional forms of social organisation, such as social class, gendered roles and political systems have weakened as they have been influenced by a multiplicity of other forces. We now live in the new world order, which as Bauman (1992) suggests is a fully fledged form of social organisation in which consumption and the marketplace now occupy the central position.

In this social formation, lifestyle and consumer choice become the ways in which freedom is expressed in a society marked by fluidity and permeable boundaries. In this market-oriented culture, projects of body shaping and forming are being undertaken by a range of agents and it is not surprising that the body has become a commodity highly sought after by various purveyors, including those of medical science. Interestingly, if one conceives of oneself as a commodity, one may care for oneself, seek help when repair work is necessary but recognise that there comes a time when one has reached one's use-by date. Thus death becomes familiar again, not in the twelfth-century sense, but in a new way we are only just now beginning to comprehend. As Eric Wilkes (1994, p. 4) noted:

> No longer can the Christian foundation for hospice work be taken for granted. It is already attenuated in a society not embarrassed by sex or death now, but immediately ill at ease at any mention of God or spiritual distress.

# From warehouse to marketplace: changing structures of modern health services

Around the middle of the nineteenth century, the modern hospital emerged as a humane response to the need to care for the large numbers of indigent sick who had flocked to cities in search of work in the wake of the industrial revolution. Following the model set by factories, hospitals came to be organised bureaucratically around principles of scientific management and the production of goods using machines. Here work was divided into discrete functions or tasks which could be undertaken by interchangeable workers on an assembly line with responsibility directed upwards to managers. The organisational structure was hierarchical, functions belonged to the domain of clearly identified units and care was provided in discrete geographic units.

By the early part of the twentieth century, and particularly in the context of the Depression of the 1930s, hospitals opened to a greater number of people. Medical science developed dramatically, particularly following World War II, and the idea of hospital or institutional as opposed to home care became very influential. Thus it is not surprising, particularly in a cultural context of death avoidance, that the site of death shifted away from home to the institution. However, in a context where death was increasingly seen as medical failure, people who died in institutional settings tended to be given minimal attention. When nothing more could be done, they were isolated and simply left to die in a situation which has been described as the 'warehousing' of death and dying (Sheldon, 1961).

The hospice movement arose as a reaction to this, and as James and Field (1992) note, was unashamedly reformist, 'fired by the radically disruptive intention of altering the tenor of British society's care of the dying' (p. 1363). It obviously met a felt demand and quickly spread to other parts of the industrialised world. The term 'hospice' was deliberately chosen by the originators of this movement to evoke the mediaeval way-station for travellers and to differentiate it from hospitals. Work done within hospices, as Saunders said, was 'in obedience to the Christian imperative' (Stoddard, 1979, p. 74). It thus set out from the outset to proclaim its Christian roots and values, and to focus on the importance of holistic care of the unique individual rather than on the treatment of a diseased body. Over time, the term hospice was argued to be a philosophy rather than a place, and the hospice philosophy extended to community- and home-based terminal care. In Australia particularly, it has become secularised into palliative rather than hospice care, and remedicalised with the emergence of the medical specialty of palliative medicine and debates about whether it should be a specialised or generalist service.

These developments are occurring in a context in which we are observing a massive shift away from the industrial, bureaucratic and medically dominated model of health care, which was so pervasive around the middle of this century, towards one based on the market-place and notions of commodification, consumerism and accountability (Parker, 1996). Shaped by global economic, technological and demographic imperatives of the late twentieth century, today we are witnessing an increasingly commercially driven approach to health care. This approach facilitates an understanding of health as a quantifiable commodity to be bought and sold rather than as an inherent and intangible value to be cherished.

The consumerist orientation results in people who seek or receive health care being defined as customers rather than as patients. The term 'patient' implies an inherently unequal relationship which is bridged by trust in a context of care. The term 'customer', by contrast, implies a commercial relationship based on the principle of 'let the buyer beware'. Indeed, in commercial transactions, there is an explicit assumption held by the customer of self-interest on the part of the seller.

The requirement for accountability in health care is clearly linked to the need for cost containment in the context of greater consumer demands for services. Advanced information and communication technologies facilitate sophisticated systems of data retrieval and tracking, and permit analysis of the relationships between health outcomes and costs incurred. Standards and protocols for patient care can be established using tools provided by computerised clinical support systems. Hence the current push to mainstream all essential health services, including palliative care, so that they can be incorporated into the cost equation.

Within this approach to care, new flattened structures are being put into place aimed at the delivery of 'patient focused' services and the provision of 'seamless' care through a co-ordinated and integrated approach which breaks down the traditional boundaries between institutions and also between the hospital and the home. While in the 1930s there was a massive shift away from the community towards institutionalised health care, we are now witnessing a major swing towards home- and community-based care which is, however, linked through sophisticated communication systems to mainstream healthcare provision.

Palliative care is now viewed as an integral part of a co-ordinated system of care designed to cross previously discrete boundaries and link services across settings. It is now becoming clear that palliative care will only be legitimated through the establishment of performance indicators of improved outcomes. Costs can then justified. The research gaps identified earlier in the area of symptom control will thus need to be addressed, so that the provision of palliative care services can be legitimated on the basis of the quality of the outcomes.

## Challenges for palliative care

There are many challenges now for the hospice philosophy and the palliative care movement as it becomes increasingly absorbed into mainstream healthcare services. In choosing the mediaeval term 'hospice' to flag an approach to death and dying that was in marked contrast to the medical approach, the innovators of this system of care were no doubt also invoking the mediaeval sense of death as familiar and known, and the embeddedness of the dying person in a community of shared values. Mainstreamed palliative care services evoke a remedicalised approach to care, albeit in a more sophisticated and consumer-oriented manner. However, in postmodernity there are many orientations to death and a multiplicity of ways in which bodies are constituted.

Today we cannot turn to one system that represents shared community values. The global and homogenising forces of the marketplace paradoxically generate diversity and variability. While some of us may long for a return to the easy familiarity with death as was manifest in the middle ages, our current social formation is about multiplicity and difference; it comprises diverse traditions, ethnicities and lifestyles. It brings together many cultures which jostle against, challenge and rub off on each other. Our configurations can be no more than provisional, partial and incomplete. This suggests that the key values which led to the emergence of the hospice movement are today but one stream of influence among many in a very different societal formation.

How then do palliative care providers respond to the human need for care and community in a mainstreamed market-oriented service? Bauman (1992), I believe, offers a useful way of thinking about this in our complex and culturally diverse culture. He writes about the skills of the philosopher or intellectual in postmodernity, but I would suggest that these are also the skills required of the palliative care practitioner. Bauman suggests that in contemporary postmodern culture, the philosopher can be an interpreter, a mediator and a broker between many different lifeworlds and cultures. Within this multiplicity, skills can be mobilised with the function of facilitating communication between communities and traditions. It seems to me that a useful response to the competing demands upon palliative care practitioners within postmodernity would be to position themselves between the imperatives stemming from mainstream palliative care services and those stemming from the traditions and cultures of the people they are caring for. Productive hybrids of practice can then be constructed which attend to and respect a variety of traditions and which are also able to mobilise the positive instrumental benefits of the mainstreamed services.

## Issues raised

This book attempts to come to grips with many of these pressing concerns. In Part I, Rumbold's chapter deals with some of the issues surrounding the mainstreaming of palliative care services and the emergence of the medical specialty of palliative medicine. Rumbold is concerned that the two approaches of active treatment and palliation are incommensurate. He argues that technical expertise and holistic awareness must be kept in creative tension and expressed through co-operative practice if the ideals of the hospice movement are to be carried forward into services dominated by palliative medicine.

Aranda tackles some of the issues surrounding the espoused principles of palliative care, which, she suggests, mask the complexity of many practices in this area. She highlights tensions that may be manifest between the ethics of individual palliative care practitioners and the expectations of patients and their families. She argues that palliative care practitioners need to work not from an ideological base reflecting the principles of palliative care, but rather from a responsive base, working with individuals and families to identify what they want and responding to these wants. Kanitsaki tackles some of the issues raised by Aranda by noting that palliative care is a cultural practice which is a product of the mainstream culture and therefore has its basis in British culture and traditions which may not be appropriate for immigrant and refugee cultures. She points out that definitions of palliative care do not make explicit reference to cultural variability and warns that while people will acculturate, the experience of a health crisis can force them back into old and familiar ways of coping. She calls for a philosophy and practice of palliative care that responds to and reflects the needs of a multicultural population.

Ashby discusses some of the issues surrounding palliative care as a medical specialty. He points out that medical expertise is pivotal to palliative care. However, he argues that expertise in this domain does not involve an exclusive knowledge domain. It is rather a unique attitude, knowledge and skill mix which requires learning and experience. Both Ashby and Aranda make the case for the palliative clinical specialist (doctor and nurse) based on the unique contextualised blend of knowledge, skills and attitude or approach to care. Ashby argues that the specialist versus generalist debate is not helpful. What is required is education aimed at changing the way the medical profession deals with death and dying.

Calder provides a very useful overview of the funding context in which palliative care is about to be mainstreamed in Australia. She maintains that because of its early isolation from the healthcare reforms of the 1990s, palliative care is now positioned to lead the way in the development of policy and funding arrangements for integrated health service delivery to Australians requiring co-ordinated care services. Street argues that in the changing milieu of health reforms and palliative medicine, nurses need to be clear about the effects of these changes on patient care, and to use this knowledge in the formation of strategic alliances with their clients to advocate strategies that retain the key values of palliative care.

Thus Part I provides a broad overview of some current issues facing the provision of palliative care services within a turbulent healthcare milieu that is being shaped in part by changes in health policy and funding arrangements. Exploration of some of the tensions surrounding the mainstreaming and remedicalisation of palliative care services, discussion of contradictions between principles and practices of palliative care and consideration of some of the complex issues surrounding provision of culturally sensitive care open up many important areas. These all point to the need for professional care providers to have a sound grasp of the wider policy context in which palliative care is being structured and to use this understanding in working strategically and responsively with clients.

Part II deals with how practitioners respond to many of the painful personal and professional issues that surround working with dying people. English tells us spirituality is about listening to the rumor that there is hope, and that jokes, laughter and the goodness of others give us hope. He suggests that the nurse's role in palliative care is to look to oneself, to be well and to be there. Then, in the words of Juliana of Norwich, 'all shall be well, and all shall be well, and all shall be very well'. Yates points to the need for a supportive work environment and suggests that workplace culture needs to evolve further so to facilitate the personal and professional development of palliative care workers. Wilkes points out that nurses may have ideas of what constitutes a good death that are in marked contrast to what patients may want. Thus a more responsive approach to care can be helpful not only to the patient and family, but also to the nurse who can learn not to impose his or her own values upon a situation.

Chapman suggests that a critical issue for nurses who care for dying patients is that they often forge close relationships, the loss of which they then have to deal with. Nurses' closeness to death can affect their relationships with other people and they often feel alone and unable to share their experiences. Some find they question aspects of the meaning of life as they cannot simply put death behind them. Sherson reflects on the inevitability of death and the strategies we may adopt to avoid this knowledge, and the consequencs this can have for both the people going through the process and those attending them.

Hunt argues that the hospice movement has been linked to the church and notions of the right to life and a comfortable death, which has over-simplified many problems surrounding the dying process. He points to the similar interests that drive both the hospice and the euthanasia move-ments and notes that the topics of terminal care, euthanasia and death are no longer taboo. He believes that these topics should be addressed from the wishes and interests of each and every patient. O'Connor and Menon, however, in considering the euthanasia debate argue that there is still too little understanding of the symptom relief that can be effected by experi-enced and skilled palliative care practitioners.

Abbey maintains that in the context of dementia the philosophy and practices of normalisation suppress discussion of and preparation for death. Like Yates, she points to the need for changed work practices and suggests that because of habit, hierarchy and obligation there is a continu-ation of nursing care based on body maintenance rather than a considera-tion of issues involved in preparing for death.

Part II thus builds upon some of the ideas surrounding the importance of responsive care and explores issues that need to be managed and dealt with in this extraordinarily demanding field of practice. Caring for one-self, dealing with loss and grief, confronting the reality of requests for euthanasia and confronting work practices which suppress discussion of the reality of the omnipresence of death are all issues to be dealt with on a daily basis by palliative care practitioners.

Part III turns to a discussion of some of the specific issues surround-ing the various contexts in which palliative care is practised. Redpath explores the key factors involved at the turning point of negotiating the end of active treatment and the beginning of palliative care. She examines some of the barriers that may need to be confronted and identifies factors involved in a successful negotiation of the turning point. Turley considers some of the challenges involved in facilitating referrals to palliative care agencies and how the tensions between the various models of care are managed. She points out that if continuity of care is to be achieved and the unique needs of clients are to be met, there is still much work to be done. Lee studies some of the issues surrounding specialist and generalist pal-liative care services and argues that both are required if the cause of palliative care is to be advanced.

White discusses the role of the nurse consultant in the provision of palliative care in the hospital setting and deals with issues surrounding collaboration between specialty areas, role conflict, territorialism, nurse referrals and education. She points out that for a role such as this to succeed a high level of acceptance within the organisation is required. Noone discusses the complex issues surrounding life-threatening illness and the death of a child in a culture that believes that such an event goes against the natural order of things. She emphasises the importance of family-centred care and the need for support of parents, siblings and grandparents. Manias turns to a consideration of the extent to which palliative care is possible within the critical care environment and explores somes of the tensions between curative and palliative approaches to care. Panek-Hudson follows this vein as she considers the issues surrounding the transition from cure to palliation when patients undertake a potentially curative procedure that fails.

Parsons examines palliative care for AIDS patients and points out that the historical and political context of AIDS has had a profound influence on contemporary health services and policy debates. Stigma and discrimination have influenced reason and have ensured that the experience of this disease is markedly different from that of other diseases. Austin addresses issues concerning palliative care for incurable and progressive diseases such as motor neurone disease and considers the role of the clinical team, how symptoms are best managed and the most appropriate setting for end stage care. Breaden also explores issues surrounding progressive disease and focuses on the challenges facing nursing in the palliative care of people suffering from Alzheimer's disease. Finally Hudson and Richmond focus on the issues surrounding meaningful care for people dying in a residential aged care setting. They consider issues such as the need for staff debriefing and the closure of the patient record.

The various sets of tensions and contextual challenges that are explored in Part III suggest that there are many hurdles to be overcome in the mainstreaming of palliative care services if responsive care is to be achieved in the many settings in which people die.

## Conclusion

This chapter has explored how notions of death avoidance and the medicalisation of death developed within western culture and how these resulted in the warehousing of death and the subsequent emergence of the modern hospice movement three decades ago. It has suggested that in the contemporary social formation of postmodernity, hospice care is becoming secularised, mainstreamed and remedicalised as palliative care in a market-oriented approach to health policy and funding, with demands upon it for accountability and cost containment. This book therefore tries to come to grips with many of the complex issues surrounding how to respond to the human need for care and community when people die in the context of these imperatives.

# References

Ad Hoc Committee on Cancer Pain of the American Society of Clinical Oncology. Cancer pain assessment and treatment curriculum guidelines *J. Clin. Oncol.*, 10, 1976–1982.

Ariès, P. (1974). *Western attitudes towards death from the middle ages to the present* (Trans. P.M. Ranum). Baltimore: Johns Hopkins University.

Bauman, Z. (1992). *Intimations of postmodernity*. London: Routledge.

World Health Organization (1990). *Cancer pain relief and palliative care: Report of a WHO expert committee*. Technical Report Series No. 809. Geneva. WHO.

Gorer, G. (1956). The pornography of death. In Phillips, W. and Raliv, P. (Eds.), *Modern writing*. New York.

Illich, I. (1975). *Medical nemesis*. London: Calder & Boyans Ltd.

Illich, I. (1986). Body history (unpublished paper).

James, N. & Field, D. (1992). The routinization of hospice: Charisma and bureaucratization. *Social Science Medicine, 34*, 1363–1375.

Kastenbaum, R. We covered death today. *Death Education 1*, 85–92.

Kübler-Ross, E. (1969). *On death and dying*. London: Macmillan.

Leder, D. (1990). *The absent body*. Chicago: University of Chicago Press.

McGivney, W.T. & Crooks, G.M. (1984). The care of patients with severe chronic pain in terminal illness. *JAMA 251*, 1182–1188.

Parker, J.M. (1996). A perspective on CQI and nursing education. In *Society of Nursing Education 10th Anniversary Publication*. Hong Kong: Hong Kong Society of Nursing Education.

Stoddard, S. (1979). *The hospice movement*. London: Jonathon Cape.

Williams, M. (1966). Changing attitudes to death: A survey of contributions to *Psychological Abstracts* over a thirty year period. *Human Relations, 19* (4), 405–422.

Sheldon, J.H. (1961). *Report to the Birmingham Regional Hospital Board on its geriatric services*.

Wilkes, E. (1994). Introduction. In David Clark (Ed.), *The future for palliative care: Issues of policy and practice*. Buckingham: Open University Press.

# Part I
# EXPLORING PALLIATIVE CARE

# 1

# Implications of Mainstreaming Hospice into Palliative Care Services*

## B.D. Rumbold

The modern hospice movement commenced in the United Kingdom in the late 1960s, spreading to North America in the mid-1970s and Australia at the beginning of the 1980s. Most hospice programs were new—although in a few instances existing terminal care services were reformed according to hospice principles—and most were initially at the margins of mainstream health services, funded by local communities or charitable trusts rather than from government health budgets. In recent years nearly all hospice programs have developed co-operative relationships with mainstream health systems, creating palliative care services.

While there is clear continuity between today's palliative medicine and the hospice movement which gave it birth, significant conceptual shifts have taken place as well. These have been in part a consequence of co-operating with other health services, and in part a product of the radical change to all health systems which has coincided with the convergence of hospice with mainstream services. Co-operation has required the hospice movement to shift from emphasising its distinctiveness, as it did in its inaugural period, to focusing on the ground held in common with other services. The new context of health care has increasingly required that hospice and palliative care services be accountable according to mainstream criteria of effectiveness, efficiency and competitiveness.

The literature of hospice and palliative care reflects these shifts. Initially, published material was non-technical and anecdotal, aimed at inspiring the community groups that would establish hospices in local communities. The technical literature that existed then was unpublished, and circulated through networks of personal contacts. Technical literature in both monograph and research article form began to be published toward the end of the 1970s. The hospice evaluation study in the United

*This chapter is based on a paper presented to the National Hospice and Palliative Care, Melbourne, October 1993.

3

States in the early 1980s (Mor, Greer & Kastenbaum, 1988), along with similar evaluation studies in other countries, generated a number of papers in major medical and social science journals. By the end of the 1980s several specialist journals for hospice and palliative care had commenced. Thus there is a development from popular literature focusing on the basic concepts and institutional expressions of hospice care, to an exploration of the convergence between hospice care and mainstream medicine, to a specialist literature in palliative care and palliative medicine. These are three major phases in the process of mainstreaming, and will be used as a framework for the following discussion.

In introducing first hospice care, then palliative care, and in initiating reforms to the health system, Australian practitioners and policy-makers have drawn on overseas developments, adapting them to the Australian context (Lickiss, 1993). Any discussion of Australian experience must therefore take account of overseas experience, while bearing in mind that because of contextual differences, insights and outcomes from overseas are not necessarily directly transferable to the local scene. Further, because the structure of health services varies from state to state within Australia, palliative care services assume somewhat different forms in different places, co-operating and expressing their accountability in ways appropriate to their particular context. The detailed ways in which hospice programs in Australia have found a place within the mainstream are thus complex. However, the broad issues raised by mainstreaming transcend the complexity of local variations, and it is on the broader issues that this chapter focuses. A central contention is that, in negotiating a place within the mainstream, palliative care has conformed itself to mainstream practice in ways that may compromise deeply held tenets of the hospice movement.

## The hospice movement: an alternative approach to care

The primary motive for developing hospice care was to offer an alternative to the institutional terminal care then available through the healthcare system (Hillier, 1988; Magno, 1992; Vandenbos, De Leon & Pallack, 1982; Wilkes, 1981), with an emphasis on good pain control, open communication between staff and patient, and a return of social management to patient and family. Hospices attempted to assist people in 'living until they died' by attending to individuals' needs in a 'home-like' atmosphere, providing active support for each patient's friends and family, and ensuring a measure of privacy and self-determination despite the institutional context. Reviews of the hospice approach to care usually articulate principles and values more than specific strategies for care (see for example Buckingham, 1983; DuBois, 1980; Ewens & Herrington, 1983; Hamilton &

Reid, 1980; Hodder & Turley, 1989). Variants of the phrase 'hospice de-notes a philosophy rather than a facility or institution' (Hodder & Turley, 1989, p. 2) are common.

The first British hospices, which were free-standing charitable institu-tions, initiated home-care programs from their institutional base early in the 1970s, recognising that hospice principles should be extended into the wider community. American programs which began in the 1970s were for the most part community-based and staffed by volunteers, emphasising home care and the 'right to die at home'. (Indeed, many of them had no institutional backup.) Canadian programs in contrast began in teach-ing hospitals, using the term 'palliative care' in preference to 'hospice care', mainly because the meaning of 'hospice' is confounded in their bilingual culture. Thus hospice care developed differently in each coun-try. British programs demonstrated their alternative approach to terminal care under the broad umbrella of the British medical system, gradually winning acceptance and funding within that system (Wilkes, 1981). Canadian programs established continuity of care with oncology, offering palliative care as part of the general management of cancer patients, and accepting greater responsibility for management once curative efforts were at an end (Scott, 1981). American programs tended at first to empha-sise their distance from mainstream care, in many cases minimising or even rejecting the role of medical practitioners in hospice programs to create a clear contrast between 'hospital' and 'hospice' care (Fulton & Owen, 1981). Australian programs in the early 1980s reflected this variety, ranging from hospital-based programs supported by existing healthcare services to local, autonomous, community-based programs operated by volunteers.

The appeal of hospice care to the wider community was its claim to offer a 'good death' as compared with the options for dying provided by the mainstream health care system. A good death in hospice terms saw an alert, socially functioning patient whose pain was controlled, who was able to maintain selected intimate relationships to the end, to say fare-wells, and to die at peace (Lamerton, 1973, pp. 43–61). Death in the hospice was solemn, dignified, and openly acknowledged—the strategies for isolation of dying patients and concealment of dead bodies found in public institutions (Glaser & Strauss, 1965; Sudnow, 1967) had no place in the hospice approach. Attention was paid to patients' illness experiences, not merely to the disease process taking place within them. Care was understood holistically, taking account of physical, emotional, social and spiritual dimensions of need. Focusing upon each patient's perspective permitted hospice care to be flexible in its approach, frequently incorpo-rating modalities such as massage, diet and meditation more often re-garded as 'alternative' approaches by the wider healthcare system (see for example Sims, 1988). Physical care focused upon palliation of symptoms, especially pain. Emotional care was provided primarily through the quality of relationship and open communication offered by workers. The social dimension was acknowledged by identifying 'patient and family' as the focus of care (where 'family' is interpreted as the network of relationships significant to the person). Spiritual care was understood not in narrowly sectarian or even exclusively religious terms, but in the sense that spiritual concerns are a fundamental aspect of human existence. This stance reflected the religious vision that motivated many of the early hospice programs, and continues to motivate many palliative care practitioners today.

Recognising the diversity of a dying person's needs meant using a range of professional disciplines to address this spectrum of need. Hospice models emphasised teamwork among healthcare workers, and the need for relationships within the team to be egalitarian rather than hierarchical. Thus no single discipline was necessarily dominant, but the team could respond flexibly to a variety of needs. The team structure was also intended to provide for the support of carers (Mor et al., 1988). In some cases, volunteers and/or family members were included as members of the team, which meant continuing the commitment to care after the patient had died. Prior to the death the hospice assisted family and friends in their anticipatory grief. Following the death the hospice program offered bereavement follow-up through a visitation program, grief support groups or bereavement counselling (Hodder & Turley, 1989, pp. 128–36).

This set of characteristics constituted a new discourse about dying which challenged the existing mainstream medical discourse. Advocates of hospice care did not see these characteristics as limited to hospice or even palliative care models, but as a revival of humanitarian values needed by the health system in general (Gunz, 1989). They wished to distinguish hospice care from mainstream care, yet also influence (in fact, reform) this care. The hospice movement was thus both progressive in being counter-institutional and conservative in appealing to its continuity with western caring tradition (Abel, 1986).

Initially hospice care pursued legitimation through developing a strong base of community support which was more concerned with perceived effectiveness than with hospice care's commensurability with mainstream medicine. This perceived effectiveness of hospice care has maintained community pressure to establish hospice programs despite the lack of clear scientific data proving their effectiveness—or rather the presence of data which fails to do so. This process parallels that described by Willis (1984) in considering the persistence of some alternative or complementary therapies. Community-political legitimation alone however has not been enough to ensure the longer-term survival of the hospice movement. Hospice programs have needed to seek legitimation within the medical community as well. This has been pursued through justification of hospice care in terms of mainstream criteria, particularly those of outcome measures and cost-effectiveness.

The inherent dualism of hospice ideals created ambiguity as hospice care converged with mainstream services. The conservative wing emphasised the medical insight and skills developed in the hospice movement, and encouraged the incorporation of hospice knowledge and skills into mainstream medical discourse. The progressive wing was concerned about aspects of this new conservative palliative care such as the narrowing of discussions of effectiveness to considerations of 'scientific' cost-effectiveness and outcome measures which neglected less tangible values of care (Mount & Scott, 1983; Vladeck, 1984).

# Palliative care: a convergence of hospice care and the health system

Once independent hospice programs were established, various forms of negotiation with existing health services began. From the hospice side, gaining access to the health budget was recognised as essential for long-term survival of programs and for hospice-style care to become a genuine option for the whole of society. There was also the hope that hospice values would influence mainstream care: as Saunders said, 'we moved out [of the NHS] so that attitudes and knowledge could move back in' (Saunders, Summers & Teller, 1981, p. 4).

## *Evaluation*

Through much of the 1970s, the advocates of hospice care simply assumed that the quality of care and the cost-effectiveness of hospice programs would be demonstrably better than mainstream care. Specifically, they assumed that costs in the 'high-tech' acute hospital environment would be higher than for the 'low-tech' domiciliary or in-patient hospice programs, and that the idealism and commitment of hospice staff would result in a much better quality of care. These commonsense assumptions did not stand up under scrutiny in the 1980s: clear-cut advantages in quality of care and in cost-effectiveness were not found. While there are variations due to different models of both hospice and hospital organisation, costs are on average comparable, as are the results of quantitative outcome studies. The major difference shown by these studies is that 'satisfaction' for both patient and family is significantly higher for hospice care than for comparable groups receiving hospital care (Higginson & McCarthy, 1989; Mor et al., 1988; Seale, 1991a). Seale's survey in particular shows little difference between hospice and hospital care on a range of criteria, either because research has failed to demonstrate difference, or because no research has yet been carried out. Perhaps the clearest distinctions are in bereavement studies, where survivors cared for by hospice programs appear to show better resolution of grief after a year has elapsed (Ransford & Smith, 1991; Seale, 1991a) although even here Kane, Klein, Bernstein, and Rothenberg (1986) found no such effect.

These evaluations were carried out for the most part according to mainstream criteria, and debate continues about the relevance of the evaluation criteria employed (Higginson, 1993), and about the logistical and ethical implications of applying standard evaluation tools such as randomised controlled trials to palliative care programs (Ling, Hardy, Penn & Davis, 1995; Mason, 1995; McQuay & Moore, 1994; McWhinney, Bass & Donner, 1994; Gilbert, 1995; Rinck et al., 1995; Wilkes, 1995). For example, evaluation based on outcome measures is unlikely to be adequate when 'in palliative care the form and mode of delivery is often more important than the outcome of care' (Clark, Neale & Heather, 1995, p. 1197).

Hospice care's inability to demonstrate a clear cost advantage over hospital care, particularly in the case of hospice programs with an in-patient facility, has dispensed with arguments that government should fund further free-standing hospices. To obtain recurrent funding traditional hospices have had to adapt their approach, while new funding tends to be directed toward co-operative programs which introduce hospice principles into existing healthcare services (Seale, 1989, p. 551). Traditional hospice care is being superseded by palliative care.

## The mutual influence of hospice and hospital care

Changes to hospice programs under the influence of mainstream management practices are clear. From the informal local networks of the formative years, hospice programs worldwide have increasingly become structured according to accreditation requirements and standardised management procedures (Magno, 1992). Unlike the diverse forms taken by programs in the early years of the hospice movement, today's palliative care programs are very much alike. Accountability to government has also had the effect of reducing accountability to the local community. The community groups that established and funded projects are now becoming more like the auxiliaries that support mainstream institutions (Ford, 1992). Resources shared between hospice programs and other services, particularly staff resources, also reduce the distinctions which existed between hospice and mainstream medical services. Further, the availability of government funding has in a number of programs increased the proportion of paid professional staff and consequently reduced contributions from volunteers.

Less easy to identify are ways in which contemporary hospital practices may have changed under the influence of hospice care. Parkes and Parkes (1984) compared hospice and hospital care in 1967–69 and 1977–79 through the perception of surviving spouses. They found that the differences observed in the 1960s had diminished significantly in the 1970s due to an improvement in hospital care. This improvement, they suggested, might be due to the terminal care training provided through the hospice to the staff of regional hospitals involved in the study. In a similar study, Kane et al. surmise, like Parkes, that hospice may have done its job by alerting conventional practitioners to the previous inadequacy of their care, and that they have now 'lifted their game' (Kane, Wales, Bernstein, Leibowit & Kaplan, 1984). An improvement in communication between hospital doctors and terminally ill patients is noted by Seale (1991b). Comparative studies of physicians' policies on disclosing terminal prognoses show a reversal from 1961 when only 12 per cent of a sample of 219 doctors were prepared to 'tell' to 1979 when 98 per cent of a matched sample of 264 would usually do so (Seale, 1989). (This says nothing about the effectiveness of such communication, bearing in mind McIntosh's (1977) findings that stereotyping of interactions, as much as the content, is the major barrier to doctor–patient communication.)

The products of this convergence are palliative care systems that incorporate hospice programs and link them in fresh ways with other community-based and hospital services. Ideally this palliative care intersects with primary care (Kenyon, 1995), and is supported further both by dedicated palliative care programs which bridge between hospital and community, and by specialist consultants based in hospital or hospice (Finlay, 1994).

## Palliative medicine: a new medical speciality

It was quickly clear that acceptance and legitimation by the medical community in general was needed if hospice programs were to be funded through government health budgets. While the data from comparative evaluations of hospice and hospital care were not available until the mid-1980s, a more conciliatory attitude toward mainstream care could already be seen at the beginning of that decade. Hospice documents of the period downplay aspects of hospice care that might be seen as critical of, or deviating from, mainstream practice, emphasising instead the need for evaluative research, co-operation with medical services, and the leadership responsibility of the medical director.

The detailed process by which legitimation has occurred varies according to context, but the process in the state of Victoria is illustrative. The earliest Victorian hospice programs were independent of the state health budget, but by 1986 six programs operated: two funded independently, two funded by a mixture of state and federal grants and private donations, one funded by a mix of state grant and private donations, one funded entirely by federal grant. These different models were linked together through their membership of the Victorian Association of Hospice and Palliative Care (VAHPC), an active multi-disciplinary body.

The convergence of hospice care with mainstream services was, however, a political process mediated predominantly by medical practitioners. First the Victorian Co-operative Oncology Group working group issued a report on palliative care in Victoria (1984), proposing a program which drew upon hospice care principles but developed them within networks based on existing hospitals. In this report, hospice care was treated simply as one sub-category of palliative care. Next, the Ministerial Review of Cancer Services 1985 incorporated the oncologists' recommendations into its report, while a Health Department of Victoria discussion paper (1986) endorsed the recommendations and proposed that the model be explored further by a Palliative Care Council in which the majority of members were to be appointed by hospitals; that is, the VAHPC would be a minority voice. The Social Development Committee of the Victorian Parliament (1987) picked up the recommendation to form a Palliative Care Council, and the Minister for Health commissioned this body later that year. The Victorian Palliative Care Council report (1989) recommended that palliative care adopt a regional model co-ordinated out of major hospitals, and that palliative care be developed as a medical speciality, arguing that specialist medical education and a career structure for palliative care physicians was necessary if palliative care was to be recognised by the medical community.

This latter recommendation was based upon British experience. In November 1987 palliative medicine was recognised by the Royal College of Physicians as a new sub-speciality of internal medicine (Hillier, 1988). The effect of this, as intended, has been an increase in the status of palliative care physicians, shown by an increased willingness of other medical practitioners to consult on matters of symptom control. Moves to increase the speciality status of hospice physicians in the USA through the Academy of Hospice Physicians have produced a similar increase in referrals from the wider medical community, although as yet the sub-speciality has not been recognised in the USA (Magno, 1992). In 1993 the Australian and New Zealand Society of Palliative Medicine was established (Maddocks, 1993; 1994). These specialist bodies, supported by medical school palliative medicine curricula (Smith, 1994), provide professional formation for palliative care physicians. While the new speciality is still in its beginnings, some hospice practitioners claim that already the balance of power within the multidisciplinary teams offering care is shifting from nursing care, central to the hospice model, toward the medical practitioners who provide the expertise required for the increasingly sophisticated symptom control used in the palliative care model (Kearney, 1992).

# The process of change
## Medicalisation

The process of mainstreaming outlined above demonstrates that the political legitimation required to gain access to government funding is associated with medicalisation, for increasingly palliative care is becoming synonymous with palliative medicine. Medicalisation or medical dominance denotes a perspective that deems biomedical services to be of primary importance (Conrad & Schneider, 1980). This perspective determines priorities for care, shapes the ways in which relationships between professional bodies are organised, and influences the nature of government interventions. It privileges an understanding of illness in terms of disease, valuing outcomes in terms of cure or remission, promoting a reductionist view in which care is expressed through a series of modular services. A linear relationship between these services is assumed; that is, an emotional, social or spiritual service is assumed to be identifiable and deliverable in the same way as a physical service. Because biomedical services are given priority, other services are subordinated, or limited, or excluded. Typically, nursing care is subordinated, and 'alternative' practices are limited or excluded (Willis, 1989). This approach has particular strengths in curative medicine, but its inadequacies in chronic illness and terminal care were the primary motivation for developing hospice care in the first place.

Speaking of the new speciality of palliative medicine, Balfour Mount says 'the primary goal is not to medicalise dying. We see the need for a speciality only because the needs of the dying require equal consideration with other health care needs at the shrinking budgetary table' (Hamilton, 1995, p. 336). Nevertheless there are risks as well as benefits associated with medicalisation. Medical specialisation increases the possibility that palliative care will be conformed to contemporary medical practice, either by becoming a sub-branch of oncology or gerontology—the two specialities which at present tend to make claims on palliative care—or by aligning itself with these others as a discrete medical speciality. This is a major concern as medical dominance historically is associated with constraints on the skills and underutilisation of the resources of other healthcare practitioners.

## Managing care

The transformations undergone in hospice care in the 1980s and 1990s reflect fundamental shifts in the culture of healthcare systems during this period. Early in the 1980s the focus of interest was largely on the professional relationships within which care was offered, and management was mostly concerned about providing resources that allowed professionals to carry out their work as effectively and efficiently as possible. The relationships professionals had with their clients, and the actual personal care they offered, were a matter of concern to all parties. Soon however new approaches to healthcare management began to focus on the specific services offered by professionals. Management now monitored the products of professional practice, and relationship concerns became less prominent, with attention turning to measuring tangible outcomes of the various services provided. Contemporary management systems are now shifting attention to the purchase and management of those services with the aim of minimising risk; that is, the goal of managed care is to ensure that problems are solved with the least outlay of resources, utilising the lowest level of technology and professional expertise possible. Further, these new systems increasingly manage professional practitioners as well as the services they provide (Roberts, 1996).

The new management approaches are designed to bring about a change from provider-defined to purchaser-defined services (Holliday, 1995). There is a sense in which this change of culture should suit palliative care, for the hospice vision of a good death has always enjoyed community support. In practice, however, the purchasers of palliative care services are not local communities but primary care providers (in the UK), or care management plans (in the USA), or in Australia the government itself, all of them parties with fiscal interest in the contractual process (Clark et al., 1995; Jost, Hughes, McHale & Griffiths, 1995; Stoelwinder, 1994). This sort of market makes it difficult to include a contribution from volunteers, who are less likely to support a for-profit service, while a contractual approach to minimising the use of resources means that the palliative care product (a good death) becomes a compromise between the needs of the patient and the needs of the service (McNamara, Waddell & Colvin, 1994). When purchaser and provider are different arms of the one government department, for example, the financial interests of taxpayers in general constrain the interests of those few taxpayers who are clients of the service. Further management factors are the pressure for through-put and economies of scale which undermine social and emotional support because of the extent to which these aspects of care rely upon creating community between staff and clients. The apparent freedoms of a market structure for care provision may mean less, rather than more, manoeuvrability than in the past (Clark, 1993, p. 176).

## Benefits and costs

The benefits of mainstreaming for hospice care programs are access to specific recurrent funding, plus in some cases the status that comes with being identified as a centre of excellence in palliative care. Co-operation should encourage more effective and efficient use of the community's health resources, provide access for hospice programs to a wider range of therapeutic and supportive services, and make palliative care services more widely available in the general community. Mainstreaming also has the potential to provide better continuity of care (MacDonald, 1993; Prior & Poulton, 1996). While hospice care focused on the end of life, a palliative care perspective connects the active treatment and palliation aspects of a person's illness experience, removing the administrative barriers that currently limit access to expert palliation. Hospital-based palliative care should be able to work co-operatively with active treatment programs in the hospital as well as in the community, whereas previously hospice programs often received referrals only after active treatment possibilities were exhausted (Victorian Department of Human Services, 1996b). Many people require palliation—pain control in particular—well before the terminal phase of disease.

There are indications, however, that such benefits are being undercut by the new management strategies being introduced, particularly the purchaser-provider arrangements which can place oncology and palliative care in competition (Calman & Dobbs, 1994). Such competitiveness created is likely to be inimical to hospice-derived practice. As we have seen, hospice practice assumes a therapeutic community in which professionals can affirm the central focus of their disciplines yet work co-operatively. In the current climate professionals can spend considerable time and energy defending their boundaries within a health system where professional autonomy and competition for resources are emphasised, perhaps to compensate for the overall constraints being placed upon professional autonomy in managed care systems (Roberts, 1996).

Mainstreaming palliative care means conforming palliative care to a management approach which de-emphasises values which have been at the heart of the hospice movement. Managed care establishes an hierarchy of services in which management and medicine share—or compete for— dominance. Professional autonomy rather than co-operation is inherent in management models which require a clear separation of services. Attention to contextual issues—the quality of relationships between a professional and a client, the relationships between the various professionals involved with any given client—is minimal. The very concept of a team which can support and implement a particular vision of care may be undermined by management structures which permit 'teams' composed opportunistically to meet particular client needs (Victorian Department of Human Services, 1996a). In such teams consultancy links with palliative medical and nursing expertise will be mandatory, but actual nursing care may be provided under contract from existing nursing services, while other allied health functions can be purchased as the client requires. Palliative care services need no longer provide services themselves, so long as they ensure that the client has access to services. A consequence of these proposals is that medical expertise is again placed at the centre, followed by nursing, while toward the margins some caregivers, notably those focusing on emotional, social and spiritual dimensions of care, may have no significant commitment to or association with the practice of palliative care and little appreciation of a palliative care ethos or of collegial practice. This valuing of technical expertise effectively marginalises care; there is no concept of a team functioning as a therapeutic community.

A mainstream response to this critique could be that current management practices do not ignore or seek to devalue care, they simply assume it to be inherent in good professional practice and concentrate on constructing a system that will conform that practice to current social requirements. To adopt such a position is however to ignore systemic realities: qualities and practices which are not supported or nurtured will be marginalised within a system. It is probably true that care can be de-emphasised in many areas of today's healthcare system without great detriment to outcomes: most patients do not remain in the system for long enough to require major personal support from practitioners, and community support networks are adequate for most curative procedures. However, the situation is different for severe chronic illness and for protracted terminal illness. A case could be made for palliative care to be retained in a co-operative rather than assimilated form in order to draw attention to the value of care within the system as a whole.

## Conclusions

Hospice and palliative care are at present in crisis, facing both risk and opportunity. The opportunity is that of bringing the insights and practice of hospice care to bear within the new horizons offered by the emerging discipline of palliative care. The risk is that this very process of mainstreaming hospice care will rob it of its essence, leaving palliative care with the forms, but not the substance, of hospice care.

A fundamental problem in integrating hospice care with mainstream healthcare systems is the incommensurability of the conceptual bases of these two approaches to care. A particular difficulty is the lack of a systemic perspective in the biomedical thinking that shapes mainstream care. It is for example frequently assumed that specific techniques developed by hospice care can readily be transferred to mainstream practice. However, such an assumption ignores the way the effectiveness of a given strategy may depend critically upon its context in the system of caring relationships provided by a hospice care team, and upon the professional formation and collegial commitment of the team members.

Hospice care continues to be an anomaly within a healthcare system shaped to meet acute care needs. Its caring practices are not easily reduced to discrete services, nor is its goal of a good death for each client easily described in objective terms. Hospice care is consistent in its values and its process, but its outcomes cannot be standardised, for a good death is a highly contextualised 'product'. For this reason, a few believe that hospice care should preserve its independence and refuse to be structured into the mainstream in the form of palliative care services. To choose this option, however, means operating as a voluntary service and relinquishing any hopes of influencing mainstream practice.

Certainly there appear to be significant imperfectly examined costs in the shift from 'hospice' to 'palliative care'. The shift is clearly associated with medical dominance through the political process; and the extent of the subordination, limitation and exclusion of certain disciplines and aspects of hospice services is yet to be seen. To spell this out a little, there are parallels between the medical dominance of midwifery and palliative medicine dominance of hospice care: a largely male medical structure has moved to take control of a largely female system of care and realign its goals in the direction of medical interest. As was the case of midwifery, nursing again is likely to be the discipline subordinated. Ironically, this is in direct contrast to the actual interest displayed by the professions involved. The investment that nursing has in palliative care is clear from the number of training programs which already exist, while there is still only cursory acknowledgment of palliative care in formal medical training. Thus it is possible that holistic practice will be undermined because some services will be identified as marginal or ancillary to core medical services, and will not receive appropriate recognition or funding. This is most likely to happen to the dimensions of practice that create and support a context for care. Outcomes of emotional, social and spiritual support are less easily quantified or framed in delivery terms, and are thereby marginalised in health management systems. Relegating social and spiritual discourse to the margins effectively discounts discussion of value frameworks and beliefs, exactly the sort of discussion that is needed for an ongoing critical review of professional practice.

Conformation of palliative care to the wider healthcare system, together with an increasing focus on symptom control through the use of medical expertise, may well lead to the types of shifts in focus set out in table 1.1. These shifts are being driven by the value ascribed to technical expertise and specialisation over emotional, social and spiritual dimensions of care. If palliative care is to retain continuity with its roots in the hospice movement, it must continue to define its speciality in terms of a multidisciplinary integrative approach distinguished not by its narrowness of interest or uniqueness of content, but by its focus upon expert palliation across a range of disciplinary interests. Such a different approach to specialisation will not be easy either to communicate or to maintain. For some, palliative care simply identifies an area that has

Table 1.1   Areas of focus in hospice and palliative care

| Hospice care | Palliative care |
|---|---|
| Holistic care | Symptom control |
| Systemic perspective | Service delivery perspective |
| Nursing the core discipline | Medicine the core discipline |
| Egalitarian organisation | Hierarchical organisation |
| Patient active in directing care | Patient increasingly a consumer of medical expertise |
| 'Bottom-up' development of care in small unit, reflecting community context | 'Top-down' direction of care in large institution, reflecting large-scale political and managerial priorities |

been given insufficient attention in the past, and therefore merits a high profile today, but will make its contribution and depart. 'I hope that palliative care will be a transient phenomenon of the 1990s, and that by the time the 2000s begin, it will have been absorbed wholly into the mainstream of medicine', writes Allbrook (1989, p. 65). If palliative care were simply specialist information and a transferable set of strategies, this could indeed be the case. But if palliative care is about reform of the mainstream medical discourse, a mere ten-year transition was hardly realistic.

The constraints imposed by new management practices have also been noted. The paradigm shift from a service-delivery to a risk-management approach to care which underlies managed care (Howe, 1994) is likely to have major implications for palliative care in the years ahead. For example, in recent years an alternative and (presumably) cost-effective model of a good death, doctor-assisted suicide, has become prominent and may well receive social legitimation. Consumer perspectives, cost-effectiveness, and the ethics of care will be in significant tension as purchasers decide which version of a good death should be funded. A fundamental issue for palliative care is to find ways to participate in and to influence the new managerial discourse, for in the healthcare field at present policy is less and less determined by consultation with practitioners or clients, more and more by management ideologies which fail to discern that care cannot be packaged and marketed like other commodities.

Nevertheless, current political wisdom is that hospice care should be integrated with mainstream services. The challenge before hospice practitioners making the transition to the new palliative care services is to find creative ways to bring about this integration, for it appears that developing a palliative care approach that remains true to its origins in hospice care will provide a crucial test of both the biomedical and managed care models that dominate contemporary health systems. It also appears that nursing is the discipline best placed to maintain the process-based systemic perspective needed to resist an uncritical assimilation of care to these dominant models, for nursing continues to combine technical expertise with an holistic concern for care. The test for nursing as a discipline in the new palliative care will be to avoid emphasising either aspect at the expense of the other; focusing on technical aspects of the nursing role and ignoring or minimising emotional, social and spiritual aspects of care, or taking responsibility for all these aspects if they are given inadequate attention, thus diffusing the nursing contribution. Technical expertise and holistic awareness must be kept in creative tension and expressed through co-operative practice. Given the directions that palliative care appears to be taking, nursing will be the key discipline in ensuring that emotional, social and spiritual dimensions are addressed, not just through nursing practice but through consultation with and referral to colleagues with expertise in these other dimensions of care.

Such a countervailing perspective provided by nursing is essential if hospice ideals are to be integrated appropriately within palliative care practice, and will require nurse practitioners to be engaged in reflective practice and ongoing conceptual analysis of their contexts—no easy task given the immediate demands imposed by the changing healthcare scene. It is also essential that the hospice contribution go beyond mere resistance to influencing mainstream practice. It is important from a hospice perspective that clinical studies pay systematic attention to quality of life issues as well as to matters such as quality assurance (George & Jennings, 1993, p. 433) so that, for example, research focuses not only on whether a given treatment reduces tumour size but also whether such clinical remissions are associated with improvement in patient well-being (MacDonald, 1993, p. 31). Nursing research is well placed to attend to this dimension of clinical practice, while holistic nursing practice is needed to keep alive and apply creatively the values of a hospice approach to care.

# References

Abel, E.K. (1986). The hospice movement: Institutionalizing innovation. *International Journal of Health Services, 16*, 71–85.

Allbrook, D. (1989). Who should be trained in palliative care in the medical profession? In Woodruff, R. (Ed.), *Palliative care for the 1990's* (pp. 61–66). Melbourne: Asperula Pty. Ltd.

Buckingham, R. (1983). *The complete hospice guide.* New York: Harper & Row.

Calman, F.M.B. & Dobbs, H.J. (1994). Access to specialist palliative care: Purchasers come between complementary specialities. *British Medical Journal, 308* (6929), 656.

Clark, D. (Ed.) (1993). *The future for palliative care: Issues of policy and practice.* Buckingham: Open University Press.

Clark, D., Neale, B., & Heather, P. (1995). Contracting for palliative care. *Social Science and Medicine, 40* (9), 1193–1202.

Conrad, P. & Schneider, J.W. (1980). *Deviance and medicalization: From badness to sickness.* St Louis: C.V. Mosby.

DuBois, P.M. (1980). *The hospice way of death.* New York: Human Sciences Press.

Ewens, J. & Herrington, P. (1983). *Hospice: A handbook for families and others facing terminal illness.* Santa Fe: Bear & Co.

Finlay, I. (1994). Setting standards for palliative care. *Journal of the Royal Society of Medicine, 87* (3), 179–181.

Ford, G. (1992). Palliative care: A wider horizon. *Palliative Medicine, 6,* 91–93.

Fulton, R. & Owen, G. (1981). Hospice in America. In Saunders, C., Summers, D.H., & Teller, N. (Eds.), *Hospice: The living idea* (pp. 9–18). London: Edward Arnold.

George, R.J.D. & Jennings, A.L. (1993). Palliative medicine. *Postgraduate Medical Journal, 69* (812), 429–449.

Gilbert, J. (1995). Evaluation of palliative care: Patients must be told that treatment will be randomised. *British Medical Journal, 310* (6972), 125.

Glaser, B. & Strauss, A. (1965). *Awareness of dying: A sociological study of attitudes to patients dying in hospitals.* London: Weidenfeld and Nicholson.

Gunz, F. (1989). The facilitation of future development. In Woodruff, R. (Ed.), *Palliative care for the 1990's,* (pp. 83–88). Melbourne: Asperula Pty. Ltd.

Hamilton, J. (1995). Dr Balfour Mount and the cruel irony of our care for the dying. *Canadian Medical Association Journal, 152* (3), 334–336.

Hamilton, M. & Reid, H. (Eds.) (1980). *A hospice handbook: A new way to care for the dying.* Grand Rapids: Eerdmans.

Health Department Victoria (1986). *Palliative care: Discussion paper.* Melbourne: Health Department Victoria.

Higginson, I. (1993). Palliative care: A review of past changes and future trends. *Journal of Public Health and Medicine, 15* (1), 3–8.

Higginson, I. & McCarthy, M. (1989). Evaluation of palliative care: Steps to quality assurance? *Palliative Medicine, 3,* 267–274.

Hillier, R. (1988). Palliative medicine—a new speciality. *British Medical Journal, 297,* 874–875.

Hodder, P. & Turley, A. (Eds.) (1989). *The creative option of palliative care: A manual for health professionals.* Melbourne: Melbourne Citymission.

Holliday, I. (1995). *The NHS transformed.* Manchester: Baseline Books.

Howe, D. (1994). Modernity, postmodernity and social work. *British Journal of Social Work, 24,* 513–532.

Jost, T.S., Hughes, D., McHale, J., & Griffiths, L. (1995). The British health care reforms, the American health care revolution, and purchaser/provider contracts. *Journal of Health Politics, Policy and Law, 20* (4), 885–908.

Kane, R., Klein, S.J., Bernstein, L., & Rothenberg, R. (1986). The role of hospice in reducing the impact of bereavement. *Journal of Chronic Diseases, 39,* 735–742.

Kane, R., Wales, J., Bernstein, L., Leibowitz, A., & Kaplan, S. (1984). A randomised control trial of hospice care. *Lancet,* 21 April.

Kearney, M. (1992). Palliative medicine—just another speciality? *Palliative Medicine, 6,* 39–46.

Kenyon, Z. (1995). Palliative care in general practice. *British Medical Journal, 311,* 888–889.

Lamerton, R. (1973). *Care of the dying.* London: The Care and Welfare Library.

Lickiss, J.N. (1993). Australia: Status of cancer pain and palliative care. *Journal of Pain and Symptom Management, 8* (6), 388–394.

Ling, J., Hardy, J., Penn, K., & Davis, C. (1995). Evaluation of palliative care: Recruitment figures may be low. *British Medical Journal, 310* (6972), 125.

MacDonald, N. (1993). Oncology and palliative care: The case for co-ordination. *Cancer Treatment Reviews, 19* (Supplement A), 29–41.

McIntosh, J. (1977). *Communication and awareness in a cancer ward.* London: Croom Helm.

McNamara, B., Waddell, C., & Colvin, M. (1994). The institutionalization of the good death. *Social Science and Medicine, 39* (11), 1501–1508.

McQuay, H. & Moore, A. (1994). Need for rigorous assessment of palliative care. *British Medical Journal, 309* (6965), 1315–1316.

McWhinney, I.R., Bass, M.J., & Donner, A. (1994). Evaluation of a palliative care service: Problems and pitfalls. *British Medical Journal, 3009* (6965), 1340–1342.

Maddocks, I. (1993). Australian and New Zealand Society of Palliative Medicine. *Medical Journal of Australia, 159* (1), 72.

Maddocks, I. (1994). A new Society of Palliative Medicine. *Medical Journal of Australia, 160* (11), 670.

Magno, J.B. (1992). USA hospice care in the 1990s. *Palliative Medicine, 6,* 158–165.

Mason, B. (1995). Evaluation of palliative care: Patients should be randomised at time of diagnosis. *British Medical Journal, 310* (6972), 125.

Mor, V., Greer, D.S., & Kastenbaum, R. (Eds.) (1988). *The hospice experiment.* Baltimore: John Hopkins University Press.

Mount, B. & Scott, J. (1983). Whither hospice evaluation? *Journal of Chronic Diseases, 36,* 731–736.

Parkes, C.M. & Parkes, J. (1984). 'Hospice' versus 'hospital' care—re-evaluation after ten years as seen by surviving spouses. *Postgraduate Medical Journal, 60,* 120–124.

Prior, D. & Poulton, V. (1996). Palliative care nursing in a curative environment: An Australian perspective. *International Journal of Palliative Nursing, 2* (2), 84–90.

Ransford, H.E. & Smith, M.L. (1991). Grief resolution among the bereaved in hospice and hospital wards. *Social Science and Medicine, 32,* 295–304.

Rinck, G., Kleijnen, J., van den Bos, T.G.A.M., de Haes, H.J.C.J.M., Schade, E., & Veenhof, C.H.N. (1995). Trials in palliative care. *British Medical Journal, 310* (6979), 598–599.

Roberts, C. C. (1996). Redefining the health care paradigm. *Hospital Topics, 74* (2), 16–20.

Saunders, C., Summers, D.H., & Teller, N. (Eds.) (1981). *Hospice: The living idea.* London: Edward Arnold.

Scott, J.F. (1981). Canada: Hospice care in Canada. In Saunders, C., Summers, D.H., & Teller, N. (Eds.), *Hospice: The living idea* (pp. 176–179).

Seale, C. (1989). What happens in hospices: A review of research evidence. *Social Science and Medicine, 28,* 551–559.

Seale, C. (1991a). A comparison of hospice and conventional care. *Social Science and Medicine, 32,* 147–152.

Seale, C. (1991b). Communication and awareness about death: A study of a random sample of dying people. *Social Science and Medicine, 32,* 943–952.

Sims, S. (1988). The significance of touch in palliative care. *Palliative Medicine, 2,* 58–61.

Smith, A.M. (1994). Palliative medicine education for medical students: A survey of British medical schools, 1992. *Medical Education, 28,* 197–199.

Social Development Committee of the Parliament of Victoria (1987). *Inquiry into options for dying with dignity.* Melbourne: Government Printer.

Stoelwinder, J. (1994). Casemix payment in the real world of running a hospital. *Medical Journal of Australia, 161* (Supplement), S15–S18.

Sudnow, D. (1967). *Passing on: The social organization of dying.* Englewood Cliffs: Prentice-Hall.

Vandenbos, G.R., DeLeon, P., & Pallak, M.S. (1982). An alternative to traditional medical care for the terminally ill. *American Psychologist, 37*, 1245–1248.

Victorian Co-operative Oncology Group (1984). *Palliative care in Victoria: Report of a sub-committee*. Melbourne: Anti Cancer Council.

Victorian Department of Human Services (1996a). *Palliative care in Victoria: The way forward*. Melbourne: Department of Human Services.

Victorian Department of Human Services (1996b). *A study of the financial feasibility of a palliative medicine ward in an acute hospital under casemix funding* (Palliative care service development series 2). Melbourne: Department of Human Services.

Victorian Palliative Care Council (1989). *Palliative care services in Victoria: A report to the Minister of Health Victoria*. Melbourne: Health Department of Victoria.

Vladeck, B. (1984). The limits of cost-effectiveness. *American Journal of Public Health, 74*, 652–653.

Wilkes, E. (1981). Great Britain: The hospice in Britain. In Saunders, C., Summers, D.H., & Teller, N. (Eds.), *Hospice: The living idea* (pp. 184–186).

Wilkes, E. (1995). Evaluation of palliative care: Important factors are hard to measure. *British Medical Journal, 310* (6972), 125.

Willis, E. (1984). The role of alternative health care in Australia. In Tatchell, M. (Ed.), *Perspectives on health policy* (pp. 311–323). Canberra: Health Economics Research Unit, Australian National University.

Willis, E. (1989). *Medical dominance*. Sydney: Allen & Unwin.

# 2

# Palliative Care Principles: Masking the Complexity of Practice

## S. Aranda

To many involved in palliative care it may, on the surface at least, seem passé to include a chapter on palliative care principles in this book. When discussing the issue of principles in recent years I have been commonly admonished for a wasted effort—comments being made that these things are now taken-for-granted aspects of practice that we all understand and operate from. With respect to those who believe this, I offer a challenge to that view and seek to explore the basis of palliative care by rendering problematic these taken-for-granted principles which underpin palliative care practice.

My objective, as a staunch supporter of the achievements of palliative care in Australia over the last 15 years, is to begin both to make visible the evolving knowledge base from which this care is practised and to reveal the complex reality of caring for the dying that is rendered invisible by the philosophical principles of early hospice care.

## What is ideology and is it relevant to PC philosophy?

Ideology, in its modern usage, is used to denote the ways in which our adherence to certain rituals or beliefs is grounded in emotional safety. 'Ideologies may be seen as justifications which mask some specific set of interests' (Bullock, Stallybrass & Trombley, 1988). Thus we tend to stick to beliefs or behaviours whose meaning and consequences we may not fully understand.

How palliative care philosophy might be seen to be ideological and how it therefore masks the reality of current palliative care complexity is the focus of this chapter. My argument is essentially that the modern hospice movement, pioneered by people like Cecily Saunders, was based on a set of beliefs and values that were established in opposition to the perceived inhumane treatment of the dying at that time. However, palliative care practice has undergone dynamic and ongoing changes while the original philosophy remains largely unchanged and unexplored. I do not argue to abandon the original philosophy; rather I would seek to unmask its ideological elements that render silent the skill and knowledge of contemporary palliative care. I would also encourage palliative care practitioners to consider the complexity of their practice and its relationship to early hospice philosophy.

## Principles of palliative care

While every palliative care service articulates the essential principles of palliative care in different ways, for the purposes of this chapter I have chosen to address four main principles that encompass the general view that palliative care:

- is an approach to care emphasising living and acknowledging death as an intrinsic part of life;
- is centred on the patient and family as client and emphasises the client's role in the direction of care;
- utilises a multidisciplinary team in recognition of the need to offer care that is holistic and meets the complex needs of the dying patient and family; and,
- focuses on comfort and the full relief of symptoms rather than cure of disease.

### An approach to care emphasising living and acknowledging death as an intrinsic part of life

The principle that palliative care is an approach to care emphasising living and acknowledging death as part of life signifies that palliative care is a style of care rather than a specific organisation or site of care. As such it is frequently portrayed as a generalist concept able to be utilised in any care situation and by any professional. The focus is on assisting the patient and family to live life to the full despite the limitations imposed by the disease, while at the same time acknowledging the need to work through issues associated with dying and bereavement. Dying is portrayed as opening the potential for growth and ongoing social contribution in stark contrast to the idea that dying should be done as quickly as possible.

This principle works against palliative care in subtle and undermining ways. Portrayal of death as a time of growth does not reflect the plurality of views in a multicultural society such as ours, often limiting the ways in which palliative care services respond to divergent beliefs and values.

Foremost are criticisms that palliative care romanticises death, dying and suffering; such criticisms are often linked to associations with the church and religion. This criticism is often articulated in the euthanasia debate when advocates of euthanasia dismiss the belief in the potential in dying as religious idealism. The euthanasia debate has illustrated the tensions that exist between a philosophy that honours the beliefs and values of people while also finding it difficult to accept someone's wish to hasten their death.

In reality, palliative care practitioners work daily with the diverse values and beliefs of all people, managing this complexity in effective ways, with a skill level that is hidden by adherence to an ideological view of this principle. A recent example illustrates how this tension is worked with in practice.

> A nurse recently undertook an assessment visit to a client who made it clear that she wanted help in dying rather than palliative care. The nurse was able to explain her inability to honour that request while also helping the lady access the information she wanted from the voluntary euthanasia society. The nurse and palliative care team continued to provide care for this woman while she pursued her other options. The voluntary euthanasia society informed her they could not help her and were not really interested in ongoing contact with her. However, the palliative care team did not abandon this woman and continued to provide care until her death.

The palliative care service responded to this woman's needs in ways that were helpful to her but did not run counter to their own beliefs and values. There are of course limits to what any service can provide. However, the hallmark of this example is that the palliative care service did not abandon this client when it became clear that they could not fulfil her expectations. Rather, the staff helped this woman clarify her options, pursue them and remained committed to her care when she was let down by the people from whom she sought help.

The notion that dying always offers potential for growth and positive living also sets ideals for the practice of palliative care that may be inappropriate. The ideology portrayed is represented in this quote from Ariès:

> Death should simply become
> a discrete but dignified exit
> of a peaceful person
> from a helpful society
> without pain or suffering
> and ultimately without fear . . .

> (Ariès, 1981, p. 614)

If palliative care practitioners work from this ideal they are doomed to failure and, I would argue, cut themselves off from many people for whom they care. Much of the skill in palliative care practice rests in our ability to be with people in their pain, suffering and fear and in our acceptance that for some, to 'rage against the dying of the light' is an appropriate and acceptable approach to death. While dying may indeed by a part of life, it is often untimely, degrading and both physically and emotionally challenging for all involved. Nowhere is this seen more than when the person suffers gross physical breakdown. Nurses working in palliative care rarely talk about this aspect of their practice with others and even among themselves they speak in a shorthand of shared under-standing that does not require description. Fungating tumours, brain herniating through previous burr holes and the devastating effects of cachexia defy the idea that pain, suffering and fear can always be relieved and highlight that for some death is a happy release. The real challenge for palliative care rests with casting off the ideology present in Ariès' prose and developing our ability to articulate the realities of specialist palliative care practice. This articulation includes our ability both to demonstrate how a person fearful of dying was able to let go of this fear and to show how it is possible to provide useful assistance to a person who fights death until their last breath.

Perhaps the most important idea arising from generalist conceptions of palliative care is that it can be practised by anyone in any setting. This raises to the fore the differences between generalist and specialist pallia-tive care settings. It is indeed a worthy goal of proponents of palliative care that all health professionals have basic palliative care knowledge and skills. However, there will always be a continuing need for specialist palliative care services to ensure both the advancement of the knowledge base in areas like symptom management and the care of people with complex and difficult palliative care needs. Current principles emphasise the generic nature of palliative care and fail to articulate expertise in palliative care practice; thus it becomes impossible to differentiate be-tween generalist and specialist practice. Indeed specialist practitioners frequently downplay their own expertise in an effort to encourage all health professionals to take a role in palliative care. Thus there is a tension for proponents of palliative care between the expansion of generalist palliative care and the advancement of a specialist knowledge base and improved care of the dying that is not clearly defined.

Additionally the generalist model does not take account of the compet-ing tensions for the professionals who would be asked to take on the responsibility for palliative care in addition to their normal duties. In the acute care sector, high levels of patient acuity, the push for rapid through-put and reduced staffing levels, particularly in the supportive care areas, make the ideal of all staff taking a palliative care approach more difficult than ever.

# Centred on the patient and family as client and emphasises the client's role in the direction of care

The principle that palliative care is client centred picks up the idea that holistic care of the person and their family is the focus of palliative care and is offered at the direction of the client, the client being the patient and family. The suggestion is that palliative care practitioners approach service delivery from the perspective of the person's understandings, values, beliefs, needs and expectations of a palliative care service and of their dying. Often this type of care is spoken about as supportive care; that is, supporting the patient and family to live and die in a manner appropriate for them and supportive of the decisions and directions for care that they make. Underlying this is the idea of patient autonomy, alien to many in our communities, and the ideological view that, given appropriate information, people will make the 'right' decision. Also inherent is the ideological assumption that all dying people come from loving and supportive families. Several challenges arise from these ideas.

## Expectations for care

Other than those people who have survived catastrophic illness or accident, most people die only once. While the patient and family may have experienced the deaths of others, this has very often been a negative experience. In an evaluation study of Melbourne Citymission Hospice Service, I found that most clients had few expectations of the service offered and often equated care needs to symptom management and assistance with daily activities as offered by the nursing members of the multidisciplinary team (Aranda, 1993). Few had clear visions of what could be offered in terms of pastoral care or counselling aspects of the service and often equated the former with religion and the latter with an admission to psychological or psychiatric problems. Several also asked why palliative care had not been involved in previous family deaths, indicating that they had not known such services were available to assist families to care for their dying relatives.

## Decision-making

The notion of supportive care suggests that palliative care practitioners need to accept and support all the decisions a patient makes. The obvious example where problems may arise is when a patient believes in and requests euthanasia. Few would argue that a palliative care practitioner should be compelled to honour the patient's request for euthanasia despite accepting the person's right to make such a request. From a legal perspective, the practitioner is unable to support or honour the patient's request in most countries of the world and from a moral perspective should not automatically be asked to accept a perspective that goes against their own moral judgments. On a daily basis, palliative care practitioners work with the competing demands of their own moral position, the law, and the needs and expectations of patients and families.

Additionally, palliative care practitioners develop expertise in caring for those who are dying and bereaved and are often required to assist and direct the client's decision-making. The concept of autonomy, especially when seen as an individual construct, has major limitations as Kanitsaki explores in chapter 3. It is also unrealistic to expect people to always be able to make decisions at a time when they are sick and often vulnerable. Palliative care practitioners frequently guide and direct the decision-making of patients in ways that are not paternalistic and that respect the individual values, beliefs and needs of that person and family. Street explores some of these ideas further in chapter 6.

The role of the family in decision-making is also an important consideration for palliative care practitioners, with many families and patients seeing their situation in conflicting ways. Such conflict occurs in loving families (e.g. when the person wants to die in hospital to relieve the burden on a family member who wants to facilitate a home death), as well as in families in disharmony. Palliative care practitioners are very skilled in the negotiation of meaning and care direction with clients and families, and yet this aspect of practice is rarely articulated. The concept of supportive care often described underplays the skills of palliative care practitioners in negotiating care that meets the needs of people with divergent and often conflicting perspectives.

## Choice of site of dying and death

Finally, a word about choices regarding site of care that have been the hallmark of modern hospice and palliative care, and emphasised in the idea of client direction of care. Initially, the choice of care site was between hospital and hospice; later, in response to some people's desire, home became an alternative. In Australia multiple home-care services have developed in response to community needs. However, recent reductions to in-patient acute hospital beds and rapid through-put of patients to meet hospital casemix targets have resulted in increased pressure on patients to choose a home death. The lessening of availability of acute beds limits opportunities for hospital death or respite care that requires a corresponding availability of palliative care beds, distributed according to local needs. In Victoria, the 1996 palliative care plan acknowledges this requirement (Department of Human Services, 1996).

A further parameter of concern to palliative care practitioners is the difference between site of dying and site of death. Many families and patients desire to be cared for in their own homes up to but not including the moment of death. Desire to die outside of the home environment is complex, often relating to previous experiences or the wish for the home to not be associated with death. The palliative care team is often required to make fairly close call judgments about the timing of death and choice in this area is often both difficult to predict and to facilitate.

## The multidisciplinary team recognises the need to offer care that is holistic

The use of a multidisciplinary team reflects the emphasis taken in palliative care on caring for the person and family's physical, psychological, sociocultural and spiritual needs. The basis of this principle is that care needs during dying and death are frequently complex and cannot be met by one discipline. An underlying assumption of this principle is that it is possible to know a dying person and their family holistically. This principle also draws attention to an emerging distinction between multi- and interdisciplinary practice. 'Multidisciplinary' applies to teams of professionals who each set goals for the patient independently, are rarely co-located and do not establish a co-ordinated approach to care. In interdisciplinary practice, the team would be co-located, work together to establish a plan of care and jointly work towards its implementation. Interdisciplinary practice also necessitates a high degree of professional respect and trust.

### Limits to knowing the patient

The goal of holistic care has significant merit in that it acknowledges that each person is a total being and that dying often challenges the person on a number of levels. However, failure to explore the limits of our ability to 'know' those for whom we care is problematic in that:

- the dying person has a reducing world where aspects of who they are as a person are contracting (even though new growth may also occur);
- the dying person is limited in their capacity to lead their usual existence by the effects of advanced disease;
- the family of the dying person is often larger than that to which the care team is exposed;
- the dying person and their family have become who they are now through a lifetime of experience that we are only able to access in limited ways.

These issues are important to palliative care practice. First, the acknowledgment that the dying person's world is contracting helps the palliative care practitioner to understand why they become such an important part of the person's world at this time. It allows the practitioner to avoid an inflated sense of their own importance to this person and family, and assists with the transition away from palliative care after death when the family's world again expands.

Second, acknowledging the contracting world of the patient and family during terminal illness can help us to understand why it may not be appropriate for all members of the care team to provide care directly to the patient. Many patients and families feel overwhelmed by the numerous people involved in their care and may refuse to accept specific aspects of care for that reason. In some instances, a patient will refuse care from the counsellor and only accept nursing visits. In multidisciplinary practice such refusal would mean the patient has no access to the care the counsellor would usually provide. However, with interdisciplinary practice, the team would assist the nurse and counselling team members to work together on a plan of care that is then implemented by the nurse. Such care ensures that the patient and family's needs are met wherever possible despite limitations on access.

## Holistic care

It is important to recognise the difference between having complex care needs and having a need to receive direct care from a multidisciplinary team. One of the essential problems with the mainstreaming of palliative care services is the belief that care needs can be met by loose arrangements between members of various disciplines. In specialist palliative care practice, the relationship that develops between the members of varied disciplines lies at the heart of their ability to provide care that takes account of the person as an holistic being. This care does not divide the person up into spiritual, cultural, psychological and physical bits, each hived off to the appropriate professional. Rather it allows the understanding and expertise of these varied practitioners to be utilised in providing appropriate, relevant and effective care regardless of which discipline primarily delivers that care. The relationship between professionals that lies at the heart of interdisciplinary practice develops slowly and painfully but consists of shared understanding of various disciplinary roles, professional trust and an ability to share practice boundaries with minimal professional jealousy. Demonstrating the expertise that has developed in interdisciplinary palliative care is yet another challenge facing palliative care.

## Focus on comfort and the full relief of symptoms rather than cure of disease

The palliative care principle of comfort and the full relief of symptoms rather than cure rests on the assumptions that full relief of symptoms is possible and that the patient will want this relief. Additionally, the focus on comfort rather than cure suggests that dying people accept that they are dying and happily abandon attempts to prolong life. Biswas (1993) suggests that there is a clear distinction between palliative care and terminal care, i.e. that terminal care accepts death as inevitable. Biswas argues that using the term 'palliative care' presents a danger that 'people may stop talking about and confronting the fact that the individual is going to die' (p. 135). This statement is largely ideological. It suggests that to achieve a good death, the person must confront the realities facing them and talk about them. What might be wrong with this?

Even when it is accepted that death is approaching, many people continue to fight for length rather than quality of life. Accepting that death is inevitable does not always equate to the person embracing the idea with open arms, nor does it equate to a desire to talk about it. I have certainly heard more accounts of dying people being brutalised to talk than complaints about not having the opportunity to do so. Work done by Arblaster, Brooks, Hudson and Petty (1989) placed talking about dying as a least desired expectation of terminally ill patients. I have also looked after many patients who continue to enrol in clinical trials of new cancer treatments on the off-chance that there may be a slight survival benefit in doing so. Does such a decision suggest death has not been accepted as inevitable and is this a less worthy choice than that of the person who decides not to pursue further treatment?

Perhaps most importantly, palliative care professionals need to acknowledge that considerable work remains to be done in the area of symptom relief. While it may be possible to relieve many symptoms, this is often at significant cost, e.g. narcotic-induced sedation. Expertise in the area of pain relief is enormous and growing; however, many other symptoms of terminal disease remain sources of significant distress to patients with few interventions available. Fatigue is an almost universal problem in advanced disease of all aetiologies yet little is known about its pathophysiology or management. The effects of cachexia are so accepted in terminal illness that they are largely ignored in practice. Fungating lesions, faecal incontinence and odour from necrotic wounds all plague our patients and are often present in the stories of those who call for euthanasia. The challenge to palliative care lies in researching and exploring interventions for these and other symptoms that continue to cause dying people distress.

## Responsive care

A useful concept to begin to articulate the way in which palliative care practitioners work with clients to negotiate care that is reflective of their values, beliefs and expectations for care may be *responsive care*. This con-

cept suggests that the palliative care practitioner/team spends considerable energy working with the patient and family to determine their specific care requirements and then respond in ways that allow these needs to
be met. The idea of responsive care also allows the practitioner to take
divergent approaches to care in various situations and even within the
same family. One nurse I recently spoke to explained that sometimes she
will stand beside a family, working with them in care decisions. At other
times the family will take the lead and she will move to the background in
a role supportive of what they are doing. At other times she will move into
the lead on decision-making because of a crisis or impasse in the dying
process. The relationship that she builds with the family allows her at
times to take risks in care, responding to unexpressed needs such as the
need to complete unfinished business or to acknowledge that death is
close at hand. Such risks are often taken without the direction of the client
but in ways that allow the client to refuse to take the path that is being
presented.

The idea of responsive care suggests that sometimes the most important
care decision will be to forget the bath and have a cup of tea with a dying
person's wife or husband. When we ask what kind of care this palliative
care service provides, the specific answer is 'it depends'. Here palliative
care practice moves away from the care demands suggested in the Ariès'
quote, which depicts the need to move the patient towards a peaceful and
accepting death, to the tailor-made service that is in reality often delivered. Responsive care accepts that sometimes the person will choose to be
in pain rather than have their senses dulled by increased doses of drugs
and acknowledges that acceptance of death is not always the goal. Such
care also raises dilemmas in practice when patients and families choose to
refuse the best of our expertise and to die in ways that we would not
choose for ourselves.

## A word about the future

Palliative care is a relatively new specialisation in health care and it owes
a great debt to those early hospice visionaries who created the possibility
of skilled and expert care of the dying. However, the early hospice ideals
mask the complexity of palliative care practice and silence the knowledge
and skill in care of the dying that has developed and continues to grow.
Today's palliative care must acknowledge the complexity of decision-
making at the end of life, grapple with symptoms that defy current therapies, act to protect the interdisciplinary nature of care delivery, and work
within the political context of mainstreaming, outcome measurement
and competitive funding. To do all this, while keeping alive the vision of
hospice care where there is respect for the person and a genuine commitment to improve their care, palliative care must remove its ideological

mask. Palliative care practitioners need to vigorously pursue greater understanding of their practice and to articulate it clearly to policy-makers and funding bodies. If an ideological perspective of palliative care continues, there is a real danger that the specialisation of palliative care will cease to exist and become a generalist tag-on to the roles of all health practitioners, with the possible exception of palliative medicine. The emerging knowledge base will end and care of the dying will lose out to the competing demands for healthcare funding.

# References

Aranda, S. (1993). *What is the relationship between palliative care philosophy and care received by dying clients and their primary caregiver? A qualitative evaluation of the Melbourne Citymission Hospice Service.* Melbourne: Melbourne Citymission Inc.

Arblaster, G., Brooks, D., Hudson, R., & Petty, M. (1989). *Terminally ill patients and their expectations of nurses.* Hawthorn, Victoria: Victorian Nursing Council Publication, Oxley House Press.

Ariès, P. (1981). *The hour of our death* (trans. from the French by Helen Weaver). New York: Alfred A. Knopf.

Biswas, B. (1993). A nurse's view. In David Clark (Ed.), *The future for palliative care.* Buckingham: Open University Press.

Bullock, A., Stallybrass, O., & Trombley, S. (Eds.) (1988). *The Fontana dictionary of modern thought,* 2nd edn. London: Fontana Press.

Department of Human Services (1996). *Palliative care in Victoria: The way forward.* Melbourne: Services Redevelopment Unit, Aged, Community & Mental Health Division, Victorian Government.

# 3

# Palliative Care and Cultural Diversity

## Olga Kanitsaki

Palliative care, like all areas of health, care and medicine, is a product of the mainstream culture. Assumptions behind ideas, beliefs and values central to palliative care (e.g. the meaning of terms such as 'individual', 'independence', 'autonomy', 'quality of life', etc.), which underpin certain practices and actions, may not be held by all individuals in society, including those outside the mainstream. It will be contended that immigrants and refugees constitute a large group of 'outsiders' within the Australian society, and that even immigrants and refugees who are more or less 'assimilated' will maintain certain ideas and perceptions from their original culture. When these ideas and perceptions are at odds with mainstream assumptions about hospice and palliative care, pain, dying, and grief, problems may emerge. Health professionals need to recognise that mainstream cultural assumptions, when applied uncritically, help them to maintain their power and cultural centrality while they disempower and further alienate their clients. Health professionals offering mainstream palliative care services thus need to question:

- whether the style and philosophy of care as advocated by palliative care is *relevant and appropriate* to all who need it;
- whether, in its present form, palliative care is *accessible* to all who need it; and
- specifically, whether mainstream palliative care services in Australia are relevant, appropriate and accessible to the people of diverse cultural and language backgrounds who now comprise a significant part of Australian society.

In this chapter an attempt will be made to answer these questions. Examples will be given to demonstrate that in order for the stated philosophies, values and beliefs of palliative care (see Australian Association for Hospice and Palliative Care, 1994) to be translated into practice in a way that is meaningful and therapeutically effective for all people living in a multicultural society like Australia, they must be culturally informed and relevant. As a 'cultural practice', palliative care reflects the values and beliefs of the mainstream culture from which it has emerged. Although benevolent in intent, palliative care also stands as an instance of *culture in action* which creates a *set of power relationships* which may not necessarily benefit or advantage all those who need or receive palliative care. In addressing these issues, suggestions will also be made on what the nursing profession can do in order to *empower* people from different cultural backgrounds and assist them to maintain their identity, dignity, family and community embeddedness/connection, self-respect and quality of life while living with cancer and other life-threatening illnesses.

## The meaning and power of 'mainstream Australian culture'

Culture is comprised of practised (as well as abstracted) values, beliefs, knowledge, ideas and lifeways. Those cultural values, beliefs, knowledge and practices considered important, usually by the powerful in a particular society, are systematically structured and institutionalised. Culture is embodied and manifest in a variety of ways. For instance, it is embodied in objects (for example, furniture, buildings, artefacts, and so forth), in the structure and function of institutions, in human beings operating in conscious and unconscious ways, and in the constructions and expressions of gender and class. It is interactive, creating meaning and significance, and creating networks of power relationships in a living interconnected and experiential world. Culture is not static, but is the subject of constant change in relation to time and place. Culture, human beings, society and social systems all interact and interconnect in a dynamic and mutually dependent way. Thus culture, is always 'in action' at all social levels and in all social spheres.

The mainstream culture of Australia has its roots in the culture and traditions of Great Britain. Many of Australia's institutions and public services such as those related to hospitals, health care services, education, legal services and social security reflect the culture from which they arose and which binds mainstream groups of people. Central to Australia's mainstream culture are values and beliefs which emphasise:

- individuality and sovereignty of the individual (expressed through institutionalised respect for individual autonomy and independence, and other individual rights);
- control and being in control;
- the structure, centrality and sanctity of the nuclear family as opposed to other forms of family (the traditional extended family, the single parent family, and the homosexual family);
- working for material gains;

- future orientation; and
- positive regard for science and technology.

The mainstream or dominant culture has become so well internalised and embodied by most people in Australia that it is perceived as being 'natural'. It is perceived as being the norm, a benchmark and even the only correct lifeway. Anyone who fails to uphold or subscribe to this lifeway risks being labelled as 'odd', 'different', 'inferior', 'other', 'difficult' and even 'a threat to social cohesion'.

## Mainstream Australian culture and the health professions

Each health profession, like the health system itself, is a product of the culture and society from which it has emerged. Further, each health profession has its own (sub)culture which, although differing in significant ways, is nevertheless reflective of the dominant culture from which it has emerged. Consider, for example, the different cultural fields of medicine, nursing, and physiotherapy, and the ways in which these interact with each other as well as with the different institutional cultures of hospitals, other healthcare agencies and settings where they are practised. The mainstream health professions and the institutions in which they operate are extremely powerful since they are the product of, are legitimised by, and in turn reinforce the dominant values, beliefs, skills and knowledge of the mainstream culture and, more particularly, those who subscribe to and are empowered by it. Members of the dominant culture, by virtue of their place within it, are in a position of advantage over those who do not belong and whose knowledge, values and beliefs do not therefore have the same legitimacy or power. The implications of this for immigrants and refugees needing palliative care and the health professionals responsible for delivering this care are extremely serious. This is particularly so in healthcare contexts where given health beliefs, values and practices are 'taken for granted' by mainstream practitioners and held to be the norm irrespective of cultural background and the culturally variant ways in which these norms might otherwise be interpreted.

## Immigrants/refugees in Australia—implications for palliative care

Australia's population is characterised by cultural diversity and language differences. About 23 per cent of Australia's population are born overseas. Of these 5 million people, 13 per cent are from non-English-speaking countries (McLennan, 1996).

Almost 3 million people in Australia are aged over 60 years, and of these over 500 000 were born in non-English-speaking countries. Different ethnic communities have different proportions of elderly people, depending on past migration patterns (Australian Institute of Multicultural Affairs, 1986). As people get older, they are more likely to acquire cancer-related and other chronic debilitating diseases and illnesses (Victorian Cancer Registry Statistical Report, 1989). Thus some ethnic groups may have a disproportionately higher number of their population affected by diseases and illnesses that require palliative care than other groups from time to time.

## Intercultural dynamics and power relations— immigrant experience

What do the 'immigrant experience', being *labelled* 'an immigrant' and experiencing *living as an immigrant* involve?

Immigrant and refugee people left their countries for various reasons, but always to find a safer and better place to improve their life chances and the general quality of their lives. On their arrival in Australia, these people brought with them their past histories, identities and experiences as individuals and as members of families, communities and nations. In other words, these people arrived as culturally constructed beings. Inevitably, living in Australia, and having to rely on its social systems in order to fulfil survival needs, brings with it new experiences and changes, not all of which are positive or good. They may be painful, involving 'culture shock' (which is typically manifest by physical and psychogenic shock reactions to an environment which is culturally unfamiliar), and being positioned in social locations that marginalise them which, in turn, seriously undermine their life chances and compound their distress. Many find themselves and their families being torn apart by the demands of the mainstream (but otherwise foreign) cultural values, beliefs and institutional practices of their new country which compel them to 'fit in' in order to receive needed services.

Disrupted, dislocated, labelled and marginalised, some immigrant and refugee people face barriers that prevent them from participating fully or meaningfully in the mainstream society, from influencing this society in any significant way, or from creating a personal sense of meaning. Problems of the overseas-born may go unrecognised by those who have little or no knowledge of the damaging and sometimes life-long impact that the 'immigrant and refugee experience' can have. Chief among these problems are feelings of isolation, marginalisation and disempowerment.

Culture shock, and other negative experiences, gradually lessen for many refugees and immigrants as they either assimilate or acculturate to the new culture and society and find a socio-cultural space within which they can survive and create a new life. It would be wrong to stereotype all immigrants and refugees as being intolerably burdened by their immigrant experience. For many, this is not the case. Yet, even for those people who have apparently assimilated and acculturated to mainstream Australian society, a major health crisis, and the need of specialised health care services such as palliative care, could unexpectedly thrust them back into the realm of 'old and familiar' ways based on past cultural values, beliefs and practices, as a means of coping.

## Cross-cultural variability of palliative care services

The generally accepted philosophy, values, beliefs and purposes of palliative care have been created by health professionals who have contributed to founding, developing and practising in the field in western countries. Palliative care as it has been developed and practiced in the western world does not, however, have universal interpretation or application. Indeed, there is considerable cultural variability around the world in terms of how palliative care is viewed, interpreted, practised and accepted (Olweny, 1994; Kerr, 1993; Zenz, 1993; Brasseur, 1993; Tawfik, 1993; Mystakiou, 1993; Dezso, 1993; Setharamaia Vijayaram, 1993; Laudico, 1993; Lickiss, 1993; Fumikazu Takeda, 1993a, b; Goh, 1993; Pongparadee Chaudakshetrin, 1993; Nguyen, 1993; Kanitsaki, 1996a). This variability is due to a range of culturally mediated factors including: a lack of resources, lack of appropriate pharmaceutical products, fears relating to the use of opiates, a lack of appropriately qualified health professionals, a lack of scientific knowledge by the public about life-threatening disease and illness, a lack of awareness and knowledge about the aims and benefits of palliative care and, not least, different cultural attitudes towards death and dying.

When people have no understanding of the potential and purpose of palliative care, demand for such services remains subdued. In Japan for example, massive communication activities were organised to teach medical professionals and lay people about cancer and pain management using the World Health Organization's (WHO) method for pain control. Following public education, substantial demands were made for the use of WHO's method to control cancer pain. These demands were made by professionals, cancer patients and their families alike (Fumikazu Takeda, 1993a).

It is estimated that 70–80 per cent of persons needing palliative care around the world suffer from cancer. Two thirds of the world's cancer patients live in developing countries with less than 10 per cent of the resources committed to cancer care (Olweny, 1994, p. 18).

Under the auspices of the World Health Organization, countries around the world are attempting to establish palliative care services. Some countries have succeeded more than others and their relative success seems to depend upon the country's culture and resources. In France, for example, palliative care developments are resisted by some health professionals, and inadequate palliative care service developments in Germany has been attributed to severe legal restrictions in the use of opiums (Zenz, 1993; Brasseur, 1993).

It is suggested that, in China, Chinese resist surrendering to diseases. Palliative care services in China, therefore, are developing in a way that is acceptable to the population. Such care services are given culturally relevant and meaningful names and are practised in a way that reflect cultural beliefs, understandings and perceptions. Palliative care in this instance incorporates active treatments, such as NGT nutrition, IV fluids, antibiotics, blood, and oxygen. Sometimes surgery and CPR is requested by patients and such requests are respected. Traditional medicine and accupressure for the relief of pain is used, and 70 per cent of Chinese who suffer from cancer are not told of their diagnosis (Kerr, 1993).

Countries such as Greece, Egypt and Hungary have developed home care networks and train family members to care for their sick members. It is estimated that 90 per cent of Greek people die at home. In Egypt and Hungary trained relatives care for their sick family members, even when they have spinal and/or thoracic and cervical catheters in situ for the introduction of analgesic drugs (Tawfik, 1993; Mystakidou, 1993; Dezso Embey-Isztin 1993).

In Australia a recent cross-cultural qualitative research study with persons diagnosed with cancer revealed some variations in knowledge, understanding and beliefs about cancer (Kanitsaki, 1996b). People from four ethnic groups were interviewed: 20 Greek born, 20 Italian born, 8 Chinese born and 20 Australian born from Anglo-Saxon-Celtic backgrounds. Participants were suffering diverse cancer diagnoses and were in different stages of their illness. The study found that strong beliefs were held among Greek and Italian participants about cancer's fatal outcomes and a number did not believe that early detection would make any difference to their survival. Perceptions of cancer included its classification to male and female categories, (see also Gifford, 1991) particularly when referring to breast cancer. It was believed that male cancer was not malignant and therefore curable, while female cancer was fatal.

Participants differed widely about whether and how they should be told of their cancer diagnoses. Significant differences existed between the different cultural groups, and to some extent, between individuals within the participant groups. Disclosure of cancer diagnosis was expected as a *right for self determination* by Australian-born participants from

Anglo-Saxon-Celtic backgrounds, while the expectations of the other groups varied. For example, the Greek-born participants clearly indicated their beliefs and wishes in regards to disclosure of a cancer diagnosis. They identified the following three preferences:

- the majority preferred a discretional judgment to be made in the first instance by the family and subsequently by the doctor; it was expected, however, that the doctor's discretional judgment would be guided by members of the family and by their intimate knowledge of the patient's personality (i.e, whether the client could cope, or would give up and die on receiving the information);
- three participants strongly preferred to be told of their cancer diagnosis; and
- two participants believed strongly that they should *not* have been told their cancer diagnosis and were extremely angry that they had been.

Rationale for such preferences was based on beliefs of what may cause harm or be of benefit to them.

Greek participants believed that the doctors/nurses who disclosed a cancer diagnosis without discretion were 'cruel', 'without compassion', 'indifferent', and 'did not care'. Disclosure was not perceived in terms of a right to self-determination and autonomy. What the Greek born (and Italian and Chinese born) considered important was whether the actions taken were (according to their judgment) to benefit or harm the client. Participants who wished to know their diagnosis believed that it would be obvious to them and it would be rather stupid of the doctors to try to hide the diagnosis. They wished to know their diagnosis because they could then employ all measures (medical and non-medical) to protect themselves from perceived threats to their health, promote their health, and secure a cure.

Beliefs and preferences of Chinese-born participants in regard to the disclosure of a cancer diagnosis were identified:

- cancer disclosure is not acceptable when it involves the elderly; and
- disclosure of diagnosis is acceptable for those belonging to the younger generation.

The Chinese-born relatives and family members of participants indicated that elderly people should not be told of a cancer diagnosis because they were brought up in a culture and time when no treatment was available for such a disease. These elderly had seen people with cancer dying quickly and painfully. Informants indicated that because of this, elderly people had strong fears about cancer diagnosis and believed that once a cancer diagnosis was made, they would die quickly. Family members believed therefore that once a cancer diagnosis was discussed with their elderly relative, the relative would give up and die quickly rather than fight the disease. To prevent the quick death, they believed that the patient must not know the diagnosis. Other Chinese informants indicated that the diagnosis of cancer is not known by many Chinese who have little education and who are from certain parts of Asia (including some rural areas). When told of the cancer diagnosis, they have no idea of the implications, and may have no fear at the time of diagnosis.

Italian-born participants had beliefs similar to those of the Greek-born participants. A greater number of Italian-born participants, however, believed that a cancer diagnosis should not be disclosed. They also believed that it was a very private issue and many would not share it with their close relatives and family members. They certainly would not talk about it to members of their ethnic community. Significantly, unlike the Greek-born participants, they did not describe the doctors who disclosed to them their cancer diagnosis as cruel, indifferent or without compassion.

Other findings indicated that participants and families felt that nurses who attempted to discuss with them death and dying were negative, insensitive, and transmitted to them a sense of hopelessness. Patients felt that nurses who were accepting and telling them they were dying were giving up on them, and feared that nurses would stop 'caring' for them.

Participant–nurse relationships with people from different cultural and linguistic backgrounds were portrayed as extremely weak and technical in nature. Striking differences in the quality of communication and nurse–patient interactions emerged between the Anglo-Celtic-Saxon Australian-born participants and those of the Greek-, Italian- and Chinese-born participants. Meaningful interactive communication was regarded as important for positive relationships to be established, but the majority of the Greek-, Italian- and Chinese-born participants did not establish a meaningful interactive relationship with nurses. Reasons which they provided for such a lack of interaction were:

- the apparent lack of ability or willingness of nurses to establish and maintain effective and meaningful communication, interactions and relationships;
- constant changes in nursing staff prevented participants and nurses from getting to know each other in a meaningful way and thus prevented effective communication between them;
- language barriers;
- shortage of nursing staff;
- nursing staff being too busy; and
- lack of sharing a common meaningful past, history and experience.

Greek- and Italian-born participants indicated that the best, most satis-fying and caring relationships they developed were with trained expert nurses who cared for them continuously and with nurses who spoke their own language and understood their background.

Some Italian- and Greek-born participants perceived that in some hos-pitals patients are given 'excessive' morphine for pain relief. They viewed these hospitals/wards as euthanasia or 'killing houses', and expressed fear in being referred to such care settings. The majority of Greek-, Italian- and Chinese-born participants, however, were unaware of palliative care services and their functions.

Cultural understandings, beliefs, values, perceptions, knowledge and practices about cancer and palliative care have not been researched ad-equately overseas or in Australia. What cross-cultural information is available, as it relates to palliative care, is superficial and inadequate yet is vital to the development of palliative care which is acceptable and hon-ouring to people who need such care services. Health professionals must reflect critically on palliative care concepts, which are commonly taken for granted, before these concepts are translated into practice in our multicultural society.

Because palliative care has existed only a relatively short time, it has not had time to expand into all institutions, nor has it fully penetrated public consciousness. For those whose language is other than English and whose access to mainstream information is very limited, the potential for receiv-ing incorrect and or mixed messages is especially high. Some immigrants and refugees may arrive in Australia (and may remain) with little or no conception of what modern-day palliative care services have to offer, and may view palliative care as overwhelmingly foreign and threatening. The need to survive and escape these perceived threats may, paradoxically, drive people away from seeking palliative care services.

## Making palliative services cross-culturally meaningful and caring

The World Health Organization (WHO) (1989) defines palliative care as:

> the total care of patients whose disease is not responsive to curative treatment. Control of pain, of other symptoms and of psychological, social and spiritual problems is paramount. The goal of palliative care is achievement of the best possible quality of life for patients and their families. (cited in Knowles, 1995, p. 5)

The Australian Association for Hospice and Palliative Care (1994) defines palliative care in similar terms, noting that it should provide 'co-ordinated medical, nursing and allied health services for people who are termi-nally ill . . . physical, psychological, emotional and spiritual support for patients and support for the patient's families and friends' (cited in Knowles, 1995, p. 5).

Such definitions reflect palliative care values, beliefs and standards that guide the practice of health professionals in the field. While driven by humanistic ideals and values, however, these definitions do not go far enough in terms of giving stated recognition to the social, cultural and political realities of multicultural societies like Australia. For example, neither of these definitions includes the term culture nor seems to recognise the role that culture and related social conditions might play in influencing the nature, quality and accessibility of palliative care services available to an individual, family, group or community.

The humanistic and benevolent intent of definitions and standards of palliative care is vulnerable at the point of access and interpretation. For example, notions of quality of life, enhancing client choice, how best to relieve symptoms such as pain, providing for physical, psychological, emotional and spiritual support and facilitating the expression of grief, will all be interpreted in ways that reflect the cultural values and beliefs of the doctors and nurses providing palliative care services and the dominant institutional culture in which they function. Unless nurses and doctors consciously and consistently take nothing for granted and, critically examine all assumptions, palliative care values, standards and principles will inevitably be interpreted and applied in ways that might not always be culturally relevant and meaningful and hence therapeutically effective for people of non-English-speaking and culturally diverse backgrounds.

Consider for example the commonly used terms: 'individual', 'independence', 'capacity to decide and make informed choices', 'terminally ill', 'respect', 'compassion' and 'quality of life', which are often used in definitions and philosophies of palliative care and in statements about what practitioners 'ought' to do to ensure quality care for their clients. While commonly used, such terms are not culturally neutral. They reflect the values and beliefs of the dominant culture, and are understood and practised in a specific way by health professionals who have grown up and who have been educated within this culture. The notion of 'independent individual' reflects a particular form of individual, that is, the lone individual of the liberal state who, it is assumed, is autonomous and self-determined, well informed, confident and free to choose in a way that maximises his (and less frequently her) preferences and self-interests, and who has the power to choose to access relevant options and resources and determine the quality of his/her life. This notion of the 'independent individual' fails to take into account the social–economic–political realities of many people, such as those who do not speak English and who are located in a socially marginal position, who are not always fully informed about the treatment options available to them, or given relevant options from which to choose. Such people can have their autonomy undermined and their ability to choose freely in ways that will maximise their self-interest and authentically reflect their individuality as *they* perceive and experience it and not as others *think* they experience it. Lacking the power to challenge or change the status quo, they may be forced paradoxically to depend on the very people and the system whose lifeways have inadvertently rendered them powerless and vulnerable in the first place.

It is not being suggested that the notions of 'individual', 'independence', 'control', 'self-determination', 'quality of life', and so on, should be abandoned. Rather, it is being suggested that the meanings of these terms should not be taken for granted, and practitioners need to find out what these terms might mean to people from different cultural backgrounds, and what impact the use and interpretation of these notions might have on the provision of palliative care services. As well, 'other' client realities need to be allowed to surface and be identified, defined and given meaning by the clients themselves and in a way that is familiar and empowering for them. The client's perceptions and meaning of 'family' (not just of 'individual'), 'freedom', 'dignity', suffering and pain, 'meaning of life' (not just of the 'quality of life'), care and what constitutes 'therapy', what constitutes 'letting die' and 'living while dying', and other related notions, must all be explored, clarified and made known to all professionals involved in the client's care. Health professionals must realise that any judgments and decisions they make about their clients' individuality, quality of life, the experience and meaning of suffering and pain, care, treatments, and expectations, must never be assumed but must all be verified by the client and their families. All such concepts are culturally bound and may inevitably differ cross-culturally and intra-culturally.

## A way forward to cross-cultural palliative care

How then can palliative care services be made more meaningful, relevant, therapeutically effective and accessible to Australia's multicultural population?

Improving the cultural relevance and appropriateness of palliative care services can be achieved in a number of ways, and requires initiatives such as those listed here.

- Qualitative research should be undertaken into how people, both as cultural beings and as clients of Australia's healthcare system, experience the system and understand, cope with and experience severe illnesses, care, dying and death. Research that has as its focus the kinds of care that culturally different people find helpful, meaningful, authentic and wish to receive will be useful.

- Cross-cultural research should also be undertaken by bicultural and bilingual researchers. It is essential that these researchers hold leading positions in order to avoid mainstream/dominant colonisation and misrepresentation of the 'outsider' the 'other' views, beliefs, knowledge and experiences.

- Multilingual and multicultural public education should be provided on palliative services and care with the aim not only of informing people about the nature and purpose of palliative care, but of demystifying its practices.

- A multicultural workforce, including transcultural nursing experts and staff, should be established. The number of bilingual and bicultural nurses, doctors and other health professionals (not merely health interpreters) in palliative care should be increased. These health professionals should not, however, assimilate entirely into the dominant culture as this could defeat the purpose of involving them effectively in delivering the services in question to Australia's multicultural population.

- Nurses in palliative care will also make a difference by taking the appropriate action to help empower their clients to live so that their dignity, integrity, well-being and personal sense of meaning are enhanced in the way that *they* (the clients) perceive and understand these things. This is not an easy thing to do, however, and requires professional and systemic infrastructure support which aims to improve the *acceptance and legitimacy of cultural variations* and to reduce social inequalities and injustices. It includes not just the development and implementation of social, public and healthcare policies, but a committed program of cross-cultural education including discussions on ethnocentrism and racism, research and other initiatives aimed at educationally preparing nurses to provide culturally informed and relevant care to clients from diverse cultural and language backgrounds.

- Institutional systematic structural changes should reflect a multicultural approach to the development and implementation of policies, regulations and practices in palliative care settings.

- Nursing staff should be rostered in such a way as to ensure continuity of carer and care.

- Services should be integrated so as to ensure that people will not 'fall between the gaps' when requiring and receiving palliative care services.

- Health professionals should collaborate closely with ethnic communities and organisations in determining the relevance, appropriateness and adequacy of palliative care services.

- A multidisciplinary university chair should be established in the area of cross-cultural health and illness, the activities of which should inform public and social health policy including the area of palliative care. The establishment of a distinct chair would give due recognition and draw the necessary attention to this complex and underdeveloped area. If cross-cultural issues in palliative care remain a part of the mainstream concerns, cross-cultural palliative care developments may well remain in the margins.

## Conclusion

In this chapter an attempt has been made to illustrate that the taken-for-granted assumptions that health professionals as cultural beings unconsciously use for interpreting and giving meaning to life and social events in palliative care settings may not be shared by all clients in a multicultural society. These mainstream cultural assumptions of health professionals permeate implementations of core palliative care concepts in ways that can disadvantage, violate and harm clients' sense of being and meaning when they are at the end of their life. This chapter offers a number of suggestions as to how health professions and the health system can develop a more equitable, just, relevant and effective palliative care delivery service to a multicultural society.

## References

Australian Institute of Multicultural Affairs (1986). *Community and institutional care for aged migrants in Australia*. Melbourne: Australian Institute of Multicultural Affairs.

Brasseur, L. (1993). France: status of cancer pain and palliative care. *Journal of Pain and Symptom Management, 8* (6), 412–415.

Dezso, Embey-Isztin (1993). Hungary: Status of cancer pain and palliative care. *Journal of Pain and Symptom Management, 8* (6), 420.

Fumikazu Takeda, F. (1993a). Japan: Status of cancer pain and palliative care. *Journal of Pain and Symptom Management, 8* (6), 425–426.

Fumikazu Takeda, F. (1993b). Papua New Guinea: Status of cancer pain and palliative care. *Journal of Pain and Symptom Management, 8* (6), 427–428.

Gifford S. (1991). The role of public health nursing in breast and cervical cancer screening: a case study of older Macedonian-Australian women. *Proceedings 6th Nursing Research Forum*. Exploring women's health: Where do nurses stand? Bundoora, Vic.: Continuing Education Unit, La Trobe University Department of Nursing.

Goh, C. (1993). Singapore: Status of cancer pain and palliative care. *Journal of Pain and Symptom Management, 8* (6), 431–433.

Kanitsaki, O. (1996a). Euthanasia in a multicultural society: Some implications for nurses. In Johnstone, J-M. (Ed.), *The politics of euthanasia: A nursing response*. Canberra: Royal College of Nursing Australia.

Kanitsaki, O. (1996b). Care and nursing caring in a multicultural society: A critical examination. Paper presented at the 18th Annual International Association for Human Caring Research Conference, Patterns of caring: universal connections. Rochester, MN: Mayo Foundation.

Kerr, D. (1993). Lin Zhong Guan Huai: Terminal care in China. *The American Journal of Hospice & Palliative Care, 10* (4), 18–26.

Knowles, R. (1996). *Palliative care in Victoria: A vision.* Report of the Palliative Care Task Force to the Minister for Aged Care. Melbourne: Health and Community Services Promotion Unit.

Laudico, A.J. (1993). The Philippines: Status of cancer pain and palliative care. *Journal of Pain and Symptom Management, 8* (6), 429–430.

Lickiss, J.N. (1993). Australia: Status of cancer pain and palliative care. *Journal of Pain and Symptom Management, 8* (6), 388–394.

McLennan, W. (1996). *Migration, Australia 1994–1995.* Catalogue no. 3412.0. Canberra: ABS.

Mystakidou, K. (1993). Greece: Status of cancer pain and palliative care. *Journal of Pain and Symptom Management, 8* (6), 419.

Nguyen, Ba Duc. (1993). Vietnam: Status of cancer pain and palliative care. *Journal of Pain and Symptom Management, 8* (6), 440–443.

Olweny, C.L.M. (1994). Ethics of palliative care medicine: Palliative care for the rich nations only! *Journal of Palliative Care, 10* (13), 17–22.

Palliative Care Advisory Council (1991). *Caring for people with terminal illness. A manual outlining Victorian palliative care standards and guidelines.* Melbourne: Health Department Victoria.

Pongparadee Chaudakshetrin (1993). Thailand: Status of cancer pain and palliative care. *Journal of Pain and Symptom Management, 8* (6), 434–436.

Setharamaiah Vijayaram (1993). India: Status of cancer pain and palliative care. *Journal of Pain and Symptom Management, 8* (6), 421–422.

Tawfik, M.O. (1993). Egypt: Status of cancer pain and palliative care. *Journal of Pain and Symptom Management, 8* (6), 409–411.

*Victorian cancer registry statistical report* (1989). Melbourne: Anti-Cancer Council of Victoria.

Zenz, M. (1993). Germany: Status of cancer pain and palliative care. *Journal of Pain and Symptom Management, 8* (6), 416–418.

# 4

# Palliative Care as a Medical Specialty

## Michael Ashby

'Dying is not a subspecialty of medicine; it is our common lot . . . the aim is not a set of rigid structures committed to their own survival and enlargement, but a concentration of effort on achieving lasting change on the circumstances of death in post-industrial societies.' (Alistair Campbell, 1990)

'The world is come full circle; I am here.' Edmund. *King Lear*, 5.3.174.

Many people express surprise that a doctor would want to work with dying people ('it must be so depressing'), but all doctors have to at some stage in their careers. All interns, residents, registrars, many specialists and all general practitioners look after dying people. Those who do so effectively will tell you how professionally and personally satisfying it can be. As with most aspects of practice, doctors derive satisfaction from things they do well and, in order to do them well, some preparation and training is necessary. Historically, in regard to caring for dying people, this has been lacking, and students and doctors have tended to be cynical about the value of formal learning in this area. After all, people have always died and doctors have looked after them, so what is the problem? Until recently, most doctors had to teach themselves by 'learning on the job'; some did very well, but many struggled and patients suffered.

## Social movement

This chapter is written with a background assumption that the Weberian charismatic social movement analysis proposed by James and Field (James & Field, 1992) is a reasonably accurate description of the social context and issues at play in the evolution of palliative care services in countries where the model is already well developed (Elsey, 1996). The opening of St Christopher's hospice in Sydenham, south east London in 1967 is usually taken as the start of what has become known as the modern hospice and palliative care movement. Cicely Saunders and colleagues felt that they had to start up a specialised free-standing institution, on a 'green field' site, quite separate from the National Health Service in order to bring about a real change in the way dying people were cared for in Britain. She gathered around her a small group of dedicated supporters and, together with other pioneers in the field such as Robert Twycross (Oxford) and Derek Doyle (Edinburgh), developed a decidedly charismatic approach as a response to the enormous task which lay ahead. What was new about the approach of Cicely Saunders and co-workers was the focus on medical care, teaching and research. The movement developed as a response to the neglect of dying people in modern healthcare systems which evolved after World War II in developed countries. Medicine throughout the twentieth century had become focused on cure as medical technology had progressively opened up new therapeutic options. The stunning achievements of medical science in an age of scientific optimism had led to a level of expectation in the community that often significantly exceeded reality, particularly in common solid tumour oncology. Healthcare professions came to feel that death was medical defeat. At best perhaps, their contribution to the care of dying people was to know when to stop treatment aimed at cure. More often it seemed that they felt clinically, morally and perhaps legally bound to treat with curative intent no matter how poor the chances of achieving a favourable outcome. Palliative care has emphasised the need for the doctor to be able to 'accompany' a dying person, to be comfortable with the inability to provide a cure and with the uncertainty inherent in terminal illness—and to recognise that there is a significant medical contribution to the care of dying people.

The early developments in the United Kingdom consisted mainly of free-standing hospice and home-care programs together with the Macmillan nurse and medical initiatives. Over the next three decades there has been a remarkable growth in the number of specialist services for the care of dying people. The model spread first to the larger (culturally eurocentric) members of the old British Commonwealth (Canada, Australia, New Zealand in particular), then to a few pioneer programs in the United States, mainly outside mainstream academic medical circles, followed by rapid developments throughout Europe. By the late 1990s most countries of the world have attempted to address the issue in some way or another. Hand in hand with the development of services has been a trend towards professional sub-specialisation, notably in medicine and nursing. However, it is only in the United Kingdom that palliative medicine has achieved full specialty status and a recent bid in Canada has failed (Macdonald, N. 1996, personal communication).

## Australian background

Originally most new initiatives in Australia attempted replication, to varying degrees, of the early stand-alone British hospice and home-care model. When palliative care services started to grow rapidly in Australia in the early 1980s, the area was dominated by a few large traditional hospice programs in capital cities, mostly with origins in established religious denominational healthcare facilities. These pioneering institutions mainly addressed the needs for terminal care (Briggs, 1992). Medical staff, including medical directors and specialists, came from general practice and a variety of specialist backgrounds (psychiatry, anaesthetics, medicine, oncology, surgery and several more). During the 1980s, there was considerable growth, with a wide variety of service configuration and models developing across the country, according to local needs, wishes and history (Allbrook, 1991). The medical role in these diverse hospital and community settings is well summarised by the medical leaders in the field in the late 1980s (Gunz, Kramer, Dwyer, Cavenaugh, Redpath, MacAdam et al., 1989). Although the issues raised were by no means uniquely Australian, these authors established a broad agenda for medical endeavour in teaching hospitals, home-care services, hospices and rural settings across the whole profession, with a strong emphasis on education, for the Australian context. There was a consensus of support among them for the establishment of a medical sub-specialty of palliative medicine.

The 'separatist' beginnings have been followed by a process of re-integration of palliative care initiatives into mainstream clinical services which James and Field argued was inevitable. Thus palliative care services are now seen as being in a continual dynamic state of development *within* health systems, which are themselves in a state of instability and rapid evolution. Higginson has shown that this process is well underway in Britain, where the hospice model always emphasised education and outreach, acknowledging that only a small proportion of patients actually die in specialist hospice units (Higginson, 1993). Australia has not built as many free-standing hospices as Britain and charitable funding support for services has been less. Palliative care units have been set up in a variety of different locations: general hospitals, private hospitals, nursing homes, other aged-care facilities. This pattern has influenced the way appointments to medical positions are made, with many of them in the mainstream public hospital and aged-care system. This process was also influenced in the same mainstream direction by federal funding allocations in 1988 (Medicare Incentive Packages (MIP)) and 1993 (Palliative Care Programme (PCP)). The result is that Australia appears to have avoided a phase of large investment in independent hospices (a 'big hospice' phase) and, consequently, fewer specialist positions have been created than in the United Kingdom. Most of the present leaders in the area made a 'lateral entry' from other disciplines because no specialist training was available, or because the prospect of physician training in mid-career was unattractive. The drive for palliative care to be a separate specialty has also been less pronounced, and even now the pluralist background and lateral entry culture of Australian palliative medicine seems set to continue.

Maddocks' (1994) triangular model of home–hospital–hospice/in-patient palliative care unit is being widely implemented so that all dying people have access to optimal care to meet their needs. Location of care is not seen as being a competition between home (desirable) and in-patient sites (undesirable) but a (seamless) network of services where patients move from one setting to another depending on their needs and wishes. Access to beds is important because of the expertise and complexity of care that is sometimes required. It is also clear that where social and family supports are absent, there are serious limitations to home care, no matter how good and available the professional services are. In metropolitan Adelaide, a good level of access to palliative care expertise developed through the generic domiciliary nursing agency during the 1980s, with 56 per cent coverage of registered cancer deaths in 1990 by a hospice service (Hunt & McCaul, 1996). However, the rate of home deaths remained around 14 per cent between 1981 and 1990. The main change was the availability of hospice beds and deaths there rose from 5 to 20 per cent (Hunt, Bonnett, & Roder, 1993; Lickiss, 1993b; South Australian Cancer Registry, 1995). For some communities (particularly in non-metropolitan areas), the palliative care beds and the team will be designated rather than dedicated, with access to advice and back-up from larger designated services when required. The ratio of designated to dedicated staff in palliative care teams will usually vary according to the population served, ranging from a part-time co-ordinator and all other staff contributing on a sessional or as-required basis in a low population rural area, to a fully dedicated multidisciplinary team in metropolitan locations.

## Palliative care as a medical specialty

The medical profession has an in-built response to new or redefined healthcare needs. Initially pioneers within the generic system take a special interest in the area. If service and academic needs appear to justify it, a process gets underway to form a separate specialty or sub-specialty. There is usually professional resistance to this budding off of a new specialty, but if the demand is there, official and academic recognition eventually occurs. The advantage of this is that a pool of expertise and research develops and (presumably) patient care improves. The down-side is that the specialty has a tendency to self-perpetuation, with professional agendas of its own—in identifying with its patients' needs and wishes, it becomes substantially dedicated to its own professional agenda of self-preservation and expansion. It also tends to focus attention (and resources) on medical challenges, often the more difficult and unusual problems. A palliative care specialist is more likely, for instance, to find a challenge in neurogenic pain than improving carer support pensions. Specialisation can also be a disadvantage in any discipline by the encouragement of over-involvement with the area and the cause of the patients, with consequent loss of objectivity and context. In the complexities and stresses of modern healthcare systems, this can be problematic.

However, the need for medical expertise in palliative care is pivotal and unquestioned. For example, one of the commonest requests from nurses practising palliative care in the community is for improved general practice education in this area. Nurse consultants have played an enormous part in the improvement of the care of dying people. Frequently this has been a demanding and at times uncomfortable role for the nurses concerned and the doctors they work with. Over the last decade or so, these palliative care nurses have had to shoulder too much of the responsibility of palliative therapeutics and decision-making. Consequently some degree of medical sub-specialisation has been a necessary part of the medical response to patients' needs in terms of providing leadership, consultative support, education and research initiatives.

In Australia a watershed era has now arrived in which questions are being asked about the future of palliative medicine. While there are now four chairs established (at Flinders, Newcastle, Monash and Melbourne universities) and programs centred around most of the teaching hospitals, the number of doctors entering specialist training is low. The Australia and New Zealand Society of Palliative Medicine (ANZSPM) was founded in 1993 (Maddocks, 1994) and the Royal Australasian College of Physicians (RACP) offers an Advanced Training Programme in Palliative Medicine with its own Special Advisory Committee (SAC). This program of three years of supervised training at registrar level, with obligatory terms in palliative medicine, oncology and research or other approved elective activity (Lickiss, 1993a, b), has so far, been taken up by only a small number of doctors. There are significant difficulties in recruiting specialists for large and small programs alike, partly due to the absence of training posts. Until now there was only one registrar training program in Australia, run by Norelle Lickiss in Sydney (Lickiss, 1993a, b). Young trainees are not attracted to an area with such limited training posts, absence of clear career pathways and National Specialist Qualification Advisory Council recognition. The possibility is being explored of creating a Faculty of Palliative Medicine under the auspices of the Royal Australasian College of Physicians which would allow multiple track entry with a final common pathway of clinically based supervised training.

Finlay and Jones have described three distinct but interconnected aspects of palliative care: the *palliative approach*, which should be a core skill-base of all clinicians; *palliative interventions*, which are often carried out by other medical or allied health specialists (e.g., radiotherapy, surgery and physiotherapy); and *specialist palliative care*, which is delivered by specialist clinicians in the context of a dedicated multidisciplinary team.

> The *palliative approach* is relevant to all patients with incurable conditions. It emphasises the importance of considering psychosocial and spiritual aspects as well as the purely physical. It includes consideration of family and domestic carers. Most specialities and all general practitioners look after patients with life threatening disease; attention to the patients' concerns and fears can guide management and ensure appropriate interventions. A palliative approach should be a core skill of every clinician, who may seek expert specialist help to ensure the best possible quality of life for the patient. (Finlay & Jones, 1995, p. 754)

This subdivision of palliative care is valuable insofar as it defines this core approach. But it might be read to mean that excellent care cannot be delivered by anyone other than a specialist team; this neglects the fact that the bulk of effective care is given by general practitioners and community nurses, particularly in rural areas, and this interpretation is not presumably intended by these authors.

It is clear that, given the diverse nature of service models required in a country like Australia, general practitioners will continue to provide the backbone of service delivery, including more specialised consultative support to colleagues, particularly in non-metropolitan areas. This role of general practitioners needs continued recognition in two respects. First, the vast majority of general practitioners want to be equipped and resourced to look after their own dying patients as a normal, integral part of general practice. Second, some general practitioners will elect to take a more than average interest in the area. They may look after patients in inpatient units and home-care programs on a sessional basis. In rural areas particularly, it is not uncommon to find that one general practitioner develops a special interest and assists others to care for their patients. This role has become formalised in some centres and some general practitioners have gone on to become directors of programs by this avenue. Each of these levels of involvement has different educational and credentialling requirements. Most resident medical officer posts in palliative care in Australian hospitals have been occupied by general practice trainees. In this way, the community has had access to a steady stream of doctors who have been exposed to the principles of palliative care practice. Similarly, consultative teams in teaching hospitals (Chan & Woodruff, 1991; Woodruff, Jordan, Eicke, & Chan, 1991) are an important source of support and role modelling to young doctors. The cumulative result of this activity for approximately the last decade, together with undergraduate and post-graduate education, has been to contribute substantially to the process of 'normalisation' of palliative care.

It is the complexity of symptom management, multiplicity of symptoms and inherent fluctuations and instability experienced by patients with advanced cancer that have driven the development of specialist palliative care services. Hanks has argued that one of the major modern advances in cancer treatment in recent years has been the improvement of symptom management in patients with advanced or terminal disease (Hanks, 1994). Oncologists have a large role to play in palliative care development, as do pain specialists, who have done the bulk of significant research into pain. Over 90 per cent of patients presently seen by palliative care services have cancer but oncological expertise among palliative care workers varies considerably. The core clinical business of palliative care services is cancer symptom control. This is not to say that there is no role for palliative care skills and approaches for non-malignant conditions, quite the reverse. Most of the symptom control strategies for the care of terminally ill people have been learnt and extrapolated from the care of patients with cancer.

When the attributes of the modern palliative care specialist are un-packed, it is difficult to identify any element that is exclusive to the domain. Those who are not opthalmic surgeons do not remove cataracts and nobody would think of a renal dialysis program without nephro-logists, but nearly all doctors may make a contribution to palliative care and many patients have straightforward deaths without specialist palliative care involvement. If the exclusive knowledge or skill litmus test is applied to palliative care, then it probably does about as well as geriatric or rehabilitation medicine. It is more realistic to view it as a unique attitude–knowledge–skill mix which requires both wide learning and experience but does not pretend to own an exclusive domain. Its main claim to existence is the historical neglect of dying people's needs and the need to refocus medical attention on clinical practice, educational and research issues of relevance to the care of dying people.

## The future

For nearly all doctors, there is an undergraduate deficit in both experien-tial and theoretical learning in palliative care, and practising doctors who are approximately 35 years of age or older may well have had no teaching from a palliative care physician. Such a deficit cannot be satisfactorily redressed by postgraduate education without acceptance by the individual doctor that the deficit exists. Opportunities for clinical experience have been limited, although consultation or shared care with a specialist service is probably the best way of improving clinical skills while enhancing the care of the doctor's own patients. Therefore, there clearly needs to be an urgent and sustained effort to improve undergraduate education in all medical schools, extending into the intern and resident years. Adequate exposure to palliative care in the mainstream medical system should, it is hoped, reduce rather than increase the amount of specialist palliative care expertise required in day-to-day clinical work. This would leave a nucleus of specialists who have predominantly academic and leadership roles.

However, it is not the goal of palliative care specialists to take over the care of all dying people, nor to appear to suggest that a terminal illness is only a medically defined event (so-called 'over-medicalisation' of death) (McNamara, Waddell, & Colvin, 1994, 1995). A commitment to a rounded multidisciplinary approach, with proper attention to spiritual and psychosocial issues, is generally accepted. The main goal of medical palliative care education should be to help doctors to become better doctors. In an ideal world, palliative care specialists would do themselves out of a job in a generation by following a consultative/educational model of activity. In reality, a core group of specialists will probably continue to be needed for many years to come. This is due largely to the time-lag between the introduction of widespread clinical activity, educational and research initiatives, and the consequent attitudinal changes within the profession and a real change in standards of practice.

A core of specialist expertise in palliative care has evolved in Australia and New Zealand in a semi-structured and eclectic manner since about 1980. This process will continue, but some form of collegiate status will probably occur in the near future. Services will most likely be developed more closely within mainstream structures, particularly oncology services. While a small number of physician trainees may elect to follow advanced training with the RACP, substantial numbers of people attracted to the area will come from non-physician backgrounds and this diversity will need to be formally accommodated within the evolving training structures. The involvement of general practitioners will continue to be central to home and nursing home care and some will develop a special interest, particularly in rural areas. Once the initial shortage of trained specialists is addressed, better general education in palliative care should lead to a diminished need for specialists over the next few decades. If this process appears to be circular, leading back into the systems whence the hospice and palliative care movement emerged three decades ago, it should not be seen as a negative result by palliative care workers. The question whether the process of 'mainstreaming' may have caused a loss of 'ideological purity', to the possible detriment of dying people, has been posed (Lickiss, 1993a). But surely the journey has not been without considerable value, in that medicine in the last part of the twentieth century has been challenged to acknowledge its limitations and resume its proper place in the care of dying people. It became temporarily alienated from this by a transient illusion that science and technology could somehow cure all human ills—or rather that if cure was not possible, doctors had no further role or responsibility. The emergence of a sub-specialty of medicine is therefore seen as the means to this end of providing appropriate care for dying people, and not the end itself.

The medical care of dying people should not then be conceptualised as a 'specialist vs generalist' struggle in which territory is demarcated and defended. Instead, the shared short and medium term goals should concentrate on helping established doctors to care for their dying patients and to know when to refer for specialist help. The longer term goals should focus on undergraduate and postgraduate training to change the way the whole profession deals with death and dying.

# References

Allbrook, D. (1991). Palliative care in the 1990s? *Medical Journal of Australia, 155*, 286–287.

Briggs, P.G. (1992). Who needs a hospice? *Medical Journal of Australia, 156*, 417–420.

Campbell, A.V. (1990). An ethic for hospice. *Proceedings of Hospice '90*. Adelaide, October.

Chan, A. & Woodruff, R.K. (1991). Palliative care in a general teaching hospital. *Medical Journal of Australia, 155*, 597–599.

Elsey, B. (1996). Hospice and palliative care as a social and educational movement. Inaugural National Conference on Palliative Care Education. Adelaide, April.

Finlay, I.G. & Jones, R.V.H. (1995). Definitions in palliative care. *British Medical Journal, 311*, 754.

Gunz, F.W., Kramer, J.A., Dwyer, B.E., Cavenagh, J.D., Redpath, R., MacAdam, D.B., et al. (1989). The role of the Australian doctor in palliative care. *Australian Cancer Society Cancer Forum, 13*, 3–31.

Hanks, G.W. (1994). Palliative medicine: Problem areas in pain and symptom management. *Cancer Surveys, 21*.

Higginson, I. (1993). Palliative care: A review of past changes and future trends. *Journal of Public Health Medicine, 15*, 3–8.

Hunt, R. & McCaul, K. (1996). A population-based study of the coverage of cancer patients by hospice services. *Palliative Medicine, 10*, 5–12.

Hunt, R., Bonett, A., & Roder, D. (1993). Trends in terminal care of cancer patients: South Australia, 1981–1990. *Australia and New Zealand Journal of Medicine, 23*, 245–251.

James, N. & Field, D. (1992). The routinization of hospice: Charisma and bureaucratization. *Social Science Medicine, 34*, 1363–1375.

Lickiss, J.N. (1993a). Australia: Status of cancer pain and palliative care. *Journal of Pain & Symptom Management, 8*, 388–394.

Lickiss, N. (1993b). Place of death. *Australia New Zealand Journal of Medicine, 23*, 239–241.

McNamara, B., Waddell, C., & Colvin, M. (1994). The institutionalization of the good death. *Social Science Medicine, 39*, 1501–1508.

McNamara, B., Waddell, C., & Colvin, M. (1995). Threats to the good death: The cultural context of stress and coping among hospice nurses. *Sociology of Health & Illness, 17,* 222–243.

Maddocks, I. (1994). A new Society of Palliative Medicine. *Medical Journal of Australia, 160,* 670.

South Australian Health Commission (1995). Trends in places of death of South Australian cancer cases by sociodemographic and tumours characteristic. In *Epidemiology of cancer in South Australia*. Adelaide: South Australia Cancer Registry, July.

World Health Organization (1990). *Cancer pain relief and palliative care*. Report of a WHO Expert Committee. Geneva: WHO.

Woodruff, R.K., Jordan, L., Eicke, J.P., & Chan, A. (1991). Palliative care in a general teaching hospital. *Medical Journal of Australia, 155,* 662–665.

# 5

# Dimensions of Change in Health Care: Implications for Palliative Care

## Rosemary V. Calder

Until the most recent times, care of the dying was regarded as an act of charity, undertaken throughout western cultures mostly by the family or religious orders with little wider societal or governmental involvement or acknowledgment of responsibility.

In this century, as public health measures reduced the rates of mortality from infectious diseases and hospitals evolved into centres of medical science, research and more latterly high technology, care of the dying was subsumed within the culture of intervention and cure—so much so that medical care is often characterised as imposing aggressive treatment beyond the point of recovery and beyond the wish and tolerance of dying patients and their families, stigmatising the death of the patient as a failure of medicine.

In Australia, religious orders had provided hospice care in some public hospitals from the early 1930s, but only in the 1960s was the modern hospice and palliative care movement launched in the United Kingdom. By the early 1980s, as the movement's focus on the control of symptoms and on the person's illness and dying experience gained acceptance in Australia, those with terminal illnesses, their carers and their families sought alternatives to hospital care. A small number of in-patient hospice and home care services and limited provision for home-based care were supported by Commonwealth funding transfers to the states.

## National reforms to healthcare financing—1983 to 1996

### Health care and hospital services financing

Reform of the financing of medical and hospital services in the early 1980s, under the federal Labor government, provided a platform for a substantial reorientation of healthcare policy and for funding reforms to institutional bed-based services, home-based care and support services, and high dependency residential care services.

In February 1984, as part of the first stage of health financing reforms, the Commonwealth government introduced Medicare to provide universal basic cover for medical services and public hospital services within a legislative framework which also aimed to reduce length of stay in acute hospital services. Shorter stays were encouraged through the reduction in payments for patients in public hospitals after 35 consecutive days hospitalisation, a parallel rapid reduction and then withdrawal of Commonwealth funding for long-stay patients in private hospitals, and the provision of some new funds to states for community health services (Deeble, 1989; Senate Select Committee, 1990).

In 1988 the Commonwealth established a Casemix Development Unit to research the introduction to Australia of a clinical classification system for in-patient hospital services. The proposal to develop casemix funding principles followed preliminary exploration by the Minister for Health of a possible trial of population-based capital payment provisions for hospital and community-based healthcare services, including general practice, through health maintenance organisation structures. This move reflected a growing concern to achieve a number of healthcare reform objectives including reduction to international benchmarks of the ratio of hospital beds to population; redistribution of hospital services towards areas of population growth; and further containment of burgeoning and projected healthcare costs. A casemix classification schema focuses on the development of clinically homogeneous classes of patients and on resource-use homogeneity within classes; a restrained classification structure maximises the differences between classes and contains the variability within each class.

The national research and development program into casemix produced an Australian adaption of the clinical classification schema Diagnostic Related Groups (DRGs), AN-DRG which was introduced in July 1992 (Eager & Hindle, 1994). The DRG system uses diagnostic categories and is designed for acute services and consequently, the AN-DRG scheme had no provision for the identification of palliative care and provided only óne category for rehabilitation. DRGs do not effectively, as yet, recognise complexity of illness, and their application within a casemix funding structure uses an average length of stay for the majority of cases as a means of price setting. Diagnosis is a poor and often irrelevant indicator of the need for complex, lower intensity and longer stay services, now collectively known as sub-acute services, such as palliative care, geriatric medical care, rehabilitation and psychiatric illness, all of which often require longer stay and multidisciplinary care. Under casemix funding principles, long-stay patients are treated as outliers and Medicare funding arrangements require that patients continuing to require hospitalisation after 35 continuous days who are not acutely ill be classified as nursing home type patients; this requirement acts as a disincentive to hospitals to provide high-quality services in palliative care and other extended stay patient care services. In 1992, the Australian Association for Hospice and Palliative Care rejected existing DRGs as a basis for casemix classification for palliative care.

## Community care planning and financing

The next stage of the reforms in healthcare financing, also announced in 1984, concerned the provision of care to frail older and disabled users of health, residential and home support services. A range of grant payments to states for home-care services were combined into the Commonwealth and state government cost-shared program known as Home and Community Care (HACC) under the *Commonwealth Home and Community Care Act 1985*, with bilateral agreements established between Commonwealth and state governments through 1985–86. The establishment of HACC followed reports and studies from the 1970s and 1980s that had highlighted a range of policy imperatives including:

- redressing the imbalance between institutional and community care which encouraged premature and unnecessary admission to institutional care;
- expanding the care options available to frail aged and younger disabled people;
- improving the co-ordination and integration of community care services;
- improving the assessment of individuals for services; and
- urgently increasing total resources for community care.

With an initial Commonwealth–state shared funding base of $172.1 million in the first year of HACC, nine main home care services were targeted for rapid expansion across the country. The services were those (such as domiciliary nursing, home help, delivered meals, laundry services) deemed to provide basic care and maintenance services designed to assist in meeting the physical, psychological, daily living and social needs of the target client group of frail aged and younger disabled people. Resources for HACC had doubled by 1988–89 to total $355.7 million (Commonwealth of Australia, 1989, pp. 1–3).

HACC explicitly excluded the provision of accommodation or related support services, and of an aid or appliance; and *limited* a range of specific services including rehabilitative services, specific disability services, post-acute care and palliative care from the program's range of services. These services, which had been provided through state grants funds when HACC was established, were restricted to 'no growth' areas within

HACC—that is, the level of service could be maintained but no new HACC dollars could be allocated to clients requiring these services. The Commonwealth government clearly perceived post-acute and palliative care services to be the responsibility of the healthcare system and expected state governments to respond to the rapid reduction in long-stay (now generally described as sub-acute care) patients in public and private hospitals. HACC-funded service providers were presumed to be appropriate providers of these services subject to the provision of funds from more appropriate sources (Commonwealth of Australia, 1989, p. 12). HACC was initially established on a 3:1 cost sharing basis between the Commonwealth and the states. The original proposal was that this would be re-balanced over a period to 1:1 funding, with growth in the program achieved through 1:1 matching of Commonwealth annual allocations of new funds by states. In the decade since the program began, states have infrequently matched all available new Commonwealth dollars and the funding ratio for the program has been set at 60:40 Commonwealth–state. The program in 1995 was estimated to provide one or more HACC services to 215000 clients in an average month, with 80 per cent of recipients more than 65 years old. Home nursing services were provided to 30 per cent of clients. No-growth services were estimated to represent 10 per cent of total expenditure, most providing post-acute and palliative care, with home nursing the major post-acute and palliative care service provided. This was estimated to account for up to 30 per cent of clients receiving home nursing (Commonwealth of Australia, 1989, pp. 24–25, 79–88).

## Residential care planning and financing

Following the introduction of the HACC program, the Commonwealth government undertook a major restructuring of residential care services to aged and disabled persons. The reform strategy was to achieve a redirection of national government investment away from residential care services, which provided care at that time to only 9 per cent of aged and disabled persons, towards provision through the HACC of the range of community care and support services shown by a major survey in 1981 (ACOTA–DCS, 1985) to be needed by up to 23 per cent of aged and disabled persons. As with healthcare financing reforms, a primary objective was to move towards lower international resource benchmarks (UK had 28 beds per 1000 of the population over 65 compared with about 50 per 1000 population over 70 in Australia) (Dept of Community Services [DCS], 1986). For a number of decades, nursing home services had been provided on an uncapped funding basis, with the Commonwealth meeting permanent recurrent and additional capital costs for organisations that raised a required capital contribution towards the construction of a nursing home or hostel. By 1985, this arrangement had resulted in the construction and maintenance of 75 281 beds at a total annual recurrent cost of $940 million.

The reform program redefined the role of nursing home care from accommodation services with clinical care to high dependency care environments with admission governed by assessment of need (McCallum, 1990, p. 227). A rudimentary casemix classification system for individual residents was introduced to attach funding to the complexity and intensity of care based on assessed client dependency levels (Dept of Community Services and Health [DCSH], 1989). The dependency funding formulae, known as RCI/CAM/SAM (Resident Classification Instrument/Care Aggregate Module/Standard Aggregate Module) provided a five-level assessment of resident dependency (RCI 1 to 5, with 5 allocated to those at the lowest level of dependency), which generated the amount of nursing and personal care funding (CAM) as per diem payments. A complex set of rules accompanied the allocation of a dependency level to each resident to limit the extent to which residents could be reclassified within a specified period. All residents of nursing homes attracted a national standard per diem amount of indirect care funding for accommodation, hotel services and for associated services (SAM). The most prominent outcome of these changes was the rapid rise in the level of dependency of nursing home residents, with the national average dependency level reaching the RCI 3 level in the early 1990s. Reduced lengths of stay in nursing home accommodation also followed and 60 per cent of all separations from nursing homes in 1994–95 were at death.

Associated with the introduction of dependency determined funding were a range of other provisions, including:

- mandatory assessment for eligibility for admission to residential care against national criteria by aged care assessment teams;
- the introduction of government-monitored outcome standards for quality assurance;
- intensive validation of operator funding claims against resident classifications and staffing ratios; and
- the implementation of resource distribution and planning ratios for nursing home and hostel services.

The ratios were initially set at 100 residential care places per 1000 people aged 70 years and over; 40 nursing home places and 60 hostel places. At the time of implementation of the ratios in 1987, the national ratio of nursing home beds was about 80 per 1000 people 70-plus (DCS, 1986, p. 113).

The RCI and Commonwealth Care Outcome Standards made no explicit reference to the role of nursing homes in the provision of terminal care to residents. The Standards of Care required that 'the nursing home must identify residents suffering from pain, investigate the cause and develop, implement and review as required, an appropriate pain management program which takes into account contemporary pain management techniques' and otherwise focus on the daily care requirements and environmental considerations appropriate to long-stay accommodation for dependent persons. The strictures attached to reclassifying the dependency level of residents seemed to militate against the provision of multidisciplinary and specialist clinical palliative care within the funding levels, and the funding structure which promoted maximum levels of occupancy (usually 98.5%) ensured that the capacity to support relatives or carers through the first stage of bereavement was severely constrained. Additionally, a high proportion of nursing homes are older, functionally inappropriate buildings providing ward-style accommodation, which also limits the capacity of nursing homes to provide effective palliative care (Dept of Human Services and Health [DHSH], 1994).

In 1989, the Commonwealth government undertook a mid-term review of the Aged Care Reform Strategy (DCSH, 1991) which led to a reorientation of some directions. In particular, the Commonwealth modified the residential care places ratio to introduce hostel level care packages as an alternative to requiring persons to enter institutions to receive care at a higher level of dependency than otherwise necessary. The Community Aged Care Packages (CACPs) were first introduced as a substitute for 2.5 hostel places per 1000 people 70+, making the national target ratios 40 nursing home/57.5 hostel/2.5 CACPs. Successive Commonwealth budgets have further amended the ratio in response to national demand so that the ratio reached 40/50/10 in 1994.

The Commonwealth government also controlled the approval of new residential care places, both geographically and in total numbers, to achieve a progressive realignment in the balance of care ratio between high dependency nursing home services; personal care, medium dependency hostel places; and medium dependency community care packages. The national strategy, however, did not take into account the distribution of and population need for substitutable services such as higher dependency community support brokerage services in the balance of care approach and excluded any consideration of the distribution of and population need for post-acute and palliative services delivered within institutions including acute hospitals and nursing homes and through services funded by the no-growth component of HACC. Various reviews of HACC continued to endorse the maintenance of no-growth provisions for post-acute and palliative care services while acknowledging the increasing demand for these services in the community (DHSH, 1995, p. xi).

## The emergence of palliative care in health policy and funding

In the wake of the impacts and interaction of the policy initiatives of the 1980s in financing and health care and hospital services, home care and support planning, and high dependency residential care planning, the Commonwealth government moved to address the gap created in provision of post-acute and palliative care services through the introduction of a targetted, trial-funding program known as Medicare Incentives Packages (MIP). MIP funding was provided to states through the Medicare agreements of 1988 to identify more cost-effective practices and to establish these as recognised healthcare practice. A specific objective of the MIP palliative care funding component was to provide palliative care in the community in order to reduce hospital stays. Total MIP funding for palliative care nationally was $37.8 million in 1988.

Various other continuing and new policy initiatives occurred in the early 1990s, further increasing the focus on palliative care. The inadequate provision of palliative care was highlighted by:

- the variable state outcomes of MIP funding for palliative care and other services;
- the continuing decrease in lengths of hospital stay;
- the introduction in 1988 of a national research and development program into casemix funding for hospital services, followed by the abrupt introduction of casemix-related hospital services funding in Victoria in 1993.

The Medicare agreements between the Commonwealth and states were signed in February 1993 for a further five years. MIP funding for post-acute and palliative care was included in the agreement. The Commonwealth budget that year allocated a $55 million over four years for palliative care. A separately identified funding program, the Commonwealth Palliative Care Program (CPCP), was to run until the end of the 1997 financial year. Funding was distributed to states on an age–sex adjusted per capita basis, with the requirement that states develop an infrastructure and an integrated network of dedicated palliative care services within the public and private sectors, with an emphasis on community-based care.

Palliative care services funded under MIP and CPCP developed within individual states in distinctive configurations.

- New South Wales provided funds through nine area health services and 23 district health services with most services providing shared primary based care with some specialist facilities.
- Victoria provided funding (from Commonwealth and state sources) to 57 community-based palliative care agencies across nine health

regions. The state established regional palliative care service development plans to foster co-ordinated care for clients across the three principal care settings of acute hospital, hospices and the patient's home.

- Queensland utilised existing community services through purchasing arrangements managed by acute hospitals, with a small number of palliative and consultative teams across the state. The state has several specialist in-patient facilities and a number of hospital outreach services.

- South Australia has metropolitan regional palliative care programs and a number of rural regional programs supported by Commonwealth and state funding. Services include hospital services, nursing services, nursing homes and domiciliary care services. Commonwealth funding expanded the range of rural services.

- Western Australia undertook a planning strategy in conjunction with the provision of CPCP funding and developed palliative care within a regional framework with the emphasis on community-based care. A model of integrated home- and hospital-based care with community services providing continuing care to patients admitted to hospital care was developed. Development of palliative care services in rural and remote areas is limited.

- Tasmania developed regional community palliative care services which provide clinical support to in-patient services. The state has one hospice service.

- The Northern Territory developed a specialist palliative care team in Darwin providing consultancy services across the Territory with a handful of identified palliative care beds in acute settings across the Territory. The Territory emphasised the development of palliative care skills within mainstream services, including those to Aboriginal and Torres Strait Islander communities, to accommodate the needs of the small scattered population.

- The Australian Capital Territory has a domiciliary nursing palliative care program, a dedicated hospice and volunteer support program.

The emergence of palliative care in health financing policy, largely as an afterthought and a correction to macro policy shifts, has highlighted a major issue for palliative care service provision within the context of the Australian health care system.

From the early 1980s, policy developments at Commonwealth level regarding the health services system radically redirected service provision from institutions to home-based care in parallel with rapid changes in clinical care and technological applications. Subsequent Commonwealth funding provisions for palliative care from the early 1990s emphasised the development of community-based palliative care services to respond to and enhance reduced hospital lengths of stay. Research undertaken in Victoria, however, supported the international view that a considerable proportion of palliative care is delivered within acute in-patient settings. Victorian data indicate that, in 1995, about half of all palliative care clients supported in the community died at home, a proportion which rose steadily from the introduction of MIP funding in 1988. About 40 per cent died in hospital, with 10 per cent dying in hospice services (Dept of Human Services, Victoria, 1996a). A Victorian survey undertaken in 1994, found that 4.5 per cent of all acute hospital beddays were used by in-patients in the palliative phase of treatment or care (DHSVic., 1996b).

The prevailing Commonwealth and state funding arrangements for palliative care thus operate with significant internal conflict. Commonwealth specific-purpose payments to states for community-based palliative care reflect a policy commitment to a continuum of care across three care settings: home, hospice and hospital. This funding supports an unknown proportion of all persons who can be estimated to need palliative care each year. Separately, the national Medicare agreement provides Commonwealth funding for acute in-patient care covering almost 1 in 20 of all in-patient beddays, while state funds support a range of community and in-patient services. The three separate funding sources offer no effective incentives to provide a continuum of care for palliative care clients and impose financial disincentives against provision of long-stay care in acute and long-term or residential care services.

Demand for palliative care can be expected to continue to increase. The majority of palliative care clients are people with terminal cancer and while cancer is responsible for the second highest number of deaths in Australia, both the number and proportion of cancer deaths have been steadily increasing since the 1940s (Australian Institute of Health and Welfare, 1992).

Reforms to the healthcare system in the 1990s have been pursued within a policy environment that has focused on increasing competitiveness and productivity in the economy generally and in public and private sector enterprises as an essential element in improving Australia's economic performance (Hilmer, 1991). Improvements in competitiveness and productivity require measurements of performance against cost, value and time productivity which reflect both leading indicators of performance and benchmark comparisons, and careful evaluation of these measurements. In the context of health services performance and financing, the National Health Strategy proposed that further reform of the hospital financing system focus on equity of finance, resource distribution and access; efficiency in distribution of resources and service delivery;

enhancement of choice; and adequacy of financing and quality of care (National Health Strategy, 1991). Key goals may be: the introduction of geographical management structures for health services; the distribution of resources on population-based funding formulae through such geographical management structures; the implementation of a price mechanism for hospital services using casemix and the introduction of purchase-provider division of responsibility.

## Future policy and funding directions

The introduction of casemix funding to Victorian hospitals in 1993, South Australian hospitals in 1994, and the planned introduction of casemix funding principles for hospital funding in other states has established the basis for fundamental reform of hospital and other health services funding. It has also established that Diagnosis Related Groups (DRGs), the clinical classification system on which casemix funding allocations are based, do not adequately recognise complexity of illness, and use an average length of stay for the majority of cases as a means of setting case–price relativities. Consequently, Victoria excluded identified palliative care and rehabilitation in-patient services from casemix funding arrangements and established an interim per diem funding arrangement. As casemix funding has been investigated, pilot studies have been undertaken to develop a clinical classification system or systems for palliative care and rehabilitation, and other clinical care now identified as sub-acute care. These studies gave rise to a National Sub-Acute and Non-Acute Casemix Classification Project (SNAP) funded by the Commonwealth Department and Health and Family Services. The SNAP project began in December 1995 with New South Wales as the lead agency and the collection of nationwide data concluded in the latter part of 1996 (DHSH, 1996). The project aimed to contribute to the development of a casemix classification for sub-acute and non-acute in-patients in hospital services and had a specific sub-collection of community-based palliative care services. Findings of the SNAP study and a similar study undertaken by the Victorian Department of Health and Community Services in 1995–96 will test the feasibility of the development of a casemix classification system and validated resource cost weights for palliative care.

The Victorian study was one of a series of research and development projects undertaken in Victoria to develop classification and payments arrangements for a number of separate streams of sub-acute care funded outside AN-DRG-based casemix funding within the Victorian hospital service system. The Victorian palliative care study comprised a comprehensive survey of patients and carers, the services provided and the costs of services in in-patient hospitals, hospices and hospice units, and through community-based home delivery of services. The study aimed to identify and develop a casemix classification system with validated resource cost weights capable of funding the full sequence of an individual patient's care from the moment that palliation was determined the most appropriate form of care. The separation of the clinical care requirements from accommodation/indirect care requirements is proposed. The concept of the sequence of care has been developed to provide a method of classifying chronic conditions and is intended to support provision of co-ordinated care across multiple settings and over prolonged periods of time. With the objective of better integration of services, the Victorian project will develop a funding arrangement that will support the provision of integrated care and will enable the purchasing of care irrespective of the setting in which the care is provided.

The Victorian work, and the parallel work through the SNAP study, fits within the new paradigm of co-ordinated patient care which has gained currency in Australian and international health policies in the 1990s. The co-ordination of patient care services to achieve gains in access, equity and choice and in cost effectiveness and cost benefit has been identified in Australia as crucial to the delivery of viable, small-scale low-volume hospital, community health and aged care services in isolated rural communities. Co-ordinated care provision, encompassing general practice, hospital and home-based care, as a strategy to restrain costs in the escalating cost areas of medical benefits, pharmaceutical benefits and hospital care for persons with chronic illness, debility resulting from advanced aged and specific high-cost health conditions, has been similarly identified by the Commonwealth government and introduced as a trial program for three years commencing in 1996 (DHSH, 1996).

Co-ordinated care, based on the clinical integration of the process of patient care, and requiring the administrative integration of delivery of care within geographic regions and at intra- and interorganisational levels, is crucial to achieving a health system capable of improving health care quality and health outcomes and of contributing to the policy requirement to deliver contained health care costs for chronic illness and long-term care support. Co-ordinated care is a response to the introduction of prospective payment arrangements for health and hospital services and to the requirement to respond to population ageing. Palliative care, as a result of early isolation from the reforms to hospital, community health and home-care support services, is now positioned to lead the way in the development of policies and funding arrangements for integrated health service delivery to Australians requiring co-ordinated care services.

# References

Australian Council on the Ageing and Department of Community Services (ACOTA–DCS) (1985). *Older people at home. A report of a 1981 joint survey conducted in Melbourne and Adelaide.* Canberra: AGPS.

Australian Institute of Health and Welfare (1992). *Australia's health 1992. The third biennial report of the Australian Institute of Health and Welfare.* Canberra: AGPS.

Commonwealth of Australia (1989). *First triennial review of the Home and Community Care Program. Final report of the Home and Community Care Review Working Group to Commonwealth, State and Territory Ministers, December 1988.* Canberra: AGPS.

Conrad, Douglas, A. (1993). Coordinating patient care services in regional health systems: The challenge of clinical integration. *Hospital and Health Services Administration, 38* (4), Winter, pp. 491–508.

Deeble, John (1989). *The Medicover Proposals.* National Centre for Epidemiology and Population Health, Working paper no. 4. Canberra: Australian National University.

Department of Community Services (DCS) (1986). *Nursing homes and hostels review.* Canberra: AGPS.

Department of Community Services and Health (DCSH) (1989). *Resident classification instrument. Guidelines for interpretation.* Canberra: Department of Community Services and Health.

Department of Community Services and Health (DCSH) (1991). *Commonwealth Aged Care Reform Strategy: Mid term review 1990–91.* Canberra: AGPS.

Department of Health and Community Services (DHCSVic.) (1993). *Everyone's future. Directions for aged care services in the 1990s.* Melbourne: H&CS.

Department of Health and Community Services, Victoria (DHCSVic.) (1995). *Aged care in Victoria: The 1995–96 Budget.* Publication no. 94/0324. Melbourne: DH&CS.

Department of Health and Community Services, Victoria (DHCSVic.) (1995). *Palliative care casemix development strategy in aged care program budget.* Melbourne: DH&CS.

Department of Human Services and Health (DHSH) (1994). *Review of the structure of nursing home funding arrangements, stage 2.* Canberra: AGPS.

Department of Human Services and Health (DHSH) (1995). *The efficiency and effectiveness review of the Home and Community Care Program. Final report.* Aged and Community Care Service Development and Evaluation Reports, no. 18. Canberra: AGPS.

Department of Human Services and Health (DHSH) (1996). National SNAP committee meets. *Australian Casemix Bulletin, 8* (1), February, 6.

Department of Human Services, Victoria (DHSVic.) (1996). *Case finding survey.* Palliative Care Publication Series, no. 1. Melbourne: DHS.

Eager, Kathy and Hindle, Don (1994). *Casemix in Australia: An overview.* The National Casemix Education Series, no. 2. Canberra: HS&H.

Hilmer, Frederick, G. (1991). *Coming to grips with competitiveness and productivity.* Economic Planning Advisory Council, Discussion Paper 91/01. Canberra: AGPS

McCallum, J. (1990). Health: The quality of survival in older age. In Australian Institute of Health, *The second biennial report of the Australian Institute of Health* (p. 227). Canberra: AGPS.

National Health Strategy (1991). *Hospital services in Australia: Access and financing.* Issues Paper no 2. Canberra:

Senate Select Committee on Health Legislation and Health Insurance (1990). *What price care? Hospital costs and health insurance.* Canberra: Commonwealth of Australia.

# 6

# Competing Discourses with/in Palliative Care

## Annette Street

Society can be analysed according to dominant and subordinate discourses; those that generally occupy the centre or norms of our life and those that are oppositional and generally marginalised (Weedon, 1987). A 'discourse' is a useful tool for analysis as it demonstrates how particular forms of language, associated practices and social institutions combine not only to structure what it is possible for us to think or do, but also to limit our potential for thinking and acting differently. These palliative care discourses are themselves intersected and disrupted by other sets of discourses framed by the interests of health economics, health policy, medicine, nursing and community. In turn these discourses are framed within philosophical, socio-ethical, legal, bio-scientific and theological discourses of death and dying. An acknowledgment of this level of complexity is a necessary basis for a reading of this chapter, although a deeper exploration of these discourses is beyond its scope.

The palliative care philosophy was structured to counter the medicalisation and institutionalisation of the dying process inherent in the prevailing discursive field of medicine. Palliative care focuses on the centrality of the person with their physical, social, emotional and spiritual needs underpinned by a number of discourses—including truth-telling, choice, spirituality, palliation and teamwork—which define the way people are cared for.

## Truth-telling

The demise of the patriarchal 'doctor knows best' discourse, with all the language structures and practices which maintained it, resulted in the emergence of a discourse of 'truth-telling'. This discourse challenged established notions of 'protecting the patient' by withholding information, proposing in its place that it was the right of each individual to know the 'truth' about their illness and prognosis. Truth-telling is a seminal discourse because palliative care decisions, practices and services are predicated on the assumption that the person is able to acknowledge their impending death and make fully informed choices about its manner. The notion of truth-telling is bolstered in the professional literature by such words as 'empowerment', 'advocacy' and the 'right to know'. In each instance the assumption is that the terminally ill person wants to know the full 'truth' about their situation. In the British and Australian palliative care tradition, truth-telling has been strongly aligned with choice but it is evident that this is not so for other European traditions who have similar western medical traditions. Kanitsaki (1989) explained that in Greek culture the practice of truth-telling to the person who has not asked for it is very cruel and is considered as removing their freedom of choice to determine just what they want to know about their prognosis. Kanitsaki (chapter 3) also makes the important point that, in family-centred cultures, the individualistic approach to conveying the 'truth' to the ill person may be inappropriate and unhelpful. The person may see that this discussion should always be conducted within a family context to provide support and participation in decision-making.

Of interest is the way that this discourse is framed to debate questions of who should tell the truth to whom and when, while leaving aside the bigger question concerning what this 'truth' means for the professional and the person. Whose truth is being conveyed and what is the effect of this 'telling'? The truth about a person's death is always framed in a particular socio-ethical context and the manner by which that context is structured depends on the discursive field from which it is comes, such as western medicine, indigenous health beliefs, nursing, counselling, chaplaincy, alternate health practices. Yet 'truth-telling' is inevitably framed discursively as if there is an agreed upon version of the truth, one which is generally framed in a medico-scientific discourse which proposes a medical prognosis of impending death. Many of us continue to be amazed at stories of how people in palliative care programs still seem to be unaware that they, or their loved one, is dying (Aranda, 1993). Why is this so if entry into a palliative care program is dependent on the acknowledgement of the inevitability of death? Who told them the 'truth'? What 'truth' did they hear? What did they want to know? These questions have not been adequately debated in the literature, nor addressed by practitioners.

## Choice

Related to the discourse of truth-telling is the discourse of choice. The discourse of choice has both a personal and a political component—it relates to manner of death and the favoured environment for the dying process. Through the truth-telling process, opportunities were created for active decision-making by the person concerning the way they wanted to live out the rest of their life. This discourse of choice was also formulated to enable the person and their family to choose the most desirable place for death. These two components of choice are influenced by many other discourses.

If we begin with the person, then choice is related to the manner by which the person can opt to 'take control' of their dying process. Again the discourses of 'empowerment' and 'patient's rights' have been central in challenging a medical and government benevolence which assumed that the person wanted to be actively treated until dying in the most techno-logically sophisticated setting. As argued by Kanitsaki (chapter 3), choice is generally focused on options for the individual but has ramifications for the family of the person. If decisions are not made in conjunction with key family members, then the person may find it difficult to discuss the impending death and options with them, particularly when family mem-bers are the children of the dying person. Yet, choice also means that health professionals need to be aware of who is considered 'family' by the person. In homosexual relationships, this may involve the gay or lesbian community rather than the natural family, or it may mean both sets of relationships. For others, friends may constitute their family of choice; and sometimes family means a range of relatives generally not considered close in our society.

Choosing to take control and be actively involved in decision-making necessitates a continual negotiation of desires as circumstances change. The discourse of the 'good death' has been undergirded by the notion that the person has the capacity and will to choose and negotiate the manner of their death. To suggest that some people may opt not to take control in this way lays the speaker open to charges of paternalism. Yet choice is about choosing to give over control as much as it is about choosing to take up control. For many professionals, the discourse of choice presupposes that a person wants the responsibility of constantly making choices; yet very ill people may not wish to be continually consulted on their preferences, nor may their saddened loved ones be able to agree on the decisions to be made on their behalf. As a man reported in a recent study (Street, 1996):

> I don't want to be constantly bothered having to talk through what to do next. I am dying. I want to spend time with my wife and friends. I don't want them arguing about what should be done either . . . I am DYING. I want one person to talk to and have them deal with all these decisions . . . it is too much . . . I don't want to talk all the time . . . I don't want all these choices.

This man made a choice: he has chosen to no longer be involved in the ongoing decision-making related to his care. Yet he reported that the professionals who cared for him had difficulties with this decision:

> . . . they come and sit beside me and talk and talk and ask me what I want to do now . . . and it is too much . . . when my son died, I wanted to be involved in all the decision-making . . . this time I have made the big decision not to have any more treatment. That is enough.

I am not advocating a return to professional decision-making for terminally ill people; indeed I have long been concerned about the exercise of power by health professionals. I want to disrupt the professional assumptions that people are offered appropriate choices and argue that these choices are framed by a particular discourse which is often applauded and rarely challenged. Do dying people have real or illusory choices? How are these choices offered? By whom? To whom? Are choices offered to the individual or the family? How? What factors influence the way these choices are presented? Are the choices culturally appropriate? It is easy to enshrine options into formulas and habitual ways of thinking, speaking and acting. It is harder to constantly question the effects of these familiar ways of thinking and being on the people we care for.

Personal choices as to the place and circumstances for the last days of life assume a range of desirable service options. Indeed the discourse of choice situates the dying person at the centre of the environment of their own choice. The emphasis on choice assumes a variety of equally appropriate options. This is rarely the case. In Australia the home has been the starting point and interventions have been minimalist and directed at creating greater comfort for the person. De-institutionalised palliative care has not relied on high technology and care has been provided as a part of home life rather than dominating it. Home care continues to be the most favoured Australian option, yet most palliative care patients are still elderly cancer patients who die in hospital for the lack of hospice beds, respite beds or 24-hour palliative team support. Why has this situation occured? Why are these choices not being supported?

Service provision is influenced by particular mainstream health economic discourses interested in costs and outcome measures which limit the services and therefore the choices people can make about services. Palliative care services have evolved to meet specific local needs and have been initiated by the competing interests of religious orders, charitable trusts and hospitals. As Calder (chapter 5) demonstrates, each Australian state has adopted a slightly different range of palliative care services and each state's focus is comparable but not the same. This situation has occured in part because government has been a late player on the scene and is now scrambling to create a bureaucratic framework to mainstream palliative care services and to address obvious service gaps. But service gaps mean that the notion of a choice of service may be somewhat illusory.

Calder argues that the marginalisation of palliative care services has left them to develop in isolation from the earlier health reforms visited on mainstream institutional and community services. She is optimistic about the role that palliative care can play in leading the way in the development of policies and funding arrangements for integrated health service delivery. Another reading of the situation might see that health reforms share common values with palliative care, but they are informed by different discourses.

Health economics became dominant at a time when the range of possible health interventions were escalating for an ever-expanding market of older people who were living longer and expecting quality health care. Consequently the economic discourses of *access* and *equity* supported notions of competition between service deliverers rather than the socially informed discourse of co-operation between services (Duckett & Swerissen, 1995). With costing allied to performance and outcomes, palliative care services have had to come to terms with a market economy which encourages competition through best practice, performance indicators and outcome measures (Tierney et al., 1994). Discourses of integration, regionalisation and de-institutionalisation are combined to structure forms of hospital and healthcare networks which are required to compete for contracts which are assessed in terms of the key criteria of the discourses of *customer service* and *quality* (Victorian Government, 1995). Customer service is described and evaluated primarily in terms of patient satisfaction, health outcomes and location, whereas quality is examined in terms of equity, access, and clinical best practice (Harvey, 1991). These concerns with quality and client-focused service are in accord with the values of palliative care on choices.

Palliative care discourses are constructed around the person as a social, familial and communal individual. These discourses are informed by social and community values of participation, choice, process, individualised care, community development—values which were reflected in the socially informed health policies. Although the health reforms also place the person and the family or local community at the centre of their policies, the interests and structures have been largely defined by a different set of values, that of health economics. As palliative care services expand through government funding, they are also being mainstreamed into structures created by the health reformers, and indeed sometimes, being asked to lead the way (Calder, chapter 5).

Yet concerns remain. The health reforms route appears to share some key discourses with palliative care, but the British experience shows that the interests which inform these discourses come from very different philosophical positions and form uneasy partnerships (Clark, 1993a). The bureaucratic and economic discourses collide with the palliative care discourses concerning what it means to provide person-centred care. They value the same thing but approach it from either a systems approach or an individualised community approach. One discourse values the manner by which the system can provide the structures to support the person whereas the other starts with the person as an individual and the ways to meet their immediate, and possibly idiosyncratic, needs. This variation suggests that although decisions on policy may be appear consistent, the actual structures and practices will frequently diverge as will the philosophical and discursive underpinnings. In this book, Rumbold (chapter 1) challenges the notion that specific techniques developed for palliative care can readily be transferred to mainstream care, highlighting the context-specific, professional nature of relationships which form the palliative care team. Do fully integrated services provide high-quality care for all people regardless of culture, desire or need?

The discourses which frame early discharge policies and hospital-in-the-home programs are the products of these reforms and are argued on the grounds of personal choice for continuity of care and 'normality' for severely disabled or chronically ill persons (Anderson, 1990). Transitions and normalisation have become the hallmarks of the de-institutionalised discourses surrounding the person, the aim being to allow the person to live as 'normal' a life as possible at home until death, in whatever way they define 'normal' for themselves.

There is little research being done on the long-term effects on families and the community of the demands of these home-care measures over an extended period of time (Simon et al., 1995). Many hospitals-in-the-home function as spokes from the hub of the acute hospital, are medically dominated, technologically driven and create a 'clinic' in the home rather than allowing the normal home routines to prevail. They are invariably set up by nurses from institutional settings who bring institutional procedures into home environments. Wellard (1996, p. 57) found that: 'nurses operated within medical, physiological and technological discourses that constructed subject positions for the patients to assume. The nursing role was to help patients conform to these subject positions through normalising strategies to facilitate "compliance".'

The mainstreaming of palliative care into institutional networks potentially provides more people with access to these services but runs the risk of changing the focus to one where the work in the home is directed by institutional and medical discourses; where person-centred approaches are rhetoric not reality. The role of the nurse is crucial in the transition from life to death and the normalisation process. Nurses can develop relations that enable the person and their family to define how they want to live and how they want to make their own transitions through the time leading to death.

## Spirituality

The emergence of a discourse of spirituality is a response to the need for the person to make their own meaning out of the circumstances of terminal illness and create their own strategies and rituals to travel the path to death. Discourses of spirituality are not restricted to 'talking therapy' but recognise also the place of the aesthetic; of art and music therapy, meditation, prayer, aromatherapy and therapeutic touch. These discourses express the sensual, intuitive and creative aspects of dying.

These reconstituted an earlier religious discourse which was connected to a theology of the salvific nature of pain. To a generation that had few resources to manage severe cancer pain, this religious discourse held explantory power concerning the reasons for pain and suffering in the dying process: the reason why the person was in uncontrolled pain was related to the way they were working out their salvation on earth. The advent of sophisticated pain management enabled theologians to rethink this supposition and to recognise a broader human need for meaning in the dying process.

Discourses of spirituality are also related to discourses of truth-telling and choice. Palliative care services have developed from a system informed by white religious, charitable and medical discourses. Little work has been done with ethnic groups to determine what meaning they make of the dying process, or what they want from palliative care services. The work that is being done is generally informed by dominant health and religious perspectives. Competing health and religious discourses are marginalised and people from those traditions are treated as 'other'. And, although her research design was structured to include Italian-speaking and Greek-speaking interviewers to explore palliative care issues with these ethnic groups, Aranda (1993) found that these Italian and Greek people did not want to participate. It appeared that some of the foundational palliative care services, such as bereavement counselling, were considered to be inappropriate as these were considered to be the role of the family.

Likewise, palliative care services that are culturally consistent with the traditions of indigenous peoples is an important but neglected area, and one that requires sensitive investigation. Anglo-Australian traditions around death and dying are reasonably explicit in the culture and there are no taboos on discussing them. Indigenous peoples, however, do not discuss some aspects of these processes with outsiders. Thus they cannot become known to other healthcare professionals and integrated into white palliative care and bereavement processes. As indigenous people are much more likely to die younger from causes other than cancer, palliative care has not been considered as vital as other health causes; however, this issue needs to be addressed by indigenous health services rather than by white government initiatives (Baker, 1996).

The discourses of spirituality have not only been focused on the terminally ill person; they have included discourses of bereavement which acknowledged the dying/after death process and the need to offer support to the person and their family or caregivers as a unit. Government initiatives to mainstream palliative care services have been structured so that these spiritual needs are met by the family, the community, local counselling services and parish churches. These initiatives assume that the members of these groups are able to effectively meet the spiritual needs of and be comfortable with dying people. Many people are not gifted to be alongside dying people: to cope with the sight and smell of deteriorating bodies and focus on the person; to offer appropriate non-judgmental support for the desires of the dying person; to facilitate different and confronting social or health practices; to allow the person to lead the way. These issues need to be acknowledged and addressed as changes are made to provide a broader, more generalised range of services.

## Palliation

A discourse of palliation has emerged that has revolutionised symptom control and enabled most people to be pain free to live well in their place of choice. This discourse privileged care practices that challenged the techno-medical discourses of cure which had hitherto shaped the approach to care of the dying (Woodruff, 1989). Techno-medical discourses of cure led either to heroic and intrusive technological interventions in the dying process or to an abandonment of the person when it was clear intervention had failed (Burns, Carney & Brobst, 1989). This discourse of palliation also challenged earlier religious discourses of suffering which supported the notion of pain in dying.

Palliation is being increasingly adopted by the medical profession and incorporated into medical curricula (see Ashby, chapter 4). At the same time it is being redefined to place more emphasis on broader care categories where the person's condition is deemed incurable and will eventually lead to their death. The role of technology and creeping medicalisation are other aspects of the debate which need continuing discussion. The low technological environment of the early hospice programs has changed as more people are given palliation for a wider range of conditions. Use of interventions such as radiotherapy to relieve pain are increasingly common activities of palliative care. The 'purists' who consider any technological intervention as an anathema are being challenged by other medical practitioners who are adamant that some patients will die in more comfort with intravenous medication (Ahmedzai, 1993). Biswas (1993) raises the concern of creeping medicalisation evident in research which shows that units with resident medical input order more invasive investigations than those without, and that there is an increased risk of these tests becoming routine practice.

The 'die with dignity' discourses of euthanasia supporters have placed pressure on the exponents of palliative care to demonstrate that they can manage symptoms to enable people to live and die well. In an Australian society where people have died with legally sanctioned euthanasia the discourse of palliation is being re-shaped in response. The desire for people to die 'pain free' can take precedence over other aspects of palliation which relate to the comfort of the person. The medical aspects can ignore the socio-ethical and spiritual aspects of the dying process. Nurses and relatives have reported concern that some people are maintained in a pain-free state but in the process lose their own identity:

> my dad was always a serious person . . . a concerned person. The doctor kept him painfree but euphoric . . . it changed him totally. He would giggle at everything and not take anything seriously. It really hurt mum and I to see him like that . . . it wasn't him at the end (Street, 1996).

Others report anger that their loved one is not pain free as has often been promised by the rhetoric of palliation.

The medico-scientific focus of discourses of palliation, with a focus on methods and drugs, are sanitised discourses. They ignore the impact and effect of the dying body when it is oozing, putrid, unsightly, disfigured, incontinent. Nursing care is often sanitised. The agony for the nurse of dealing with the depressing and dehumanising aspects of nursing are disguised in discourses of patient care and personal hygiene. Nurses are often the only people, besides the closest caregiver, to experience the physical effects of terminal illness. This intimate relationship is typified in the central nursing comfort activities of body care. Nurses need to enter the palliation debates with their own experiences of intimate care for the dying. They need to disclose the effects these intimate bodily relationships have on themselves, on those they care for and on their caregivers.

## Teamwork

Teamwork was integral to the development of palliative care services and redefined multidisciplinary team relations. This multidisciplinary team was focused around interdisciplinary relationships typified by the discourses of collaboration and co-operation between the person, their family, health professionals and volunteers. The team met regularly to discuss each case, a feat which required physical proximity and an appropriate location. Early palliative care services were marginal to mainstream health services, and required professionals to be prepared to make sacrifices to maintain the service.

Recently, the Australian government has quite rightly proposed that palliative care services should not be limited to those fortunate few who have access to a palliative care service. To achieve this there have been proposals that generalist domicillary nurses and the GP form the backbone of service delivery, rather than specially trained palliative care teams. This decision is an obvious attempt to broaden access, particularly in rural and remote areas where the domicillary nurse is an essential front-line health provider. Yet moving from specialist nurses to generalist nurses, with specialist back up, may have important implications for the quality of service provided and the future of palliative care services. Aranda (1993) argues that the role of the palliative care nurse is complex and often not well understood by bureaucrats and other health professionals. District nursing services are primarily funded as nursing services and not as interdisciplinary teams. No matter how well equipped the nurse may become to offer palliative care, they have heavy case loads and belong to a generalist nursing service. The use of general domicillary services may also serve to support the increasing dominance of palliative medicine because decisions are made by a physician and carried out by a community nurse, rather than within the interdisciplinary team context. As a consequence it is possible that the dying person may lose the holistic interdisciplinary approach because the nurses do not have the same specialised networks.

Public appeals have funded much of the work of hospices and palliative care services and volunteers have been central to their development and service provision. With the integration of palliative care services, there have been changes to the roles of volunteers. Social changes mean fewer volunteers are available for the skilled roles of working with the terminally ill. And yet, the health reforms in Australia are designed to involve the community as much as possible in the delivery of local health services. The increasing expectation that appropriate bereavement work can be done by local churches and community counsellors denies the specific expertise needed to provide sensitive and effective support to the dying person and their family provided by trained lay and professional team members.

The impact on the multidisciplinary team is instigated not only by the discourses of government health policy. Another set of medical discourses are at play. These discourses argue the advancement of palliative medicine through the academic discourses of research and teaching (Doyle, 1993). Academic appointments and research fellowships in palliative care are located in medical faculties and where there are interdisciplinary teams, they are under the direction of a medical professor and involve staff who are more focused on the medical concerns (nurses, physiotherapists) than on those involved in more psychosocial and spiritual concerns.

Nurses and other health practitioners speak of how they are invited to contribute to workshops for medical practitioners but the invitation and the leadership is provided by the doctors who organise them. While this direction continues to be led by doctors saturated in the alternative hospice values and practices, then the concern about how symptom control fits into the wider picture of palliative care is not a major concern. However, it is easy to visualise a scenario where medical students have had a few classes in symptom control, under the guise of palliative medicine, and then are expected to collaborate as team members in the provision of appropriate holistic care to terminally ill people in their practice.

As has been argued by Rumbold (see chapter 1), there has also been a change in team leadership in community-based palliative care services from nurses to doctors. Palliative care nurses have lamented the demise of teams where the nurse co-ordinated the care and have commented on the increasing leadership being offered by doctors or health administrators which has resulted in a more hierarchical style no matter how benevolent it appears (Street, 1996). Under the New South Wales registrar scheme, the doctors have argued for generalist nurses and specialist doctors, another indication of the emerging primacy of the medical role in the team.

Government policies support the primacy of the GP in the care of the terminally ill. Although many general practitioners provide an excellent service to palliative care patients at home, the increased use of GPs as the primary palliative care practitioner may also mean that the person receives a specifically medically focused service, unless the GP is linked into an interdisciplinary team. In the busy general practice, the doctor may refer to nurses but not involve volunteers or other professionals like a psychologist or chaplain.The rise of 24-hour bulk-billing medical clinics in Australia means that many people no longer have a primary GP, but see whoever is rostered on duty. This situation makes the need for co-ordinated and focused care of the terminally ill person more complex and raises many questions about the future of palliative care services.

## Conclusion

What then is the future of palliative care? Central to this question is the contention that a number of different approaches to palliative care are appearing which are shaped and informed by different discourses with different values and interests. A brief reading of some of the discourses raises many questions. Are the central tenants of palliative care being marginalised by the emergence of palliative medicine and the restructuring of health services? Can we look forward to an integrated seamless health system where the principles of palliative care lead the way (see Calder, chapter 5)? Should we be trying to maintain specialist palliative care services? What is the role of nurses? Should they be generalist staff with specialist support or specialist palliative care nurses? Have palliative care nurses had to shoulder 'too much of the responsibility of palliative therapeutics and decision-making' (Ashby, chapter 4)? Or is the demand for medical leadership, consultation, education and research part of a creeping medicalisation?

There is no way back to small individualised hospice services. We have to deal with the demands of the present to provide greater access and equity to these services in the light of a clear vision for the future which also supports other values such as choice and appropriateness of service. Calls for efficiency need to be countered with demands for effectiveness; increases in professionalism need to be balanced with volunteer and community involvement so that the values of health economics and institutionalised medicine do not derail the key values of palliative care.

Over time the palliative care movement has grown and affected mainstream health services (Maddocks, 1990). Growth inevitably brings its legacy of bureaucratic routines, structures, standards and protocols (James & Field, 1992). The tough competition for scarce resources will influence the future shape of palliative care by placing smaller individualised programs at risk. It is evident that healthcare policy, which is driven by economic concerns, may now share some common agendas with palliative care services, especially that of quality service which is person-focused and conducted in the community as much as possible. This agenda assumes that economic values should form the basis for palliative care decision-making. A case could equally be made for also addressing the non-economic values of acceptability, appropriateness of service, community participation and community development as being essential elements of the palliative care approach. But the greatest threat is that, with external chaos in the health arena and escalating demands for palliative care services, the focus of the field will be on maintaining and preserving the present rather than making informed, critical decisions about palliative care services of the future.

Another key question for the field is: is palliative medicine a partner or competitor? Palliative medicine as a recognised sub-specialty is indeed coming of age. With international associations of palliative medicine, a Royal College of Physicians formal recognition, WHO and RCP definitions and a major journal entitled *Palliative Medicine*, this direction is *firmly* ensconced in medical practice of the future (Kearney, 1992). The arguments surrounding this development are for the improvement of practice, the placing of symptom control on all medical curricula and the fostering of further research in the area. The confusion regarding the field of palliative care and the impact of palliative medicine is typified in the following comment made by a medical director of a large palliative care service.

> I know what palliative medicine is—it is symptom control—but what is palliative *care*? What is palliative care nursing? The exponents of palliative care can't define themselves but we know what palliative medicine is. We just need the resources for education and research to develop it. (Street, 1996)

This doctor has worked in the hospice movement for a long time and is well known for the holistic care he personally provides to his clients but the dilemma he raises is a real one for the field to address. The specialty of palliative medicine is not going to disappear. It brings many strengths to the area of palliative care—excellence in symptom management, possibilites for widening the focus to service a much larger group of people, further research and education opportunities, a capacity to pressure governments. The field of palliative care needs to be pro-active in challenging the assumptions, policies and structures which support the further development of palliative medicine and the alliances that are being made within the rapidly changing structures of healthcare reforms. I will let Kearney have the final say for me on this matter:

> Palliative medicine is in its infancy and yet we in palliative medicine are faced with a choice. One possibility is that we may choose to accept the roles of 'symptomatologist', one who specializes in controlling and curing symptoms be these physical, emotional or (God forbid!) spiritual. Such a choice, it has been argued, while being valuable, would nonetheless sell ourselves and the vision of the pioneers of the hospice movement, short. The other choice is one which would involve dual committment. A committment to constantly strive to improve our clinical skills while simultaneously beginning to explore what it means to approach the person's experience of illness in an intuitive as well as analytical way. (Kearney, 1992, p. 46)

Government policy can be influenced by powerful interests to redefine its priorities or to accept services that are framed within its own economic rationalist discourses. Traditionally, medicine has remained strongly aligned with government, redefining and marketing its services according to the discourses of the healthcare reforms. Therefore the values and focus of palliative care are not only challenged by the health reforms but may also be in real danger from palliative medicine.

Nurses have been central to the development of palliative care services. Yet, they are members of a discipline that has traditionally been focused at the bedside and, unlike doctors, nurses have not been politically active in advocating the directions of health policy and practice. This attitude needs to change. Nurses need to be clear about the effects on their practice of the development of palliative medicine and the proposed health reforms. They need to act politically by creating alliances with their clients to jointly advocate for policies and strategies that value patient-centred care. An understanding of the impact of the competing discourses and a questioning mind will help nurses in this quest.

# References

Ahmedzai, S. (1993). A doctor's view. In D. Clark (Ed.), *The future of palliative care: Issues of policy and practice* (pp. 140–147).

Anderson, J. (1990). Home care management in chronic illness and the self-care movement: An analysis of ideologies and economic processes influencing policy decisions. *Advances in Nursing Science, 12* (2), 71–83.

Aranda, S. (1993). *What is the relationship between palliative care philosophy and care received by dying clients and their primary caregiver?* Melbourne: Melbourne Citymission Hospice Service.

Baker, J. (1996). Personal conversation, Flinders University of South Australia.

Biswas, B. (1993). A nurse's view. In D. Clark (Ed.), *The future for palliative care.*

Burns, N., Carney, K., & Brobst, B. (1989). Hospice: a design for home care for the terminally ill. *Holistic Nursing Practice*, February, 65–76.

Clark, D. (1993a). Whither the hospices? In D. Clark (Ed.), *The future for palliative care* (pp. 167–177).

Clark, D. (Ed.) (1993b). *The future for palliative care: Issues of policy and practice.* Buckingham: Open University Press.

Doyle, D. (1993). Palliative medicine—a time for definition? *Palliative Medicine, 7,* 253–255.

Duckett, S. & Swerissen, H. (1995). Specific purpose programs in human services and health: Moving from an input to an output and outcome focus. Cilento Oration to the Queensland Branch of the Royal Australian College of Medical Administrators, Queensland.

Harvey, R. (1991). *Making it better. Strategies for improving the effectiveness and quality of health services in Australia*, Background paper x. Canberra: National Health Strategy.

Hodder, P. & Turley, A. (1989). *The creative option of palliative care—A Manual for health professionals.* North Fitzroy, Victoria: Melbourne Citymission.

James, N. & Field, D. (1992). The routinization of hospice: charisma and bureaucratization. *Social Science Medicine, 34* (12), 1363–1375.

Kanitsaki (1989). *The creative option of palliative care—A manual for health professionals.* North Fitzroy, Australia, Melbourne Citymission.

Kearney, M. (1992). Palliative medicine—just another specialty? *Palliative Medicine, 6,* 39–46.

Maddocks, I. (1990). Changing concepts of palliative care. *The Medical Journal of Australia, 152 (May),* 2.

Simon, E.P., Showers, N. et al. (1995). Delivery of home care services after discharge: what really happens. *Health and Social Work, 20* (1) (February), 5–14.

Street, A. (1996). Research interviews: Issues in mainstreaming hospice/palliative care services. Bundoora, Vic.: La Trobe University.

Tierney, A.J., Sladden, J.A. et al. (1994). Measuring the costs and quality of palliative care: a discussion paper. *Palliative Medicine, 8,* 273–281.

Victorian Government (1995). *Victoria's Health to 2050.* Melbourne: Victorian Government.

Weedon, C. (1987). *Feminist practice and poststructuralist theory.* Cambridge & Oxford: Blackwell.

Wellard, S. (1996). Family connections? Exploring nursing roles with families in home-based care. *Nursing Inquiry, 3* (1), 57–58.

Woodruff, R. (1989). Principles of palliative care. In R. Woodruff, *Palliative care for the 1990's.* Melbourne: Asperula.

# Part II
# DEATH AND CARING FOR THE DYING

# 7

# This is It! An Approach to Spirituality

## Graham English

Germaine Greer (*Sydney Morning Herald*, 16 Oct. 1996) is reported saying, 'Happiness is something to be worked for; it is hard to achieve. It is a challenge to be happy in a world that is in such a dreadful mess.' Few people would disagree with her assessment. Most people, even quite small children, have four o'clock in the morning blues or Sunday afternoon depression now and then in response to their experience that life is not always easy, and that, at the end, we all have to die. Somewhere very early in human history our ancestors had the same realisations. The world has always been in a mess and all of our ancestors, like us, had to face the ineluctability of dying. They came up with many explanations. Ulysses, as Alfred Tennyson recounts it, set out to drink life to the lees, to strive, to seek, to find and not to yield. For him life meant something if it was filled with action. Siddhartha, the young Buddha, decided that life was all about suffering and that if we could detach ourselves through meditation we would be set free. The followers of Jesus claimed that they experienced him as alive again after his death and their belief in resurrection became the central teaching of Christianity and one of the major themes of western art and religion. Some people have concluded, so their T-shirts note, that, 'Life's a bitch and then you die'.

There was once a man who was walking through the forest. He heard a roar behind him and realised he was being pursued by a tiger. He began to run but found in front of him a steep cliff which in his haste he fell over. As he fell he grabbed a sapling growing on the cliff face. Looking down he saw another tiger looking up at him. Then he noticed a rat nibbling through the sapling. Beside him there was a strawberry plant. He reached over, took a luscious strawberry, and ate it saying, 'Oh, how sweet it is.'

If you work with people who are dying, you are working with people for whom the crunch has come. 'I am going to die. What does it all mean?' And none of us knows for sure, no matter what we believe. All of us in the face of death are inadequate; others' deaths are sometimes harder to face than our own. And some of us feel more inadequate than others. What if

I don't know what to say? What if I muck somebody up? What if I don't believe anything much? What if I have no spirituality?

*Well, most people have a spirituality!* The two main aims of this chapter are to explain that claim, and to further claim that for all those involved in nursing, in fact for all people, the most important spiritual task we have is to develop and care for our own spirituality. You have to answer only for yourself! You can't muck other people up—they can only do that for themselves.

What is this spirituality that most of us have? One definition of spirituality, from Robert E. Young, is 'the overarching meanings, goals and values for both persons and communities and the actual conditions of our attainment or non-attainment of these'. Another, from Matthew Fox (1991), is 'that path away from the superficial into the depths . . . from the outer person to the inner person . . . into the deeply communitarian'. Most people have an overarching meaning. Some meanings are more profound than others but in a time of crisis, death for example, it is how the meaning is lived out that counts. Dying can push us from the superficial into the depths very quickly so that it is often only at death that we find out what we really mean. Spirituality is really tested by death. That is why anyone

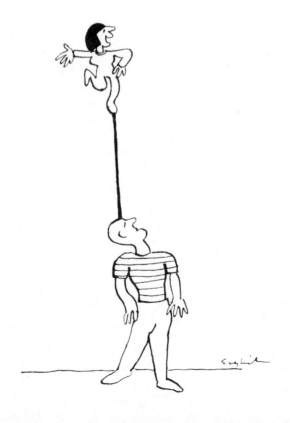

living with the dying needs to be in touch with their own spirit, their own meaning.

The sufi mystics in Islam say that a person who dies many times finds it easier to die at the end. 'Our task is to put our death behind us and our childhood in front of us', Paul Ricoeur says. The only spirituality, the only life, and the only death I am responsible for is my own. Said the rabbi Zusya, 'In the next life I will not be asked, "Why were you not Moses?" I shall be asked "Why were you not Zusya?"'

The Buddha tells the story of a man and his daughter who scraped a bare living by travelling the roads as acrobats. In each village they would spread their mat on the ground in the square and perform tricks for the few coins the villagers could spare. Their main trick was for the father to balance a long bamboo pole on his forehead, then the daughter would climb to the top of it and perform balances. One day the father said, 'Child, I am here holding you. You can trust me with your safety.' She replied that his job was to look after himself as hers was to look after herself. Then they would both be safe. This is a valuable insight. I am not the saviour of the world nor the saviour of my patients. I have to save only myself.

## Religion

Religion is the system or organisation that some people use to nurture, inform and contain their spirituality. Religion is a very useful way of being spiritual for many people because it provides a community, a moral code, a set of rituals all ready to use. It also contains leaders in the life of

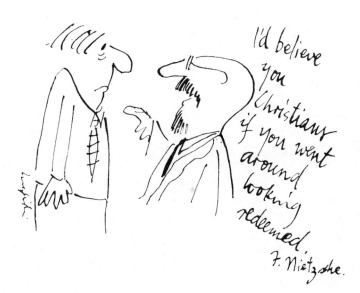

I'd believe you Christians if you went around looking redeemed.

F. Nietzsche.

the spirit, for example Buddha, Jesus, Catherine of Siena, Thomas Merton, Juliana of Norwich, Teresa of Avila, Mohammed, David, Ghandi, Hillel. Their sayings, writings, lives are a rich source of spiritual material for others to use in their own lives. But the truly great spiritual leaders transcend religions, even the ones founded in their names. There are those who use Buddha as a guide even though they are not Buddhists, others who are touched by the teachings and life of Jesus without being Christians. Martin Luther King's spirituality—he was a Baptist minister—was profoundly influenced by the Hindu Mahatma Ghandi. Today many people in their spiritual quest will take bits from here and there. And many people are spiritual without being religious at all, just as some religious people are not spiritual. For some of us, a spiritual journey might involve leaving a religion or finding another. And for some, spirituality may have nothing to do with religion at all.

## Spiritualities

The Buddha says that there are 84000 Dharma doors. What he means is that there are as many good ways of living as there are good lives. There are as many ways of being spiritual as there are spiritual people. Someone else's good life may not be the same as yours. Your only obligation about your good life is to see that you have it. For the other person, our task is to help them have their good life. Joseph Campbell says that the privilege of a lifetime is being who you are. Spirituality is, ultimately, finding out who you are and being that person. An old-fashioned term for this is 'following your vocation'. Of course that is not as easy as it sounds. Paul Ricoeur puts it, 'I want you to enjoy being I as much as I enjoy being I.' Jesus said it, 'Love your neighbour as you love yourself.' Both of these statements are loaded with dynamite if you hate being you, so the basis of spirituality is to first love yourself.

## Spiritual distress

Now what of our patients and their families and friends?

A short document called a *Nurse care planning guide* proposes some evaluation criteria or desired outcomes for nurses who have diagnosed 'spiritual distress' and set out to cure it. Spiritual distress is a condition of having a disturbance in one's belief system, hopelessness, or an inability to participate in services. It is brought on by a crisis, for example a terminal illness, that leads to 'Why me?' and 'What have I done to deserve this?' kind of questions. It can manifest itself as anger, fear, depression, guilt, despair or any number of distressing feelings. The planning guide's desired outcomes are: expressed increased acceptance of death, a statement of increased spiritual peace, and an acceptance and practice of spiritual rituals associated with the dying person's specific beliefs.

There are lots of problems with these preferred outcomes! There is also a problem with the idea of spiritual distress. The definition presumes that distress is a bad thing. Maybe that is not true. Maybe distress is just another *crisis*.

Crisis is the Greek word for 'decide' so a crisis is, literally, a time for deciding something. A crisis is a decisive moment or turning point. The overarching meaning of our life is challenged by crisis. For the Australian writer Bill Harney, the killing fields of France in the first world war were his crisis. He went away to the war an enthusiastic, naive young man. He came back a peace activist determined never to leave here again. He lost faith in the claims of the warmakers; he had a spiritual crisis because the overarching meanings of his life up until then were not enough. Some of them were wrong. He had to decide what life meant now. For an even more profound account of spiritual crisis, read some of the Jewish meditation on the meaning of the Holocaust, for example Eli Weissel's *Night*. People who are dying or who know that someone they love is dying have a time of decision, maybe the last big decision in their life. The decision could be to accept death. But Dylan Thomas did not agree with that at all. 'Do not go gentle into that good night', he urged his old father, 'Rage, rage against the dying of the light.' Crisis brings on many decisions. Be careful about having too limited a set of desired outcomes. Honour the crisis of the dying and the decisions they make. That is a spiritual response. Because death doesn't change us: it finds out who we are.

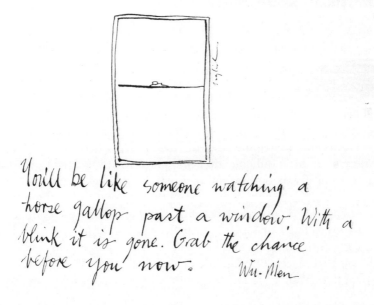

You'll be like someone watching a
horse gallop past a window. With a
blink it is gone. Grab the chance
before you now.        Wu-Men

When Dennis Potter was dying of cancer of the pancreas in March 1994, he recorded a television interview with Melvyn Bragg. It is a splendid interview and I recommend you to read or to watch it. In it he describes the blossoms outside his window:

> . . . last week looking at it through the window when I'm writing, I see it is the whitest, frothiest, blossomist blossom that there ever could be, and I can see it. Things are both more trivial than they ever were and more important than they ever were, and the difference between the trivial and the important doesn't seem to matter.

What are we to *do* then? After all nurses are helpers, doers. One of the best answers I have heard was given to me by Merlin Freeman, a palliative care nurse in northern New South Wales, 'Just hang about.' Hanging about means giving the person room to discover their spirit, or to suss you out to see if they are going to involve you in their dying, or to have room to ask you for help. Hanging about is also giving you time to find out what rituals or what people they might want. Hanging about also gives you room to learn.

The hard lesson for us, particularly if we are helpers, is that when it all comes down to it we cannot change other people, we cannot give them meaning. They have to find their own meaning for themselves. In the face of any crisis, death included, we can only be with them; a meeting of spiritualities, a meeting of meanings is all we can offer. We can only stand and watch, even if we are holding their hands and praying. As that great medieval play *Everyman* is at pains to show, we die alone even if we are surrounded by a crowd.

## Australian spirituality

As far as we can tell each of us gets only one go at life and so we get only one go at dying. Some people have near misses, for example there are those who claim that they have had near death experiences. And some religions teach that we come back over and over until we reach some endpoint like Nirvana, and that may well be right. Even then, *this life and death that a person is undergoing are the only ones they have at the moment.* If it is my one go at life and death, even if I will get many other goes before I reach Nirvana, I have the right to have the very best go that I can.

And we can be in only one time and place at a time. That is, spirituality is contextual. I was born a boy in Australia in 1944. Somewhere on the calendar in a place that I have passed by fifty-two times, there is a date that will appear on my death certificate. For me, as for each of us, 'This is it!' Sure go to India or Tibet, Lourdes, Jerusalem or Mecca. Each of these places is worth going to, and maybe they will change your life. They are very spiritual places. But the only place for us is where we are. Heaven is not over there. When we die, whatever happens next if anything does, will

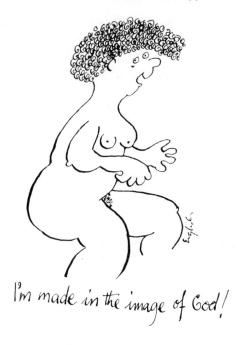

I'm made in the image of God!

happen wherever we are at the time. And it will happen to us, not to anyone else. *This is the place. This is all there is.* That is why, for each of us, growing in our own spirituality is to do with growing into who we are. Our gender is important, our body is important, our experience is critical, our place is a holy place.

But is it possible to be spiritual in Australia? Australia, some commentators tell us, is the most secular of countries. Secular means one of two things to these people. One is that for most Australians God is not the final explanation for most things. That is, we can find some human explanation for almost every event, even if it is only to be ironic or despairing. The second meaning is that religious activity does not feature very highly in Australian preoccupations. We are not very religious, most of us do not go to church regularly. The Italians, Portuguese and Spanish have saints' feastdays, the British have an established church, India has many feasts, the Moslem countries have Ramadan, and the Americans put 'In God we trust' on their money, while we celebrate the Melbourne Cup and have a cricketer and a racehorse as our patron saints. How do we have spirituality in a secular country? One answer is that it is up to us to discover what it is to be spiritual here because this is where we are. Peter Berger, in his book *A rumour of angels*, claims that there are experiences we have like jokes, laughter, the goodness of others that give us hope. He calls these 'rumours of angels'. In a way, spirituality is just that, listening to the rumours that there is hope, that it does have meaning, that we can reach heaven. So what are the rumours of angels for you here in Australia? Henry Lawson said, 'Beer makes you feel how you ought to feel without beer.' Lawson drank more than his fair share of beer seeking to feel the ecstasy that he couldn't feel unaided. That is one answer but surely we can find some answers that are less injurious to our well-being. The answer has something to do with being here, being in the present. Maybe, in the process, we will discover how to have the beer feeling without the beer.

John Keats said that the world is the valley of soul making. Les Murray says much the same in that wonderfilled poem of his 'An Absolutely Ordinary Rainbow'. We make our soul wherever we are. Soul making is just another term for spirituality. How do we make our soul? For a start, it is enough of an aim to want to live a richer and fuller life, to really hear rather than just listen, to really see rather than just observe. 'Tourists see what they came to see', Chesterton said, 'while travellers see what they see.' Travellers lead richer lives.

## Biggles spirituality

Biggles was a fearless pilot who each day went out to fight the enemy. Each evening he came back to base, sometimes with the odd bullet hole in the wing or fuselage, but always with daring exploits to recount and a tally of enemy planes shot down. His faithful mechanic would stay up late into the night painting the outline of yet another enemy plane just below the cockpit cover. Biggles spirituality, where the expert goes out collecting trophies, is for the power of the expert, not the empowerment of the person who is sick. No Biggles, no saviours, no judges. James Freeman was a Catholic priest at Darlinghurst in Sydney many years ago. One day he was in the church when a child came running in to say that a man had been hit by a car in Oxford Street. Freeman ran out and knelt beside him and said, 'I'm a Catholic priest. Is there anything I can do?' 'Yes. You can go to hell!' said the man. Then he died. People have the right to choose their own path no matter how it shocks us. Some people will not be satisfied with heaven so you have no hope of satisfying them. That is not your problem.

Some people try to use illness and death to frighten people with the future so they will be 'good' now. There is more to be said for living fully in the now, for encouraging people into the now. If our death is behind us, when it comes it will look after itself. Spirituality is not a political thing though some people try to use it politically. That is, they use others' fears and insecurities, sometimes talking of eschatology. Eschatology is the study of what happens to us after our death, for example heaven and hell. As most humans fear death or at least feel confused or uneasy by it, any religion that can promise to get you peace and happiness after you die is

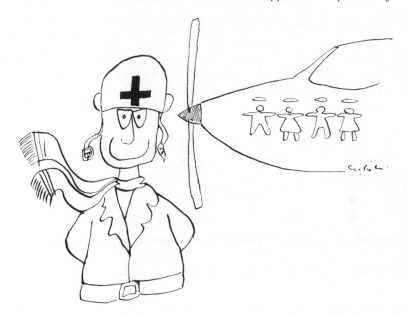

onto a winner. Assuring people you can fix it for them in the after life is a highly political act. But it has nothing to do with spirituality.

What is your attitude to death? Weddings and funerals bring out the best and the worst in families. That is, when we find out how different, or similar, the values and beliefs of family members are. That's when we find out where the power is, where the struggles are. We find out who is about power and who about empowerment. Your attitude to sickness (and of course death) will be much the same as your attitude to life. We die as we live. Grumpy young people usually become grumpy old people. So a fitting rather than a happy death might be the best result. The tug of war that surrounds some deaths is a denial of the rights of the dying person and is really about the power and the needs of the survivors. It is what the survivors believe about life and death, not what the dying person does. Sometimes the things we do to patients are the same, more about our needs than theirs. Brother Reginald was dying of a painful bone disease in 1959. Brother Martin knelt by his bed saying prayers. 'Sacred Heart of Jesus have mercy on the dying,' he said over and over and over. Brother Reginald opened one eye and said, 'For God's sake Martin shut up! I'm dying.' Leave the heroics to Biggles!

## Prayer and meditation

In the Bible, there's a story of Moses who came upon a bush in the desert. The bush was well alight but it was not being consumed by the fire. Moses heard the voice of God saying to him, 'Take off your shoes, you are standing on sacred ground.' I do not know who said it first, but there is a lot to think about in the words: 'The present moment is sacred ground.' Thic Nhat Han puts it, 'Present moment, sacred moment.' This moment is all we have, maybe we don't have even it. The past is gone, we can do nothing about it. All the *if onlys* in the world won't change a single second of the past. And the future is not here, and it mightn't get here either, for you or me anyway. What can you promise yourself? Nothing except to make the utmost of now. This living in the moment is the aim of meditation. The Buddha sitting under the Bodhi tree, the monk chanting in the chapel, the nurse doing a walking meditation as she or he goes about the ward is practising the art of living in the moment. There's a story of an old woman sitting all day in a church. The priest asks her, 'What do you do there all day?' 'Oh, I look at *him* and he looks at me.' Whether you believe in him is not the only point here. Can you, do you want to stay in the presence, stay in the moment? Gregorian chant, Budddhist chant, the wind in the trees, the waves on the shore, each of these can be a way of staying with the moment. It is the same with colours and smells. Incense and scented oils have, since humans first discovered them, been ways of affecting our space so that we are centred in it.

## Ways of being spiritual

People do odd things. Some paint their faces, some circumcise their children, some bury the dead while others expose the body to the elements. Some people wear tattoos while others pierce various body parts and wear jewellery there. Odd usually means 'not what I'd do' or 'not what I'm used to'. The meaning of 'odd' changes from place to place and time to time. People also do odd things when they are sick or dying. What these things *mean* is much more important than what they are. To find out what an action means requires a lot of hanging about. Being open to people's pain and grief is being open to their joy and power as well. The Dalai Lama speaks of the need for many religions. It is like food he says. Some of us like our food bland, others like a little spice, but for some food has no taste unless it is full of chillies. Just so there are some who need to believe that they live many lives and that death is but the beginning of a new round. Others, Christians for example, believe that there is only one life and then there is eternity. Jews say 'L'chayim, to life.' This life, every second of it, is precious. In Monty Python's *The Meaning of Life*, there is a song that begins, 'There are Jews in this world, there are Buddhists, there are Hindus and Mormons as well, and there are those that follow Mohammed, but I've never been one of them'. Knowing about other people's religious practices is part both of honouring their spirituality and, in palliative care, of helping them die with integrity. Australia has always had many spiritualities. Before Europeans came, there were Aboriginal spiritualities, how many and of what variety we can only guess. Ever since, spiritualities here have multiplied. Now wherever you nurse, you will find formal and informal approaches depending partly on people's religion or lack of it, partly on their culture. Not all Christians have the same spirituality, nor all Moslems, nor all atheists! Helping another live out the meaning of their life can involve knowing what they believe, sometimes joining in with them. A Baptist Christian I know learnt the rosary so that she could pray with a Catholic patient because this way of prayer was so important to the patient. But we don't always have to join in. Just knowing what people are doing, or why some act is special can be a gift of understanding or acceptance. It can be the patient's gift to you too.

What if their spirituality is half-baked? What if you think that it is a poor spirituality for someone to be dying with? Thérèse Martin (1873–97) was a nun in a convent in Lisieux near Paris who, despite her youth and her ill health (she was dying of tuberculosis) was wiser than most of her contemporaries when it came to talk and action about spirituality. One of the other sisters asked her why some people had a great capacity to love while others did not. Thérèse's answer was that it was like buckets and thimbles: a bucket full of water holds much more than a thimble full of water but each of them is full. Loving to our capacity is the critical thing. Probably some spiritualities offer more than others. Maybe some are better than others. I think you can make a good argument that Christianity, say, has more to say about the meaning of life than football. But an empty Christian may be in more distress than a full footballer! Satisfactory comes from the Latin word for 'enough'. A spirituality only has to be satisfactory, not for you but for the person who has it.

## Ritual

When you change your office, or move into a new house, or set up your room, what do you do? Some people will put out their photos first. 'There's Gran, and there's my photo of Murringo Gap, and then there's Amanda.' And so on. For others it is their collection of rocks, the granite from Loch Lomond, the rounded stone from the valley of Elat, the chip of limestone from Cairo. When these objects are arranged, the new space has become theirs; they have, by a simple ritual, made an anywhere into a somewhere. This is a spiritual action, this ritualising an ordinary spot into a sacred place. Again Joseph Campbell, 'To live in sacred space is to live in a symbolic environment where spiritual life is possible, where everything around you speaks of exhaltation of spirit.' Ritual can be eating. What do you eat when you are feeling blue? Rice, mashed potato, chocolate, pasta? How do you get out of the miseries? How do you reward yourself? Do you get your hair cut? Your ears pierced? (That has a limited number of times you can do it.) Your hair dyed? Do you buy a new hat? Most of these actions are rituals, they are metaphorical acts, symbols that stand for and accomplish something else. We ritualise our own lives and remind ourselves of our overarching meaning. Sometimes we do it to alter or even change our meaning. Going through a wedding ceremony, coming out as gay, cutting our hair in a certain way, wearing particular clothes; all of these are rituals. Doing them with someone else or helping another do them, helping a person with leukaemia cut their hair when the chemo has done half the job can be the most profound spiritual act. In the film version of *Dead Man Walking,* as Matthew is about to be executed, Sister Helen holds her arm out towards him. It is a sign that she cares for him. It is also a sign that he is forgiven. In some religions, an arm held out like that as a blessing can often forgive patients, lay their spirits at rest.

Ritual is simply a way that we have of telling ourselves the truth, or remembering, or marking rights of passage. With a little thought and practice, palliative care nurses can become profound exponents of ritual that can make all the difference in someone getting in touch with their spirit.

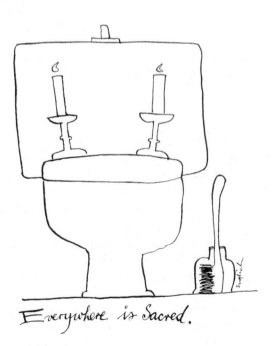

Everywhere is Sacred.

# Drawing and poetry

Go and get a packet of crayons and some sheets of paper. 'But I can't draw!' many will say. Tell me this, if you say you can't draw, were you ever in kindergarten? Yes, because everyone was once in kinder. Well, I can assure you, after a long time knocking around schools, that *every* child in kinder can draw and when you were in kinder so could you. The refrigerator doors of Australia, and every country that has refrigerators, are decorated with *really good drawings* by children. What happened to you? Someone probably told you that what you were drawing didn't look like a foot. Or a tree. Your spiritual problems had begun. What was happening was that the feet, or the trees that you were drawing did not look the way Leonardo da Vinci draws trees. They did look like how you saw feet and trees. But your critics—it might even have been self-criticism—wanted you to be someone else and you fell for it. They said, 'See, like Leonardo', which you cannot do, and so you set off on the wrong track. My painting teacher, John Ogburn, used say to me, 'Your only job as a painter is to be a first rate you. There's no point being a tenth-rate Picasso because we have the first-rate one already.' All you have to do is find out how you draw, and then be a very good you. If you are still shy, draw with your wrong hand and if someone says, 'That doesn't look like a foot,' say, 'Well, I did it with my wrong hand'. And go discovering how you draw.

Now get those crayons and paper. Go on, really. Right? Now sit quietly and draw the outline of the first house you can remember in your life. Imagine you are up in the air above it and draw the plan of it. Put in all the rooms and anything you remember. Put in the yard if there is one. Now wander around the house and remember the things that happened there. Do you get any surprises? Whom do you meet? How do you

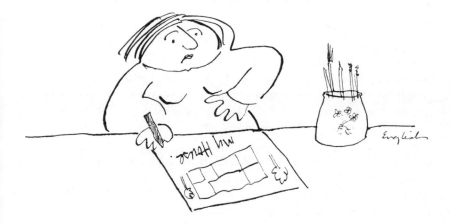

feel? Drawing is one way to discover your own story. And your own spirituality.

If they convinced you that you could not draw, what did they do to you about poetry? 'Oh, I never read *poetry*' so many people say, 'it's too hard.' No it isn't. Poetry is a wonderful place to find your spirituality. Try this. It's by Philip Hodgins who died in his thirties in 1995, from his book *Up on all fours*.

> ### Autumn of the Critic
> The days are getting shorter now.
> The leaves are falling from the trees.
> He finds complexity, somehow,
> in sentences as plain as these.

Hodgins knew he was dying of cancer when he wrote this. Notice the different meanings in the first two lines. He is not just talking about the seasons or the trees. And hear the two meanings in 'sentence'. Poetry like this is like those children dying of cancer who draw balloons cut off from their strings. Often it is the only way they can share with us their spirituality. 'I am dying, Soon I will be like the balloons. Will you share my dying with me?' Dying children seem to dive straight into their spirituality. The adults around them are not always as adept. Morris Gleitzman's book *Two weeks with the queen* is about this and it is a fine book for anyone interested in spirituality. We cannot, usually, match the skill of Hodgins or Gleitzman but, even if we cannot write poetry that expresses who we are at this moment, we can find great poets who get it just right for us. Try Adrienne Rich's 'To A Woman Dead In Her Forties' for a way of saying, 'Oh, I wish we were able to say what we wanted to say before it was too late.'

## Wellness and well-wishers

The nurse's role is to be well and to be there with the patient. 'And all shall be well, and all shall be well, and all shall be very well,' Juliana of Norwich put it. 'Well' is centred, coming from a secure centre. Well is nourishing. Well is deep and mysterious. In villages wells are where the people meet and be with each other. Effective nurses are well-wishers, people who practise mutuality. They are wellsprings. If we are well, we can water the flowers. Wellness is not necessarily a medical term. The sick can be well and the healthy can be unwell. Wellness is a spiritual term as much as it is anything else. It is linked to realising the truth of what John Dewey wrote, 'We are participants in an unfinished universe rather than spectators of a finished universe.' We are all part of this and we do not know how it will end. In the meantime we can but hope that the French mystic Bernadette Soubirous was right. As she lay dying in her late

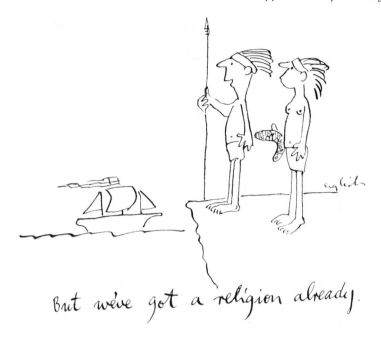

*But we've got a religion already.*

twenties, she said, '*Voyez comme c'est simple, il suffit d'aimer*': 'see how simple it is, all you need is love.'

## References and further reading

Aitken, Robert (1994). *Taking the path of zen*. New York: North Point Press.

Beck, Charlotte Jako (1989). *Everyday zen*. San Francisco: Harper.

Berger, Peter. *A rumour of angels*. Ringwood: Penguin.

Cain, Elizabeth (1995). *Grass grows by itself*. Sydney: Millennium.

*The cloud of unknowing* (1965). Harmondswoth: Penguin Classics.

Fox, Matthew (1991). *Creation spirituality*. San Franciso: Harper Collins.

Garrison, Jim (1995). *The new scholarship on Dewey*. Dordrecht: Kluwer Academic.

Gleitzman, Morris. *Two weeks with the Queen*. Ringwood: Penguin.

Harney, Bill (1983). *Harney's war*. South Yarra: Currey O'Neil.

Hodgins, Philip (1993). *Up on all fours*. Sydney: Angus & Robertson.

Kirkwood, N. (1994). *A hospital handbook on multiculturalism and religion*. Sydney: Millennium.

Murray, Les, A. (1986). *Australian religious poetry*. Melbourne: Collins Dove.

Nouwen, Henri (1986). *Reaching out*. London: Fount.

Osbon, Diane, K. (1991). *A Joseph Campbell companion*. New York: Harper Perennial.

Potter, Dennis (1994). *Seeing the blossom*. London: Faber and Faber.

Radford Reuther, R. (1985). *Women–church*. San Francisco: Harper and Row.

Rich, Adrienne (1984). *The fact of a doorframe*. New York: Norton & Co.

Sharma, Arvand (1993). *Our religions*. San Francisco: Harper.

Stockton, Eugene (1995). *The Aboriginal gift: A spirituality for a nation*. Sydney: Millennium Books.

Stuart, E. (1992). *Daring to speak love's name: A gay and lesbian prayerbook*. London: Hamish Hamilton.

Thic Nhat Han (1987). *Being peace*. Berkeley: Parallax Press.

Thic Nhat Han (1990). *Present moment, wonderful moment*. Berkeley: Parallax Press.

Weisel, Eli (1986). *Night*. New York: Bantam Books.

White, E. & Tulip, M. (1990). *Knowing otherwise*. Melbourne: David Lovell Books.

Women–Church Collective (1987–97). *Women-Church: An Australian Journal of Feminist Studies in Religion*, 1–20.

# 8

# Psychosocial Dimensions: Issues in Clinical Management

## Patsy Yates

Psychosocial dimensions of palliative care have been the focus of considerable scholarly attention during the past few decades. Numerous sociologists, psychologists and nurses have contributed to the proliferation of theories and research concerning human responses to chronic and terminal illness. More recent interest in evaluating the efficacy of various psycho-educational and supportive nursing interventions has also seen an accumulating body of knowledge emerge to guide those who provide palliative care services. This work has resulted in major changes to the philosophy and practice of care for the dying, whereby psychosocial issues have been removed from the margins to the centre of the discipline of nursing.

Despite such advances, the management of psychosocial concerns in palliative care continues to pose many challenges for clinicians. The aim of this chapter is to explore this psychosocial dimension of palliative care delivery, and to examine the management of psychosocial issues in the contemporary clinical context. The chapter will begin by exploring how dying and death are viewed in the modern world, and consider how such views influence both the dying person's experience of dying, and the frameworks nurses have adopted for managing the psychosocial concerns of their patients. This discussion will provide the context for analysing current nursing practice in this area, and for identifying the scope that exists for improving psychosocial support of the terminally ill.

## Features of death in modern society: Privatisation and ambivalence

The classic sociological studies of interactions between dying patients and hospital staff conducted during the 1960s (e.g., Glaser & Strauss, 1965; 1968; Sudnow, 1967) were notable for their emphasis on death as a social experience, rather than merely a biological event. By demonstrating how perceptions and expectations of patients, families and healthcare workers determined how people would respond during the dying process, these studies noted how an individual's experience of dying, and the way nurses and other staff conceptualise and approach management of psychosocial concerns were shaped by societal views of dying and death. To understand the nature of psychosocial dimensions of contemporary palliative care, it is important, therefore, to examine the place of death in modern society. Two particular features of death in modern society which have been the subject of increasing attention in recent literature will be discussed here: the removal of death from the public to the private world of individuals (the privatisation of death), and the ambivalent relationship that has developed between humans and death.

## The privatisation of death

It was common in many of the earlier historical accounts of death in the twentieth century for writers to claim that twentieth-century society was a death-denying society, where the subject of death had become taboo (see Airès, 1981; Becker, 1973; Gorer, 1965). Such accounts typically emphasised how increasing secularisation, loss of community, and increased reliance on science and technology in western society had radically changed humanity's relationship with death and dying (Moller, 1996). That is, since twentieth-century society no longer had the same religious or social mechanisms for ascribing meaning or for explaining suffering and death that previous societies had, dying had become a universally feared event which an individual should go to extreme lengths to avoid. More recent sociological analyses of death have further suggested that since one of the distinctive features of late twentieth-century society is reflexivity (i.e. a greater willingness to critically examine, monitor and revise one's beliefs and practices in light of changing circumstances), death today may be becoming even more isolating than before (Giddens, 1990; 1991). Death remains elusive and feared because it is unfamiliar and unknown, and with no communal framework to give it meaning, an individual must deal with such issues within the private realm of individual experience (Mellor, 1993). Arguably, this privatisation of death has made the provision of psychosocial support to terminally ill patients increasingly complex in today's world, as healthcare providers strive to find solutions for the difficult problems of meaninglessness, uncertainty, powerlessness and loss of control which characterise the modern experience of death.

However, while death has in some ways become privatised, an increasing number of scholars have noted the ambivalence that exists in the relationship between modern people and the process of death and dying (Moller, 1996; Walter, 1991). That is, it has been claimed that while there appears to be widespread reluctance to talk about death in everyday interaction, death and dying issues have at the same time become more prominent in the public sphere. The proliferation of academic and lay literature on death and dying during the 1970s and 1980s, changes to public policy to accommodate emerging hospice and palliative care programs, attempts to implement legislation concerning the rights of the terminally ill, and the media interest such legislation has attracted are just a few examples of the greater public profile now afforded death-related issues. Moller (1996) claims that this placing of care of the dying on the policy agenda is evidence of the bureacratisation of dying in the modern world.

This placement of death-related issues in the public realm has important implications for the clinical management of psychosocial issues. Spurred on by the growing individualism and consumerism that characterise the late twentieth century, there is today a much greater expectation that healthcare services will respond more effectively to the suffering and distress associated with chronic and terminal illness. More specifically, maintenance of dignity, promotion of autonomy and relief of suffering, have emerged as fundamental principles which society has come to expect will be incorporated into contemporary palliative care services.

## Challenges in the management of psychosocial issues

The emergence of death-related issues in the public domain has seen contemporary nursing approaches to the management of psychosocial issues in palliative care come to reflect the core values of preservation of dignity (i.e., death with dignity), and the promotion of personal autonomy (i.e., negotiated death) (Moller, 1996). However, while such goals are congruent with changing public expectations for care of the dying, the available evidence suggests that, for a variety of reasons, the achievement of such ideals in actual clinical situations is problematic for healthcare providers, and that practice may continue to lag behind rhetoric in this area. In this section, the way in which nurses have shaped their practice to accommodate the principles of dignity and autonomy, and the difficulties they have in applying these principles in practice will be discussed.

### *Death with dignity*

The stage theorists during the 1960s and 1970s, in particular Elisabeth Kübler-Ross (1970), have been extremely influential, not only because of the important role they have played in drawing attention to the psychosocial concerns of the dying and bereaved, but also for the way they have been able to shape how healthcare providers have come to define 'death with dignity' (Moller, 1996; James & Field, 1996). These theories have been based on the premise that, when confronted with death, people experience a range of emotions which can be seen as occurring in a series of stages. Importantly, the final stage noted in the work of Kübler-Ross is acceptance. She describes this stage as one which is characterised by dignity, and the reaching of it as being the 'final stage of growth' (Kübler-Ross, 1975).

Recently, a number of writers have pointed to the negative consequences that the widespread acceptance of stage theories has had for the management of psychosocial issues (see James & Field, 1996; Moller, 1996; Corr, 1993). These writers describe how the uncritical acceptance of the assumptions of this work has led to the adoption of a framework that identifies the nurse as a 'travel agent for the dying' who leads the patient through stages to 'a singular destination: tranquil, peaceful death' (Moller, 1996, p. 51). Death, viewed as the final stage of growth where the person has come to terms with their fate, has encouraged nurses to facilitate such a 'good' or 'happy' death (James & Field, 1996). The result has been that nurses and other healthcare providers may in fact prescribe for dying patients the way in which they should respond while dying. As such, they may consciously or unconsciously place pressure on patients and their families to conform to their own notion of the ideal death, rather than allow the patient to define this for themselves.

Researchers who have examined nurses' views of the 'good' death have provided evidence to support the contention that some nurses do in fact see the acceptance of death as being a critical element of 'death with dignity' (McNamara, 1996; Taylor, 1993). McNamara's (1996) analysis of the views of hospice nurses in Western Australia described how non-acceptance of death was problematised by nurses who saw it as their role to facilitate acceptance and eventual surrender to death. He noted how issues of non-acceptance of death were often discussed in clinical and informal meetings, and suggested that there is a fundamental assumption among clinicians that acceptance of death will somehow be beneficial. Hunt's (1992) research similarly identifies various 'scripts' for dying from analysis of conversations between nurses and cancer patients. These 'scripts' included not only that physical symptoms be controlled, but also that patients and relatives openly accepted their cancer diagnosis and prognosis and had a peaceful death at home, while they continued to enjoy life and 'fight back'.

Those who espouse the value of acceptance generally point to the opportunity for personal growth and enhancement of personal relationships that is provided to individuals who can openly discuss and reflect on life goals and aspirations (Mayer, 1989). Furthermore, such 'scripts' may in fact provide a normative framework that actually reduces the uncertainty of dying and provides some way of ascribing meaning for personal suffering. Other writers have also argued that, since the person must eventually confront evidence of progressive disease, failure to accept one's prognosis will inevitably lead to increased anxiety because of 'reality' seepage into consciousness and unconsciousness, increasing isolation from others as the person tries to avoid threatening information at all costs, delay in seeking appropriate health care as the person denies physical and emotional problems which may indicate worsening condition, and unreasonable persistence at difficult or impossible tasks which could have substantial social and financial costs for the individual (Erseck, 1992).

However, while a number of researchers have attempted to test such assertions, by addressing the questions of whether acceptance is beneficial, or denial is harmful, the outcomes from these studies have been far from conclusive. Taylor (1983), for example, has reported a study where women with breast cancer who were able to maintain illusions that they had control over their disease could actually handle it better than other women, and adapted better to their illness. Similarly, Watson, Greer, Blake and Shrapnell (1984) and Hackett and Cassem (1974) have reported that denial is associated with better adjustment to illness and less psychological distress. What is clear from the empirical work to date, however, is that people respond in many different ways to a terminal diagnosis, that they use many different strategies for coping with their situation, and that they constantly modify strategies according to changing perceptions and circumstances. The assumption that the 'good' death necessarily involves acceptance of dying is therefore increasingly being challenged. Attempting to describe what is a 'good' death for all individuals in all circumstances in the way that nurses appear to be doing is unlikely to provide us with frameworks for practice that will be flexible enough to manage psychosocial issues inherent in palliative care today.

## Negotiated death

A second goal of death in modern society identified by Moller (1996) is to facilitate personal choice and to offer individualised approaches to management of clinical problems (i.e. to enable the person to negotiate the terms of their own death). Recent studies which demonstrate the dramatic shift that has occurred over the past few decades in practices regarding the open disclosure of threatening diagnoses would suggest that significant progress has already been made toward the attainment of this goal (Williams, 1989; Novack, Plumer, Smith et al., 1979). However, while healthcare providers may state they are in favour of the principle of openness in interactions and patient autonomy, there is accumulating evidence that some have reservations about their ability to apply such principles in actual clinical situations (Kelner & Bourgeault, 1993). Furthermore, research on nurse–patient interactions over a number of decades continues to find that, in some situations, nurses appear to have difficulty with facilitating open communication with their patient, and that they find unstructured interactions with patients especially challenging. There are two main findings which have consistently been reported in these studies: first, that many nurses use what are classified as distancing or blocking tactics (i.e., they use a range of strategies for avoiding difficult situations or questions, such as cutting patients off and changing the subject when difficult issues are raised by the patient, asking closed questions, giving information inappropriately, and keeping busy and focusing on physical tasks); and second, that many nurses have poor levels of facilitative communication (i.e., they don't follow up, or they miss patients' cues which may be indicative of emotional problems or concerns, and they don't provide opportunities which would encourage patients to verbalise their feelings about their situation) (Hanson, 1994; Wilkinson, 1991; Maquire, 1985). Studies from both Australia and overseas have also noted that psychosocial issues are rarely commented on in progress notes (Hanson, 1994; Parker & Gardner, 1992).

## Evasive nurse–patient interactions

To further explore the nature of interactions between nurses and patients and families receiving palliative care, secondary analysis of interview data which was collected as part of a larger study of factors influencing the well-being of recently bereaved families was conducted (Yates, 1996). This data was collected during in-depth interviews with a convenience sample of 15 family members who were referred from a domicialiary nursing service in Brisbane and had been bereaved for less than twelve months. The primary aim of these unstructured interviews was to explore how the participant's life had been affected by caring for a relative who had died from cancer. Participants were asked to discuss their perceptions of their relationship and interactions with healthcare providers while they were caring for their relative. Any text relating to interactions between healthcare providers and patients was highlighted and analysed for recurring themes. Four examples of 'evasive interactions' (a term used by Moller (1996) to describe ways of communicating with terminally ill person and family) were identified from this data. These include:

- maintaining a pretence;
- being discreet;
- focusing on attainable aims; and
- being frank.

In the following section, exemplars from interview transcripts are presented to show these ways of communicating and the consequences they have for psychosocial care. They are not meant to depict communication styles of nurses, but rather to describe how family members have interpreted particular interactions with healthcare providers, to emphasise the complexity inherent in achieving the goal of openness.

## Maintaining a pretence

This refers to interactions where family members perceived healthcare providers simply avoided less desirable information or uncomfortable patient and family interactions. For example:

> we were just in the dark all the time, that was the problem because I knew that he was sick and we were told over the phone that he had cancer. From then on I mean when you say cancer I mean you don't think, well you just don't think of death. Well I've had cancer myself. I had a complete hysterectomy for cancer. I sort of thought 'oh yes, he's got cancer, we can get through this'. But I feel nobody sat down and had a good talk with us and told us exactly the way he was. I mean the most we ever got was that radiotherapy would help. They just seemed to avoid it altogether.

This woman went on to tell a story of how she believed that health professionals deliberately avoided talking with her about her husband's illness, and how this was a continuing source of anxiety and anger for her some eight months following her husband's death. Such interactions are similar to those described in the work of Hanson (1994) and Wilkinson (1991), and depict a context that is arguably the complete antithesis of a negotiated death.

## Being discreet

This refers to interactions where the healthcare provider selectively chooses information, and/or uses vague or ambiguous words or phrases when communicating with patients and family. For example:

> I think the whole thing was that we were in such a state of shock each time that we couldn't ask the right questions. Dr [name] I would say he was more straight. He was the one that said it was a very aggressive tumor he called it. I suppose at that stage, well, I looked at a tumor as a very different thing, like a growth say on your bowel that grows out. That's how I was thinking a tumor was, but that is not the way it is, is it. I thought it was like a growth, like your finger growing out, whereas I think of cancer as something attacking your cells. I wasn't thinking along the same lines.

This example illustrates how the use of medical jargon, or euphemisms by healthcare providers can lead to misunderstanding. Within such a context, it is difficult to see how a person could meaningfully negotiate their own death. It emphasises the importance for healthcare providers of continually reassessing the patient and family members' interpretation of interactions.

## Focusing on attainable aims

This refers to interactions where the nurse may be open to communicating about management of clinical problems, as long as this involves discussion about problems which are perceived by the nurse as being appropriate. For example:

> I suppose from my point of view there was well a couple of bad things in that I think it was the first day they overdosed him on morphine because they expected he would have a lot of pain, to the extent where he couldn't even close his eyes. He was like a zombie. I suppose I found them a bit negative. They were quite serious, yes very negative. You know sort of basically saying 'well we don't know why he's alive, but we will try to manage his pain, try to do this and that'. They didn't want to talk about whether he could possibly live a bit longer—that's what we were working towards.

While this interaction may not at first appear to be evasive in the same sense as the avoidance tactics depicted in the previous examples, it does nevertheless have the same end result. That is, by focusing on goals and attending to care that the nurse views as being of priority, the patient or family are given little opportunity to openly communicate personal care goals, particularly goals which may be incongruent with those of the healthcare provider. Comments such as these illustrate how discussions that might imply the patient or family has not accepted the inevitability of death may be particularly problematic, since they may be incongruent with the healthcare providers' goals of achieving 'death with dignity' (see the discussion earlier in this chapter). The potential for conflict between the patient and healthcare providers in this context is obvious. Opportunities for self-determination are also clearly constrained if the person perceives they are unable to freely communicate their personal wishes. In this instance, the patient's and family's emotional needs became marginalised, as the professional's opinion of what was needed became the central focus of intervention.

## Being frank

This refers to interactions where the healthcare provider presents to the patient or family what they consider to be 'statements of fact' in a direct manner. For example:

> I remember just before he died and the nurse just turned to me and said 'you know we have no hope for (my husband)' and I knew that all along, but I guess I had never really said it to myself. But I don't know why, but just those words, I almost felt it physically. I didn't let her see

that I just nodded and after I came out I was just in such shock, it was just so stark the way she had put it. She might as well have said to me 'you know he's going to die' but I didn't really need to hear that, because I knew that already. You don't need to hit me over the head with it you know.

In this instance, the nurse's approach prevents the person from negotiating their experience of death, since they appear to dismiss any alternative perceptions and feelings about the situation at hand. Instead of acknowledging that the dying person may interpret their situation in a manner different to that of the healthcare provider, the healthcare provider assumes their view of the situation is more legitimate than that of the dying person or their family. They then present information in a manner which is arguably designed to encourage the dying person and their family to conform to their superior world view. While we may espouse the value of openness in interactions, this participant's description of the impact that such an approach had on her highlights the complexity of achieving this goal in actual clinical situations.

## Explaining evasive interactions

There are a number of factors that are likely to be contributing to the continuing reports of the types of evasive interactions described by participants in this research. First, it could be argued that such an approach may be used consciously or unconsciously by nurses because they simply feel uncomfortable with difficult emotional situations, or because they need to protect themselves from becoming overwhelmed by the stress which results from continually being exposed to human suffering and distress. The existence of this type of stress in palliative care workers has been well documented in the literature (Vachon, 1995), and is clearly an area requiring attention if the psychosocial dimensions of palliative care are to be adequately addressed.

Second, it may be that some nurses choose to avoid open interactions because they do not feel confident that they have the skills necessary to make an appropriate response should the patient become distressed. Evidence from numerous surveys have supported the view that key areas of concern for healthcare providers include handling questions and conversations with dying patients, dealing with ethical and moral issues, and handling emotions (Copp & Dunn, 1993; Corner & Wilson-Barnett, 1992). Therefore, professional education programs which address such issues may also offer some potential for improving psychosocial care.

A third explanation for evasive interactions between healthcare providers and people who are dying is that the healthcare provider is able to justify such an approach on the grounds that discussing 'bad news' might cause unnecessary distress and destroy the hopes which are sustaining that person. James and Field (1996, p. 78), for example, discuss how healthcare providers may explain their diffidence about such openness by saying that 'although people say they want to know, they don't really'. They note how the constraints imposed from these types of traditional medical and nursing practices have led to major problems with implementation of policies of open disclosure.

Finally, it is also crucial to recognise the barriers and limitations created by the healthcare context. Moller (1996), for example, argues that the increasing bureaucratisation of death limits the type of spontaneity and flexibility that is necessary for negotiation of death. Since tensions will inevitably develop between the maintenance of personal autonomy and the maintenance of a functioning organisation, healthcare providers may choose to respond in these ways as their ideal is simply unattainable. A recent study of the changing stressors for cancer nurses over the past decade has noted that nurses today report that environmental stressors such as work overload, lack of resources and staff shortages are seen to be increasingly affecting their ability to provide good quality nursing care to people with cancer (Wilkinson, 1995).

Whatever the reasons for the evasive interactions described here, the bottom line is that within this interactional context, it is unlikely that a negotiated death can be achieved. Evasive interactions will inevitably place significant constraints on the opportunities for patients and families to express concerns and desires. The result for all involved may be greater emotional distress and suffering.

## Implications for practice

This chapter has focused on the psychosocial dimension of palliative care. In particular, the way in which societal views of death have shaped the philosophy and practice of palliative care has been examined. We noted from our review of death in modern society that the dying experience is typically characterised by meaninglessness, uncertainty and lack of control. We examined how prescriptive models of practice have been adopted by many healthcare providers, whereby acceptance of death is often seen as the ultimate goal. Finally, our analysis of the many healthcare provider and environmental factors that prevent the dying from being able to negotiate their death has highlighted the multifaceted and complex nature of the psychosocial dimensions of palliative care.

What do the issues raised from this analysis imply for improving clinical management of psychosocial issues? In answering this question, one must be careful not to fall into the trap of providing simply another prescription for practice which imposes the same constraints and problems that exist with current practice models. Nevertheless, it is clear that consideration must be given to how practice can be further developed if we are to facilitate a more compassionate approach to care for the dying.

The recommendations outlined in this section are therefore offered as guiding principles. They are presented to highlight some of the possible directions that might be further explored by clinicians and researchers in their endeavours to improve palliative care services.

First, the importance of being flexible and adopting a reflexive approach to practice seems to be a fundamental prerequisite for individualising psychosocial care. Individuals respond to dying in many different ways, and will have many different wishes as they proceed through the dying process. Being reflexive is therefore essential if the nurse is to assess continually the differing needs and responses of individuals, and modify management strategies on the basis of changing circumstances and needs. Adopting this more reflexive approach to practice may go some way to overcoming the prescriptive frameworks that currently appear to dominate palliative care.

Second, it seems that it is time for nurses to be more creative in how they manage psychosocial issues in palliative care, if they are to manage the realities of modern death more effectively. This will require the application of measures that will help people to find meaning, to gain control and to reduce uncertainty. Much promising work has already been done in this area. For example, a recent meta-analytic review of 45 studies on the effect of psychosocial interventions reported that 'the cumulative evidence is sufficiently strong to claim that such interventions have consistent beneficial effect on emotional adjustment, functional adjustment and treatment and disease related symptoms of cancer patients' (Meyer & Mark, 1995, p. 106). Key aspects of modern dying, such as uncertainty, have also been the subject of increasing theoretical and research interest in recent years (see Mast, 1995; Mishel, 1990; 1988), with the focus of these efforts now shifting to developing and testing uncertainty management interventions (McHenry, Allen, Mishel & Braden, 1993). The challenge now is for nurses to develop a repertoire of therapeutic supportive interventions which can be applied flexibly, according to individual circumstances, needs and the personal choices of the dying patient. The analysis presented in this chapter, however, reminds us that we must be mindful of the failure of efforts to date which have attempted to find simple solutions to complex problems. The psychosocial dimensions of palliative care are multifaceted, and effective management will often require addressing these issues on a number of levels.

While it is important to identify strategies which are effective in preventing and managing psychosocial problems in palliative care, the effectiveness of any such strategies is interpreted within a wider context and will depend on broader issues relating to the nature of the relationship between the healthcare provider and the dying person, as well as the broader healthcare environment. Since the individual's perception of their relationship with healthcare providers will influence how he or she will ultimately interpret their interaction with the nurse, the third principle proposed here is that clinicians and researchers give more attention to the meaning of such relationships in practice. The data discussed in this chapter suggest that a better understanding of the processes of communication, the factors which influence such communication, and the impact communication has on patients and families may enable one to respond with greater flexibility, and to make adjustments to how messages are delivered and received. To date, it appears that research has focused on identifying coping and support strategies, with much less attention being given to understanding the complexity of such important communication processes (Ruckdeschel, Blanchard & Albrecht, 1994).

Finally, attention should also be given to the broader context of practice if any significant improvements are to be achieved. The analysis presented in this paper suggests that there are many features of the current organisation and delivery of palliative care services that present barriers to effectively managing psychosocial issues. These require attention both at the broader public policy level and at the level of the organisation. It is clear from the data presented here, however, that traditional approaches to developing nurses' ability to provide psychosocial care through basic and continuing education programs have had only limited success. What is required, therefore, is the development of more innovative approaches to personal and professional development of palliative care workers. These programs should be designed to facilitate a greater understanding of how the context influences the practice of palliative care, and to foster the development of the skills necessary for palliative care workers to address the barriers to providing the type of psychosocial support desired by patients and their families. These programs should be offered in conjunction with programs that can foster the type of support and confidence needed for nurses to address the complex issues involved with palliative care nursing (Yates, Clinton & Hart, 1996; 1997). Recent work on peer consultation provides one example of a strategy that seems promising, since it works at addressing the culture of the workplace and the context of practice in an effort to improve practice (Hart, Bull & Marshall, 1995; Hart, Bull, Mongomery & Albrecht, 1994). As with all principles outlined here, much remains to be done. The scope for innovation and creativity is enormous.

# References

Ariès, P. (1981). *The hour of our death*. London: Allen Lane.

Becker, P.L. (1973). *The denial of death*. New York: Free Press.

Copp, G. & Dunn, V. (1993). Frequent and difficult problems perceived by nurses caring for the dying in community hospice and acute care settings. *Palliative Medicine*, 7, 19–25.

Corner, J. & Wilson-Barnett, J. (1992). The newly registered nurse and the cancer patient: An educational evaluation. *International Journal of Nursing Studies, 29*, 177–190.

Corr, C.A. (1993). Coping with dying: Lessons that we should and should not learn from the work of Elisabeth Kübler-Ross. *Death Studies, 17*, 69–83.

De Raeve, L. (1996). Dignity and integrity at the end of life. *International Journal of Palliative Nursing, 2*, 71–76.

Erseck, M. (1992). Examining the process and dilemmas of reality negotiation. *Image: Journal of Nursing Scholarship, 24*, 19–25.

Giddens, A. (1990). *The consequences of modernity.* Cambridge: Polity.

Giddens, A. (1991). *Modernity and self-identity.* Cambridge: Polity.

Glasser, B.G. & Strauss, A.L. (1965). *Awareness of dying.* New York: Aldine Publishing.

Glasser, B.G. & Strauss, A.L. (1968). *Time for dying.* Chicago: Aldine Publishing.

Gorer, G. (1965). *Death, grief, and mourning in contemporary Britain.* London: Crosset.

Hackett, T.P. & Cassem, N.H. (1974). Development of a quantitative rating scale to assess denial. *Journal of Psychosomatic Research, 18*, 93–100.

Hanson, E. (1994). An exploration of the taken for granted world of the cancer nurse in relation to stress and the person with cancer. *Journal of Advanced Nursing, 19*, 12–20.

Hart, G., Bull, R., Mungomery, L., & Albrecht, M. (1994). Peer consultation: Options and opportunities in Queensland hospitals. *The Australian and New Zealand Journal of Mental Health Nursing, 3*, 119–131.

Hart, G., Bull, R., & Marshall, L. (1995). Peer consultation: A strategy to support collegial practice. In Gray, G. & Pratt, R. (Eds.), *Issues in Australian nursing*, vol. 4 (pp. 391–405). Melbourne: Pearson Professional.

Hunt, M. (1992). 'Scripts' for dying at home—displayed in nurses', patients' and relatives' talk. *Journal of Advanced Nursing, 17*, 1297–1302.

James, V. & Field, D. (1996). Who has the power? Some problems and issues affecting the nursing care of dying patients. *European Journal of Cancer Care, 5*, 73–80.

Jeffrey, D. (1995). Appropriate palliative care: When does it begin? *European Journal of Cancer Care, 4*, 122–126.

Kelner, M.J. & Bourgeault, I.L. (1993). Patient control over dying: Responses of health care professionals. *Social Science and Medicine, 36*, 757–765.

Kübler-Ross, E. (1970). *On death and dying.* London: Tavistock.

Kübler-Ross, E. (1975). *Death: The final stage of growth.* Englewood Cliffs, NJ: Prentice-Hall.

McHenry, J., Allen, C., Mishel, M.H., & Braden, C.J. (1993). Uncertainty management for women receiving treatment for breast cancer. In Funk, S.G., Tornquist, E.M., Champagne, M.T., & Wiese, R.A. (Eds.), *Key aspects of caring for the chronically ill* (pp. 170–177). New York: Springer Publishing Co.

McNamara, B. (1996). Nursing concerns in hospice care organisations. *Cancer Forum, 20*, pp. 19–30.

Maguire, P. (1985). Barriers to psychological care of the dying. *British Medical Journal, 291*, 1711–1713.

Mast, M.E. (1995). Adult uncertainty in illness: A critical review of research. *Scholarly Inquiry for Nursing Practice, 9*, pp. 3–24.

Mayer, S. (1989). Wholly life: A new perspective on death. *Holistic Nursing Practice, 3*, 72–80.

Mellor, P. (1993). Death in high modernity: The contemporary presence and absence of death. In Clark, D. (Ed.), *The sociology of death* (pp. 11–30). Oxford: Blackwell Publishers.

Meyer, T.J. & Mark, M.M. (1995). Effects of psychosocial interventions with adult cancer patients: A meta-analysis of randomized experiments. *Health Psychology, 14*, 101–108.

Mishel, M.H. (1988). Uncertainty in illness. *Image: Journal of Nursing Scholarship, 20,* 225–232.

Mishel, M.H. (1990). Reconceptualization of the uncertainty in illness theory. *Image: Journal of Nursing Scholarship, 22,* 256–262.

Moller, D.W. (1996). *Confronting death: Values, institutions and human mortality.* New York: Oxford University Press.

Novack, D., Plumer, R., Smith, R.L. et al. (1979). Changes in physicans' attitudes toward telling the cancer patient. *JAMA, 241,* 897–900.

Parker, J. & Gardner, G. (1992). The silence and the silencing of nurses' voice: A reading of patient progress notes. *Australian Journal of Advanced Nursing, 9,* 3–9.

Ruskdeschel, J.C., Blanchard, C.G., & Albrecht, T. (1994). Psychosocial oncology research: Where we have been, where we are going and why we will not get there. *Cancer, 74,* 1458–1463.

Sudnow, D. (1967). *Passing on.* Englewood Cliffs, NJ: Prentice-Hall.

Taylor, B. (1993). Hospice nurses tell their stories abut a good death: The value of storytelling as a qualitative health research method. *Annual Review of Health Social Science, 3,* 97–108.

Taylor, S.E. (1983). Adjustment to threatening events: A theory of adaptation. *American Psychologist,* Nov., 1161–1173.

Vachon, M.L. (1995). Staff stress in hospice/palliative care: A review. *Palliative Medicine, 9,* 91–122.

Walter, T. (1991). Modern death: Taboo or not taboo? *Sociology, 23,* 293–310.

Watson, M., Greer S., Blake, S., & Shrapnell, K. (1984). Reaction to a diagnosis of breast cancer. Relationship between denial, delay and rates of psychological morbidity. *Cancer, 53,* 2008–2012.

Wilkinson, S. (1991). Factors which influence how nurses communicate with cancer patients. *Journal of Advanced Nursing, 16,* 677–688.

Wilkinson, S. (1995). The changing pressures for cancer nurses 1986–1993. *European Journal of Cancer Care, 4,* 69–74.

Williams, R. (1989). Awareness and control of dying: Some paradoxical trends in public opinion. *Sociology of Health and Illness, 11,* 201–212.

Yates, P. (1996). Surviving death: A study of the impact of the death of a family member to cancer. Unpublished PhD data, University of Queensland.

Yates, P., Clinton, M., & Hart, G. (1996). Improving psychosocial care: A professional development programme (Part one). *International Journal of Palliative Nursing, 2,* 212–216.

Yates, P., Clinton, M., & Hart, G. (1997). Design of a professional development programme for palliative care nurses (Part two). *International Journal of Palliative Nursing, 3,* 70–75.

# Reflection on the Good Death and the Nurse in Palliative Care

## Lesley Wilkes

The art of dying has always fascinated humans. In our society, palliative care is one practice area that concerns itself with this art. The picture of death that arises in much of the discourse in palliative care literature is that of a 'good death'. The meaning of this 'good death' to the patient, family and palliative care health workers will influence the outcome of this life trajectory. The nurse as a healthcare worker has been seen as integral to palliative care (Scanlon, 1989; Greene, 1984) because of, according to Greene, (1984) the emphasis on individualised care in the nursing philosophy, the nurse's position as an active rather than reactive agent in the management of patient care and because the nurse has the knowledge and skills to improve the patient's quality of life. Nurses have a definitive role when a patient is dying and therefore their perceptions of 'good death' will play a significant role in how they provide care to the dying patient. Nurses' values and perceptions of 'good death' may also cause conflict with patients and work colleagues (Wilkes & White, 1995). Thus it is important to analyse nurses' descriptions of good death and their ramifications.

A palliative care nurse's paradigm case of a 'good death':

> A man in his early 60s. He wanted to be cared for at home for the weeks prior to his death (despite being bedridden all the time). The wife was the main care giver who was very accepting of the death and took responsibility for most of the care of the client with some intervention by visiting nursing staff. The man was symptom free, except for some pain which he accepted as part of his fate. The man was nursed in the centre of the living room in the house and so was able to watch the goings on around him. There was also a large open window near the man so he had visual contact with the outside world. His grown family and grandchildren visited frequently and were nearby up until his death. After his death his family, some friends and myself sat near his body and talked about his life and the fact that he had died as he had lived—in control and very much a dominant figure in the family. (Wilkes, 1993, p. 13)

**Table 9.1   Nurses' descriptions of 'good death', 1992–96**

| Researcher/s | Study sample | Site | Research method | Nurses' criteria for 'good death' |
|---|---|---|---|---|
| Hunt, 1992 | Five nurses (all aged over 40) in a symptom control team and 54 cancer patients (the majority aged over 60) | Community in England | Case-study and ethnography; audio-taped conversations between the nurses and the patients | • Physical symptoms controlled<br>• Patient and relative accepting<br>• Presentation of hope and desire to live<br>• Keeping mobile and fighting back<br>• Enjoyment of life<br>• Peaceful death at home |
| Wilkes, 1992 | 16 nurses (aged 21–50) | Oncology, palliative care, general medical, surgical wards, acute care and gerontology in Sydney, Australia | Written narrative | • Painless<br>• Acceptance<br>• Family present<br>• Chosen environment<br>• Symptoms controlled<br>• No aggressive medical treatment<br>• Not prolonged<br>• Peaceful |
| White, 1994 | Four nurses (all over 40 years) | Hospice in Sydney | Case-study (part of larger study on ethical issues for nurses in a hospice); audio-taped focus groups and reflective journals | • Peaceful<br>• Accepting<br>• Without the indignities of tubes<br>• No agitation<br>• No active interventions<br>• Painless<br>• Patient having time to prepare emotionally for dying |

| | | | | |
|---|---|---|---|---|
| McNamara, Waddell & Colvin, 1994<br>McNamara, Waddell & Colvin, 1995<br>McNamara, 1996 | 22 nurses (aged 25–62 years) | Community-based hospice service and in-patient hospice in Western Australia | Ethnography; interviews, participant observation, field notes | • Feeling of participation<br>• Excellent standard of care<br>• Adequate pain control<br>• Patient autonomy<br>• Individual and family values accounted for<br>• Acceptance<br>• Symptoms controlled<br>• Over-medicalisation not good<br>• Supportive family and friends<br>• Not sudden |
| Taylor, 1995 | Ten nurses | Domiciliary hospice service in regional city in Victoria | Narrative, audio-taped interviews | • Family and friends provide their presence, support, love and encouragement<br>• Promises kept and wishes fulfilled<br>• Acceptance and surrender to impending death<br>• Good-byes said and messages given<br>• Support given<br>• Trust gained<br>• Effective symptom control<br>• Nurses' involvement and facilitation makes a difference<br>• No unfinished business<br>• The funeral is a fitting farewell |

This description of 'good death' typifies it as family centred, set in a chosen environment, peaceful, the family and the dying person accepting and in control. Is this view true for all nurses who care for the palliative care patient and their family?

A number of studies on nurses' descriptions of 'good' and 'bad death', and death scenes have been published in the 1990s (Hunt, 1992; Wilkes, 1993; White, 1994; McNamara, Waddell & Colvin, 1994, 1995; Taylor, 1995; McNamara, 1996). Table 9.1 summarises the main components of a 'good death' that emerged from these studies. In their studies, Hunt and Wilkes focused only on descriptions of 'good death'; in the other studies 'good death' was part of a larger context. In White's study, the major focus was ethical problems for nurses in a hospice and, similarly, McNamara et al.'s interest was the implications of the ideal of 'good death' on nurses coping in a hospice. Taylor's study described nurses' stories of 'good death' with an emphasis on how nurses could promote this ideal.

As seen in table 9.1, a number of common themes emerge in the descriptions of the 'good death' ideal. The major themes are: the compliance of the patient and family to the nurse's ideal of good dying, good death/peaceful death, symptom control but not over-medicalisation, and good death and acceptance; other themes that are elucidated in some of the studies are: preparation for death and completion of unfinished business, presence of family and farewell, and hope. Each of these will be discussed in relation to their implications for the patient, family and nurses involved in this rite of passage.

## Compliance of the patient and family to the nurse's ideal of 'good dying'

'We all die. Mortality is 100%. No-one saves lives. Death is not the problem. It never as been the problem. Dying—getting there—sometimes is' (Baume, 1995, p. 8). The problem is not limited to the patient and family. This dying can become a problem to nurses who believe that the patient and family are not compliant to the nurse's ideal of 'good dying'. In Hunt's study (1992), it is clear that the nurses thought that the patients should do what the nurses wanted. They had to enjoy life, they had to fight to the end. The person had to be compliant. If the patients decided to stay in bed and not be mobile, they weren't doing what the nurses expected. An example of this is a 24-year-old man who decided he was more comfortable in bed. This concerned the nurse who told the patient, 'you can't spend your life in this room'. The man died a week later (Hunt, 1992, pp. 130–2). The notion that the patient must comply to the ideal also came out in McNamara et al.'s study (1994, 1995, 1996). If the patient did not fit the ideal, the nurses might still acknowledge them as 'good', but shifted the responsibility for this goodness to the patient because they found it a problem. As one in-patient hospice nurse stated: 'We always seem to be looking for good death from the nurse's perspective, rather than the patient . . . what are the patient's expectations . . . we need to give people permission to make their own decisions' (McNamara et al., 1994, p. 1506).

The patient and family's concept of the ideal death may be varied and very different to the nurse's prescription. The idea that 'good death' must not be prescriptive comes out very clearly in reading popular literature written by dying patients or their families. In categorising but three of these views, Hawkins (1991), using three novels, described the journey of three couples. It can be seen that a 'good death' for one couple was a ritual death of stages, to another a victorious death which attempted to transform death into a battle victory, and to another couple an attempt to plan the conditions of the husband's dying. Many other descriptions come from literature. For example, de Beauvoir (1965) described her mother's 'easy death' (an avoidance of suffering being the key).

Contrary to this idea of compliance is the patient being in control. Patient control is emphasised in the literature not only by health workers (e.g. Field, 1989) but in studies by sociologists such as Kellehear (1990) and patients themselves. In her writings of a personal journey with cancer, Graham (1982) emphasised the importance of the need to know what was happening and to be in control.

In the paradigm case cited above, the patient's control over the place and circumstance of death were seen as important for the 'good death', with the presence of the family being particularly relevant. Nurses in the other studies reviewed supported patient control, but, at the same time, as McNamara (1996) noted, patient compliance to the nurse and the institution's wishes made patient care and dying easier and more efficient. Is this why compliance rather than patient wishes are paramount? Or is it that giving patients control over dying is against the healthcare professionals' (nurses') concept of themselves as supporters and healers (Kelner & Bourgeault, 1993)? Such ideas must be challenged, and the patient, family and the nurse need to form partnerships for a 'good death' through open communication and action.

## Good death/peaceful death

In all the studies reviewed in table 9.1, the nurses had an overriding perception that death must be peaceful and quiet in order to be 'good'. This is not a new perception—as Strauss and Glaser (1985) state, health professionals should not be disturbed by the dying patient and Fields (1984) found that nurses preferred caring for dying patients who were peaceful and accepting. Again in two studies on euthanasia (White, 1994; Wilkes & White, 1995), nurses working in palliative care may go to extreme measures with patient sedation to ensure that death is peaceful. Nurses who do not hold this view may come into conflict (Wilkes & White, 1995) with colleagues, patients and the patients' families. Are we heading for a situation where death is a symptom to be alleviated (Biswas, 1990; James & Field, 1992)? James and Field (1992) speculate that the early ideal of hospice care (palliative care) of a 'good death' has been gradually interpreted by some workers as 'death with dignity' and more recently as 'a peaceful death'. They suggest a move from the broad concept of 'good' to a prescribed type of death which is 'peaceful'. This led to another perception by nurses of 'good death' as one where there is symptom control but not over-medicalisation.

## Symptom control but not over-medicalisation

A prescription of a peaceful death which is free of pain and other symptoms comes out in all the studies in table 9.1. This concept of the 'good death' as symptom free is not restricted to nurses. It is often the foundation of the euthanasia debate. In an interesting study by Kastenbaum and Normand (1990) outlining university students' descriptions of desired death scenes, no symptoms were paramount. While we should be able to control pain and most symptoms, Morris, Sherwood, Wright and Gulkin (1988) showed that 96.3 per cent of patients have one or more symptoms (nausea, dry mouth, constipation, dizziness, fever, shortness of breath) in the week prior to death. In order to achieve this ideal, nurses need a good knowledge of the range of methods available. Two studies in Australia by Harrison (1996) and McGovern (1995) found this knowledge to be lacking. With the advent of more specialised education programs in palliative care, directed particularly at nurses, this requirement for the 'good death' can be met.

Over-treatment and over-medicalisation during palliative care is seen as detrimental to 'good death' by nurses in the studies of McNamara et al. (1994, 1995, 1996) and those of Wilkes (1993) and Wilkes and White (1995). Death is inevitable, the obligations of the health professional caring for the dying 'are not fixed by obligation to provide treatments that serve only to extend the dying process but rather by obligations to provide appropriate care in dying' (Beauchamps & Childress, 1994, p. 200). As McNamara et al. (1994, 1995) and McNamara (1996) postulate, this ideal may be challenged in today's setting and practice of palliative care. The encroachment of mainstream medicine onto the scene and aggressive interventions are abhorrent to the nurses' ideal. One nurse's description of a 'bad death' in intensive care exemplifies this:

> An aged patient (more than 70 years) with cancer and metastases
> continued having tests—daily blood tests, IV [intravenous] therapy
> (resited daily as the veins were collapsing), X-rays, sigmoidoscopy,

antibiotics (leading to mouth ulcers and diarrhoea). Nurses and medical staff not giving the patient relaxed, quality time as they were too busy doing tests. Not enough analgesia given. Patient eventually died after weeks of further tests even though she had her metastases confirmed (lymph nodes and liver). (Wilkes, 1993)

While aggressive treatments as described above are not to be tolerated, patients in palliative care who formerly would not have had invasive therapies now receive treatments made available through developments in palliative medicine and new technology. Intravenous hydration (Musgrave, Bartal & Opstad, 1996), total parental nutrition (Fainsinger, Chan & Bruera, 1992), blood transfusion (Monti, Castellani, Berlusconi & Cunietti, 1996), and chemotherapy (Byock, 1992) are but a few therapies discussed in the literature. These therapies are becoming commonplace as part of the medicalisation of palliative care. The situation of AIDS patients under palliative care who have active treatments to relieve or inhibit the development of symptoms, for conditions such as meningeal infection and retinal haemorrhage, highlights how significantly medicalisation can improve the quality of life.

While technology is developing rapidly, nurses express concern that it will not be used appropriately. This is not to deny that much of modern palliative care and its successes have come from using a full range of medical knowledge and appropriate technology delivered in a caring way, taking into account the spiritual, physical, psychological and social needs of the patient and family. There must not be a prescription for 'good death', nor a view that it can be controlled by medicine as a symptom.

## Good death and acceptance

Nurses in the studies outlined in table 9.1 see a 'good death' as one where the patient particularly, but also the family, accept that death is inevitable. Otherwise the rite of passage will not be 'right'. The nurses in Taylor's study (1995), like the other nurses, thought that it was important for the individuals in their stories to come to acceptance and surrender so that the dying person was able to face the final days with a sense of peace. Whose motivations should be obeyed? Is it the nurse or the patient or the family who demands peace and acceptance?

For some people this concept of a death of acceptance may be morally oppressive. De Raeve (1996) contests there are other modes that constitute a 'good death'. These include a rageful death as advocated by Dylan Thomas (1952): 'do not go gentle into the good night' (p. 116). A rageful death goes against the grain for nurses who believe in a good death as one of peace and acceptance, but what of the patient's desire for dignity? De Raeve (1996) sees a dignified death as one where the person is treated not merely as a means to an end but as an end in themselves. Szawarski (1986) describes dignity as pertaining to people simply by virtue of their being human and thus maintaining respect is a proper acknowledgment of this dignity. The acknowledgment of humanism and respect must be paramount for the nurse assisting the person and family towards the ideal of 'good death'.

## Preparation for death and completion of unfinished business

The nurses' descriptions of 'good death' often contained need for the person and family to have time to prepare for the death. This may include will and funeral arrangements. This preparation aspect has also been highlighted in the literature as key criteria for a 'good death' by both patients and health professionals.

In a sociological study of patients dying of cancer in Australia, Kellehear (1990) found that the major features of 'good death' included many aspects of preparation such as:

- public preparation for death (before awareness), especially regarding legal, finance, and funeral matters;
- awareness of their dying from information given by other people, particularly their doctor;
- personal and social adjustments—maintained and increased social support, talk and some informal willing;
- public preparation after awareness including ratification of existing material preparations, some religious and funeral preparation made.

These features are again highlighted in stories by people when they have a life-threatening disease such as cancer (e.g. Graham, 1982) and by people surveyed on their views of death (Williams, 1989). It is important that nurses and other health professionals provide avenues for this preparation without reducing the personal empowerment of the dying person and their family.

## Presence of family and farewell

The sense of ritual death with the family around the bed is prominent in the criteria for 'good death' set by the nurses in the studies and is also seen as important in much of the general literature (for example, see Ariès, 1974; Williams, 1989; Hawkins, 1991). It is also a feature of dying patients' descriptions of the ideal 'good death' (for example, Graham, 1982; Kellehear, 1990). However is this public death, an occasion for affirming the joy of being (Ariès, 1974, p.124), possible in this era of institutionalised death, where death has become unnameable: 'death is so frightful that we dare not utter its name' (Ariès, 1974, p. 13)?

## Hope

In this review of studies about nurses' descriptions of 'good death', the sense of hope present in Hunt's descriptions does not creep into the other studies. This is interesting as other writers talk of instilling hope in palliative care patients (e.g., Scanlon, 1989). As well, Graham (1982) describes how important hope was in her personal cancer journey. She relates how a nurse instilled hope when she was discouraged after having chemotherapy which caused her to be sick 14 days out of 28. The nurse turned it around saying she should look at it as 14 well days in every 28. Taylor (1995) talks of the nurses giving support and peace to the patients, but not hope.

Further studies on the importance of hope for dying patients are required and one is in progress in Sydney. From these nurses can learn how to facilitate this aspect of the dying patient's care.

## Conclusion

One observation that can be glimpsed from the studies of nurses' description of a 'good death' is that 'the process of dying' is more important in the eyes of the nurse than the moment of death.

In a sense there is no conclusion to this paper. Maybe the most significant feature of the 'good death' is its many and varied manifestations. A point of reflection to consider is that of Hawkins (1991):

> If death is simply the end of life, then it becomes an unknown to be confronted, not an experience that can be possessed by or assimilated into the personality . . . death may simply be the 'other side of life', an 'it'—random, inevitable and unknown. (p. 317)

If this be the case, prescribed death, a death of compliance, death as a symptom of illness to be controlled, cannot be allowed to happen. The patient's and family's ideas, feelings and expectations must be incorporated into any care given in preparation for the inevitable and unknown.

## References

Ariès, P. (1974). *Western attitudes toward death*. Baltimore: Johns Hopkins University Press.

Baume, P. (1995). Voluntary euthanasia and the liberal tradition. 9th Lionel Murphy Memorial Lecture at the State Library of NSW, Sydney, 30 November.

Beauchamp, T. & Childress, J. (1994). *Principles of biomedical ethics*. Oxford: Oxford University Press.

Biswas, B. (1990). The medicalisation of dying. In Clark, D. (Ed.), *The future of palliative care*. Buckingham: Open University Press.

Byock, I.R. (1992). Cancer chemotherapy and the boundaries of the hospice model. *The American Journal of Hospice and Palliative Care*, March/April, 4–5.

de Beauvoir, S. (1965). *A very easy death*. P. O'Brien (trans.). New York: G.P. Putnam.

de Raeve, L. (1996). Dignity and integrity at the end of life. *International Journal of Palliative Nursing*, 2 (2), 71–76.

Fainsinger, R.L., Chan, K., & Bruera, E. (1992). Total parenteral nutrition for a terminally ill patient? *Journal of Palliative Care*, 8 (2), 30–32.

Field, D. (1984). We didn't want him to die on his own—Nurses' accounts of nursing dying patients. *Journal of Advanced Nursing*, 9, 59–70.

Field, D. (1989). *Nursing the dying*. London: Tavistock Routledge.

Graham, J. (1982). *In the company of others: Understanding the human needs of cancer patients*. San Diego: Harcourt Brace Jovanovich.

Greene, P.E. (1984). The pivotal role of the nurse in hospice care. *Cancer Journal for Clinicians*, 34 (4), 205.

Harrison, R. (1996). Management of chronic non malignant pain in the elderly client: The perspective of the nurse. Bachelor of Nursing honours thesis, pp. 1–101, Australian Catholic University, Sydney.

Hawkins, A.H. (1991). Constructing death: Three pathographies about dying. *Omega*, 22 (4), 301–317.

Hunt, M. (1992). 'Scripts' for dying at home—displayed in nurses', patients and relatives' talk. *Journal of Advanced Nursing*, 17, 1297–1302.

James, N. & Field, D. (1992). The routinization of hospice: Charisma and bureaucratization. *Social Science & Medicine*, 34 (2), 1363-1375.

Kastenbaum, R. & Normand, C. (1990). Deathbed scenes as imagined by the young and experienced by the old. *Death Studies*, 14, 201–207.

Kellehear, A. (1990). *Dying of cancer: The final year of life*. London: Harwood Academic Press.

Kelner, M.J. & Bourgeault, I.V. (1993). Patient control over dying: Responses of health care professionals. *Social Science & Medicine*, 36 (6), 757–765.

McGovern, M.G. (1995). Nurses' understanding of pain control and their opinions regarding the use of morphine for cancer pain. Unpublished Masters of Nursing thesis, Australian Catholic University, Sydney.

McNamara, B. (1996). Nursing concerns in hospice care organisations. *Cancer Forum*, 20 (1), 19–29.

McNamara, B., Waddell, C., & Colvin, M. (1994). The institutionalisation of the good death. *Social Science & Medicine*, 39 (11), 1501–1508.

McNamara, B., Waddell, C., & Colvin, M. (1995). Threats to the good death: The cultural context of stress and coping among hospice nurses. *Sociology of Health and Illness*, 17 (2), 222–244.

Morris, J.N., Sherwood, S., Wright, S., & Gulkin, C.E. (1988). The last weeks of life: Does hospice care make a difference? In Mor, V., Greer, D.S., & Kastenbaum, R. (Eds.), *The hospice experiment* (pp. 173–179). St Louis, MI: CV Mosby.

Monti, M., Castellani, L., Berlusconi, A., & Cunietti. E. (1996). Use of blood transfusion in terminally patients admitted to a palliative care unit. *Journal of Pain and Symptom Management*, 12 (1), 18–22.

Musgrave, C.F., Bartal, N., & Opstad, J. (1996). Intravenous hydration for terminal patients: What are the attitudes of Israeli terminal patients, their families and their health professionals? *Journal of Pain and Symptom Management*, 12 (1), 47–51.

Scanlon, C. (1989). Creating a vision of hope: The challenge of palliative care. *Oncology Nursing Forum*, 16 (4), 491–496.

Strauss, L. & Glaser, B.G. (1985). Awareness of dying. In Galdieri Wilcox, S. & Sutton, M. (Eds.), *Understanding death and dying: An interdisciplinary approach*, 3rd edn. Palo Alto, CA: Mayfield Publications.

Szawarski, Z. (1986). Dignity and responsibility. *Dialectics and Humanism*, 2 (3), 193–205.

Taylor, B. (1995). Promoting a good death: Nurses' practice insights. In Gray, G. & Pratt R. (Eds.), *Issues in Australian nursing 5: The nurse as clinician* (pp. 209–220). Melbourne: Churchill Livingstone.

Thomas, D. (1952). *Collected poems 1934–1952*. London: Dent & Sons.

Willliams, R. (1989). *A Protestant legacy: Coping with illness, aging and death in Scottish culture*. Oxford: Oxford University Press.

Wilkes, L.M. (1993). Nurses' descriptions of death scenes. *Journal of Cancer Care, 2*, 11–16.

Wilkes, L.M., White, K., & Tolley, N. (1991). Palliative care nurses' attitudes to euthanasia. *Proceedings of Nursing Research Conference* (pp. 142–148). Adelaide.

Wilkes, L.M. & White., K. (1995). Palliative care nurses' conflict of values. *Journal of Cancer Care, 4*, 97–100.

White, K. (1994). Ethical problems experienced by four palliative care nurses working in a hospice. Unpublished Master of Nursing thesis, Australian Catholic University, Sydney.

# 10

## Nursing Dying People

### Ysanne B. Chapman

Much of our work as nurses has a strong bias towards wellness and a focus on the living. However, not all patients live, and some patients are placed in our care because they are about to die. This chapter reports on a study which was largely influenced by my own traumatic experiences with death in the clinical setting and by my knowledge that nurses have similar experiences today despite the availability of educational programs for health professionals in many aspects of care for the dying or the dead.

The study reported here, which drew upon a methodology of hermeneutic phenomenology, focuses on twelve registered nurses' reflections on their significant encounters with nursing the dying or dead patient. I hoped that the study would illuminate what it means to nurse the dying or the dead. I did not intend a 'recipe book' approach to nursing the dying. Rather, in articulating the meaning of the experience, I hoped to encourage nurses to move towards improving their practice of nursing the dead or the dying.

One of the strengths of phenomenology as a methodology is that it differentiates between appearance and essence, giving import to the interpretation of the experience as well as to the experience or action itself. After extensive work on the transcripts and tapes of my interviews with these twelve nurses, I identified four essences—connectedness, aloneness, questioning and accepting—that offered a unifying structure to the various elements of the stories.

### Connectedness

Participants regularly mentioned the multifaceted phenomenon of connectedness in the process of forming relationships with the dying person, their relatives and with other healthcare professionals. In connecting with the dying person, each participant recognised a need not only to place themselves in the dying person's shoes but also to get in touch with what it means to be dying. All participants described how being involved with the dying situation enabled them to fully utilise personal and professional resources to enhance their carative practices.

> So I tend to like to look after people, and relatives, and I tend to look after them the way I wanted to be looked after. And I remembered what helped me or if I saw the nurses doing something to my mother, that's the way I would like to do it. And again, the opposite.

Benner (1984) suggests that 'caring cannot be controlled or coerced . . . caring is embedded in personal and cultural meanings' (1984, p. 170). The participants in this study were mindful that their own personal and cultural meanings of death could not be easily put aside when caring for dying people. Their personal qualities equipped them to relate effectively to a person whose death is imminent. Spending quality time with dying people was very important for these nurses, enabling them to get to know the patient on a personal as well as a professional level, and allowing them to discover and build a patient profile regarding coping mechanisms and individual needs. In addition, this relationship helped to extend these nurses' own awareness of the dying process.

Most of the nurses agreed that it was easier for them to accept the death of an older person than a younger one. Some talked of the quality of life as opposed to the quantity of life of the dying person and how they seemed to sense that the patient wished to die. In addition, several participants described the importance of their need to 'be-with' the patient and in doing so to create an awareness of the approaching death event. Other studies (Rieman, 1986; Watson, 1987; Benner & Wrubel, 1989; Vohland, 1994) also highlight presencing or 'being-there' as central to caring for patients who may be facing death. 'Presencing' is more than the physical closeness of the nurse. It is the nature of the time spent with the dying person that is important.

'Being-with' dying people requires the nurse to be flexible in approaches to different people involved in the same situation. Being-in-the-world-of-the-patient assists nurses to identify and experience shared understanding of the patient's experience of dying. Similarly, holistic nursing practice permits this shared understanding to encompass the dying person's relatives and/or friends. Two nurses commented on the importance of spending quality time with the relatives. During such times, discussions about the impending death assisted all those involved in the interaction to connect with the death event and with the patient's sense of reality of the situation.

> I see death as being quite natural. I am also aware that for the people close to them it isn't natural at all times and it's very difficult for them, so I'd like to think that when I'm with the relatives, and patients when they are dying, that some way it is conveyed to them that it is okay for

this person to die, because they have such ambivalent feelings that they certainly don't want their loved one to go away, yet they realise that it's time.

The death environment was often described by the participants as impersonal or clinical. Some resented their inability to fashion the environment to suit the dying or dead person. However, many spoke of their need to change the dying environment from one of a seemingly clinical appearance to one of a peaceful ambience.

In the palliative care ward we put a rose on the pillow or hibiscus flower or whatever's available, freshen the room up and everything. Just because they like to spend time with them it's much nicer to have a better environment for them.

However, the difficulties of providing a palliative focus in a technological environment such as intensive or coronary care were of concern to many of the nurses. Some nurses have difficulty dealing with the tension between the care that is normally given in such an environment and the care needed in a palliative framework (Walters, 1992, p. 351). The nurses in this study discussed their difficulties in grappling with the move beyond technology towards a more humanistic focus and agree with Walters (1992) that the humanistic approach is not given the same degree of credibility as the former. This devaluing of care again creates a tension within the nurse and helps to perpetuate the notion that care of the dying is not appropriate in a 'high-tech' area. Being in a connected relationship with the patient can assist both the nurse and the patient to 'come to terms' with the change in outcomes.

Several of the nurses confirmed that as they progressed through their nursing careers, their own attitudes to death changed. Instead of feeling apart from the death experience, they learned to accept death as a part of life and thus to engage in a more meaningful manner with the death event of their patient(s). In reaching a 'professional maturity', these nurses expressed concern for those less experienced in caring for the dying. They commented upon the necessity to be aware of the emotional reactions of less experienced staff, and they realised that their role as registered nurses included making quality time available for these less experienced nurses and assisting them to vent their feelings about death.

Most notably, preparation of the body after death elicited personal responses within each nurse. Many described the differences in the laying out procedures as students and later as more experienced registered nurses. Overall, they were distressed by their initial experiences, seeing the laying out as an invasion of the dead person's body. Some noted that this procedure was carried out with a sense of urgency or indifference. This situation left them feeling that they had broken their connection with the dead person.

I felt it was a real violation, 'cause I honestly felt, 'cause I have a great belief that they're still there, somewhere, do you know what I mean, whether they're sitting above the bed or standing behind me or . . . I don't feel uncomfortable about it.

In developing a sense of connectedness, many participants spoke of being aware of the deeply personal and subjective nature of the dying experience for the person. They alluded to a 'therapeutic intimacy' they shared with their patients in their final hours of living. In short, the phenomenon of connectedness in nursing dying or dead people can be defined as a willingness to be actively involved with the dying milieu: the dying patient, the relatives of the dying patient, and colleagues. Connectedness also implies a two-way conversational existence between the nurse and the dying person in which each person has the potential to grow and change.

## Aloneness

Backer, Hannon and Russell (1994, p. 49) discuss the challenges involved in nursing dying people. They state, 'The work will never be easy. In some ways, a part of the caregiver dies with each dying patient'. In western society, death has become invisible. Nurses must face their own fears and anxieties about death, often alone. The literature speaks of the advantage of self-awareness in coming to terms with these struggles (Penson, 1990; Backer et al., 1994; Benner & Wrubel, 1989). However, the burdens nurses carry regarding their own emotional conflicts with the dying event are sometimes hidden from those closest to them (their patients and their peers). Many described their initial experience with death as disturbing: their professional inexperience and lack of personal death situations compounded these feelings of inadequacy and some felt disillusioned.

> I can still smell the smell of my own fear and illnesses that pervaded that little world. That smell was mixed with the all-pervading smell of Lysol that seemed to ooze out of the pan room and permeated the beds, screens, walls and floors. I could even smell it on myself, my hands and nails, my uniform and hair. My thoughts and impressions of what I had imagined and dreamed nursing was about, had fled.

In discussing their early experiences of nursing dying or dead people, almost all of the experienced registered nurses described how it felt to be alone with their negative emotions. These nurses recalled how it was expected that these powerful emotions somehow dissipated as they finished their shift in the institution.

> You know, when I first started nursing we were told that when you walk out the front door you leave all your emotions and feelings and what-have-you in the hospital and you go home. I have never been

able to do that. I don't honestly know that there is anybody who can do that.

Many discussed the lack of support in the work situation. Some health care agencies appear to foster a climate of horizontal violence within nursing, and the formation of a workplace that values each other's feelings is not considered legitimate. For a profession that claims to be part of a healthcare team, it is ironic that the conflict between individuals within that team may lead to factionalism and a breakdown in the communication channels which are deemed vital to maintain a strong team approach to care of the dying (Stein-Parbury, 1993, p. 303).

The older, more experienced registered nurses recognised that their individual upbringing and socialisation played an influential part in the experience of nursing dying or dead people. Many spoke freely about their childhood and how death did not feature as a high priority in their early lives. Consequently, when they faced death in their earlier years of nursing, either as a student or as a registered nurse, they were reminded of this knowledge deficit and felt abandoned. Some of the participants described their perceptions of being in a subordinate position when students. The hierarchy within nursing was well identified and students were made to feel they had to obey the rules without questioning. This position of inferiority contributed to their understanding of junior staff not having input into planning patient care or decision making, and thus to their feelings of aloneness in the death situation:

> It seemed that there was no emotion felt by anyone except me. I felt unable to express my feelings for fear of being laughed at. . . . It was important to keep a stiff upper lip and to be always in control. Showing emotion was seen as being out of control and perceived as a weakness.

Without exception, all participants noted that the death event was a sad occasion for all people involved with the dying or dead person. This sadness invariably resulted in a sense of loss as the emotional bonds between the patient and the nurse were severed.

> It's the loss. It's very selfish, I know myself, it's a very selfish thing, like, I don't want them to go. It's your loss and dealing with your loss, not so much trying to put myself in their shoes. It's totally a selfish thing—I've lost this person I love so dearly, they're no longer going to be with me.

The participants gave graphic descriptions of the setting of the death event, highlighting their own identification with the loneliness of dying in an unfamilar setting.

> His loved ones weren't there. The room was like a typical hospital room. Even though we were in the newest portion of the hospital, it was still, like, very cold and it felt very cold. It was very clinical. And

he seemed alone. It was almost as if he needed someone to take him on the passage, do you know what I mean, just that crossing over.

While encouraging family members or friends to stay with the dying person sometimes assists in making this experience peaceful, it does not alter the situation that many patients die in unfamiliar surroundings, away from their treasured possessions or pets.

When a patient dies, nurses need to come to terms with their own feelings of loss and grief. Several participants spoke of the lack of space and time within the working environment to undertake such a function. Jane poignantly remembers her behaviours, which were usually undertaken in solitude: 'I don't let go until I get home. Sometimes I go home and do lots and lots of housework, keep myself really busy. Other times I sit down and think about it, release my emotions.'

Emotional detachment was an issue for some of these nurses. The sense of loss and aloneness experienced as a result of the death of a patient was often described as traumatic and many avoided these feelings by choosing not to be personally involved with their patients. I believe staying with a dying patient during and after the death event is one activity that nurses can, and in the main do, embrace—yet, not all dying in hospital is peaceful and Helen described her feelings of abandonment for the patient and herself after such an experience:

> The lady had died and everyone, that is, everyone except the nurses, of course, abandoned her. The lady had been left in a state of disarray, tubes everywhere, machines everywhere and she was lying naked and exposed. It was awful, it was like she was a lump of meat rather than a person really. I wanted to cover her up but the nurses wanted to do the laying out quickly. It was like we had to clear her away as quickly as the other staff had left, you know?

While dying in hospital may be the preferred option for many people, hospitalisation need not imply depersonalisation.

The literature reflects nurses' needs for support in caring for dying or dead people. Parkes (1985, p. 6) states 'no seriously ill person should be cared for in circumstances that do not allow the patient and the family to share their feelings with staff and staff to share their feelings with each other'. Three people in the study commented on the minimal communication with colleagues during and after the patient's dying. This lack of interaction contributed to their feelings of ineptitude and aloneness in the death event.

> So we went to our tutor sister, who said we could always come and see her if we had any problems. So we went and spoke to her, . . . you know, about how many people had died and how this was affecting us. This tutor sister said, 'Well, they're gone and dead. You can't do anything with them. Get on with the living.' It's only been in the last few years I've really realised just what a shitty thing that was to say to

anybody. It didn't address what was happening for us. It helped to bury what was happening. If we were being affected by it we were inadequate, was really what the message was as I received that.

In an environment where the emphasis is on caring for dying patients, the care of colleagues can be overlooked. This lack of thought for others in the caring relationship may be detrimental and counterproductive. From the discussion with these registered nurses, energy put into proactive measures to assist colleagues in a trusting and supportive environment would appear to counterbalance the negative energy associated with feeling stressed or burned-out. Active listening is a valuable tool in the nurse–patient interaction and could be easily transferred to the nurse-nurse relationship. The participants in this study who risked exposing their feelings to other staff members in a supportive environment found they were able to address their perceived lack of knowledge or fears of incompetence.

In performing the rituals after death, many of the participants spoke of their own distancing from the procedure. Most reported, in graphic detail, the archaic practices associated with early experiences. Some described their experience as ghoulish, 'not real' or distressing, resulting in a non-involvement reaction within themselves. '[They] just treated the body as if it was a shell and nothing else, as if it was just like a real, reality hit for me in the sense that, you know, it's over, forget about it, let's get rid of it.'

The negative aspects of the phenomenon of aloneness in nursing dying and dead people is largely the responsibility of all nurses engaged in this type of care. Aloneness is congruent with these nurses' feelings of retreating from involvement with the dying process, either from inexperience or as a result of pressure from others to remain detached. In part, aloneness can be overcome through the development of collegiate assistance and the establishment of a supportive environment.

## Questioning

Backer, Hannon & Russell (1994, p. 49) suggest 'the struggle to find a balance and harmony in the continuation of one's own personal and professional life while being involved with another person's exiting life can be difficult'. In this endeavour nurses consistently question the meaning of life and death, as well as their approaches to, and delivery of, nursing to dying or dead people. Questioning arises from our experiences and 'we make our experience a problem to be solved as we demand an explanation for our experience' (Maturana, 1992, p. 2). By constantly asking questions such as 'what is it that we do?', 'why do we do it?' and 'can we do it better?' nurses are re-searching their experience for explanations which inform the art and science of nursing. In this study, the participants referred to persistent self-exploration and investigation of their own practice and the practice of others.

Some described their naiveté regarding death in their early years of nursing. On the other hand, some newly registered nurses were clearly questioning their own attitudes and values about nursing dying or dead people. However, common to both neophytes and experienced nurses was a constant questioning which assisted them to be better practitioners. 'I find my situation leads me to question my values with regard to palliative care and to question the impact of my personal situation on the care I provide.'

Palmer (1994, p. 1) states: 'Today's nurses, more than at any other time, are faced with an increasing obligation to evaluate and improve their practice.' In accepting this responsibility, it could be argued that the participants in this study found questioning all aspects of their approaches to caring for dying and dead people valuable in assessing their own practice and the practice of others. Building on Schon's (1991) notions of reflection-in-action and reflection-on-action, I would argue that there is also a need for questioning-in-action and questioning-on-action. Both contribute to informing practice and ultimately to the discipline of nursing. Questioning-in-action could involve all members of the health care team in the situation of nursing a dying or dead person. Questioning-on-action can be done either in a team or as an individual, for example, while journalling the experience.

Several participants described how their experiences of nursing the dying person brought into question their personal perspectives about death.

> I suppose he must have stimulated something within me because he made me think about my own beliefs. I was very judgmental and wasn't looking at things from his point of view. You know, it often takes a personal experience to put things into perspective and make us take a closer look at why we do the things the way we do.

Benner and Wrubel (1989, p. 22) state 'suffering is part of the illness experience, a part of the human world of meaning'. In her story, Sarah discussed her thoughts on suffering and continually questioned its relationship to the death experience and in turn its impact on her quest to find meaning in death and dying:

> It's the suffering that I find the hardest thing to live with. I find it the hardest thing to cope with, with death in hospitals, because it's always there, whether it's the suffering on behalf of the person physically or the suffering on the family's behalf. But the suffering is always there. I don't find the actual death to be an issue for me. Sometimes it is a release.

Many participants noted how, as they gained more experience in nursing the dying, the level of involvement with each case increased. Helen describes how she began to question her practice in greater detail after having to deal with the relatives of a dying patient:

> When I finally graduated and became a registered nurse I would often have to deal with the relatives of a dying patient. This I found more difficult than anything else as it was not so easy to 'turn off' from the situation. People, the relatives, would often ask questions and I think that my answers were often inadequate. I began to feel uncomfortable, dissatisfied with my nursing towards the dying, the palliative patient.

These nurses continually questioned the ability of the healthcare system to answer their own personal and philosophical questions about death and dying—some clearly identified perceived inadequacies within the health care system. Only two participants spoke freely about their own practice and the contentious issue of euthanasia. Both of them appeared slightly uncomfortable in their descriptions, yet both were committed to the view that nurses do not question the ramifications for health care workers of active or passive euthanasia. They advised that it would be useful for all nurses to be fully aware of the sociopolitical and legal issues surrounding the current debate. 'You should be allowed to die pain free. If that means we have to provide large doses of morphine or whatever to provide that pain-free death, then so be it.'

Some nurses described how, as students, they had looked towards other, more senior registered nurses as role models, but felt that some senior staff were not able to provide adequate explanations of how to respond to, or cope with, death. A few spoke about their relationships with colleagues and new staff. They wondered what qualities they would need in order to facilitate a caring environment for these staff members— they did not want their own experiences repeated.

> We recently had a newly registered nurse on our ward who seemed quite, almost obsessed, with dying, with death. It was very difficult to know how to handle her or how to help her. I think with newcomers to death you have to try and evaluate where that person is at.

Many discussed the professional interactions they had with the dying patient and the personal costs that could arise as a consequence of involvement with that person or their family. Gloria questioned the level of involvement necessary to give good nursing care and pointed to some potential difficulties associated with over-involvement:

> I think there is still very much a hanging onto the person—nurses becoming attached to someone who is dying and don't realise just how much energy they are using to be attached to a patient. Sure, I think that caring is great but that attachment, I think, is really sort of dangerous and difficult to deal with afterwards, when that person's gone, when there isn't a lot of debriefing after a person's died.

Reflecting upon philosophies and questioning practices is important to the development of new knowledge and improvements in nursing care.

## Accepting

The essence of accepting can be construed as being in direct contrast to the essence of questioning. That is, the nurse may choose, for a variety of reasons, not to question a particular issue in the practice of nursing the dying or the dead. On the other hand, accepting can also be defined as an appreciation of the limitations that nurses have set on themselves in feeling comfortable with nursing dying or dead people. I am not postulating that accepting in this sense is in any way negative; rather, these limitations may well have arisen from constant questioning and evaluation of self in the domain of this particular nursing work.

Accepting is part of the nurse's role in the nurse–patient interaction. As communicators, nurses learn to accept the patient's point of view without necessarily agreeing with it. This type of acceptance does not preclude nurses engaging in their own internal questioning. On the contrary, in achieving an acceptance of self, the patient, and others, the nurse may have reached an understanding based on sound holistic principles.

Nursing dying or dead people encompasses certain ritualistic practices that could be perceived as an assault on a person's body. Prior to very recent changes in these practices, nurses were asked to pack every orifice of the dead body. In addition, it is customary to cleanse the body and remove any evidence of leakage of body fluids as nurses prepare the body for transfer to the mortuary or the funeral agency. Several participants described their embodiment of these processes—some feeling distressed or disturbed as they described this procedure.

> We don't pack orifices and I wouldn't like to have to do that. I would find that unpleasant, physically unpleasant. Even cleaning up bodily fluids is an unpleasant job, there's no two ways about it.

Death awareness for some of these registered nurses was underpinned by the influence of the moral and ethical considerations they had developed as a result of being exposed to certain religious teachings. Several participants talked about their religious convictions and accepted that their beliefs about death and dying were firmly linked to their faith. 'As a Christian, death should not be seen as a failure or as the end. It is one of the few certainties of life. It is natural to grieve for the passing of life.'

Nearly all the participants described aspects of their own development regarding becoming comfortable with death. 'Well, now I am more comfortable about death. It's been very gradual . . . I think I'd have to work from being with relatives, I think that's how I became to be comfortable with actual patients.'

Nurses often place themselves in a position of conflict. Choosing to work within a particular hospital could mean accepting policies that contradict their own belief system. Sometimes the individual may not have the energy required to institute changes to accommodate these beliefs, and compromise may be the only option. Sarah disclosed how, over time, she had come to accept the discrepancies within the healthcare system.

> In looking at the units I've worked in, the style of care which is unfortunately given, when I said to you that it becomes second best, I find that a real sadness and disappointment but it's inevitable. And in saying that, that's where my belief comes that they should have a specialty area. Management. Time. Under staffing. All those awful, awful realities for patient care, full stop. That just made me hate medical wards from the beginning. It became a factor of time that, like, I used to feel, like, for example, people who were dying, like, I used to feel horrendously . . . I can remember several cases where a patient would be in real need of counsel and my being unable to afford them the full amount of time . . . I had no other support in order to give me that time . . .

Working in a team necessitates accepting the limitations of individuals within that team as well as the limitations of the team as a whole. Many of the participants in this study alluded to an awareness of their own limitations and those of the institutions in which they work. I am not arguing for complacency, but rather for the need to develop an awareness of when we have reached our personal and professional boundaries, coupled with some undertaking to share this knowledge with others.

When a patient dies in an open ward setting, it is unrealistic to expect that the death will proceed unnoticed by other patients. Yet some nurses engage in the common, rather ritualistic, practice of talking in hushed tones behind closed screens as they prepare the dead body for transfer to the mortuary. Very few nurses engage in open discussion with other patients about the dead person. As nurses become more accepting of sharing their feelings of grief, they may become more comfortable with helping patients, their families, and colleagues experience their losses. Sarah spoke about her role in helping others to discharge their anxieties in the grief response.

> . . . and there had been, like, actually lashing the chests of the relatives and with the male nurse. It was sheer distress. That was really, I think that was actually the hardest one I've ever had to deal with because of the torrid emotion that was surrounding me. And they stayed with her until the body went cold, the family, they stayed with her. That was, that was two and a half hours. I can remember some of the nursing

staff saying, 'They can't do that, they can't stay here,' and I said, 'They have every right to.'

Accepting as a phenomenon in nursing dying or dead people is established through an evolutionary process of self-understanding and reflection on each experience. Accepting is also indicative of nurses' non-judgmental interaction with those people involved with the dying process. The phenomenon of accepting can be viewed as antithetical to that of questioning. However, in the context of the participants' stories, accepting could be linked to creating a climate of being non-judgmental in caring for dying or dead people. Being non-judgmental does not imply that challenges to problematic issues in caring for the dying are unacceptable. Being non-judgmental implies that a decision has already occurred within the challenger; there is a choice. By choosing the non-judgmental approach, accepting others' choices creates an environment of mutuality and trust. In this milieu, knowledge about a particular issue or event can be respected, shared and discussed and new knowledge potentially generated.

Nursing dying people will always be a part of the world of nursing and, as the incidence of terminal illnesses increases, death will have difficulty remaining in the confines and comfort of invisibility. Death awareness may well become antecedent in the carative practices of nurses. Given the personable nature of nurses' responses, further exploration and studies with those involved in end of life care are necessary, particularly within the community.

# References

Backer, B.A., Hannon, N.R., & Russell, N.A. (1994). *Death and dying: Understanding and care*, 2nd edn. Albany, NY: Delmar Publishers Inc.

Benner, P. (1984). *From novice to expert: Excellence and power in clinical nursing practice.* Menlo Park, CA: Addison-Wesley.

Benner, P. & Wrubel, J. (1989). *The primacy of caring, stress and coping in health and illness.* Menlo Park, CA: Addison-Wesley.

Maturana, H.R. (1992). Biology of self-consciousness. Unpublished monograph.

Palmer, A. (1994). Introduction. In Palmer, A., Burns S., & Bulman, C. (Eds.), *Reflective practice in nursing* (pp. 1–9). Oxford: Blackwell Scientific Publications.

Parkes, K. (1985). Stressful episodes reported by first-year student nurses: A descriptive account. *Social Science & Medicine, 20* (9), 945–953.

Penson, J. (1990). *Bereavement: A guide for nurses.* London: Chapman & Hall.

Rieman, D.J. (1986). The essential structure of a caring interaction: Doing phenomenology. In Munhall, P.J. & Oiler, C.J. (Eds.), *Nursing research: A qualitative perspective* (pp. 85–108). Connecticut: Prentice Hall.

Schon, D.A. (1991). *The reflective practitioner*, 2nd edn. London: Temple Smith.

Stein-Parbury, J. (1993). *Patient and person.* Melbourne: Churchill Livingstone.

Vohland, D.J. (1994). Dying in hospital: The lived experience of the bereaved. Unpublished Bachelor of Nursing (Honours) dissertation, School of Health, University of New England, Armidale.

Walters, A. (1992). The phenomenon of caring in an intensive care unit. Unpublished PhD thesis, Deakin University, Geelong.

Watson, J. (1987). Nursing on the caring edge: metaphorical vignettes. *Advances in Nursing Science*, October, 10–18.

# 11

# The Inevitability of Death: Some Personal Reflections

## Susan Sherson

There can be no reflective nurse who does not regard death with awe and wonder. From their first encounter and the amazement that comes with realising that a person can be 'of this world' one moment and gone from it the next, they progress through countless different and maturing experiences.

One quickly learns that death is not always kind. It does not always come as a friend in the night when we are old and enfeebled, but may take a child on the brink of life or an adult in their prime. It can be deeply distressing, even devastating, but no matter how we push back the frontiers of science and technology, it is inevitable.

Recently, and particularly in response to the euthanasia debate, there has been renewed consideration of some of the issues that surround the inevitability of death. Many of these have short- and long-term implications which need to be recognised and examined by health professionals, particularly those working with people with a terminal illness.

One morning, while in the middle of writing this chapter, I turned on the computer screen and read the following daily message: 'Health is merely the slowest possible rate at which one can die'. It reminded me of a resource allocation forum I attended at the University Hospitals of Cleveland in 1993. The speaker, a nurse on the hospital's Ethics Consult Team, told of hearing an English intensive care physician answer a question from an American colleague by saying, 'you American interventionists are the only people in the world who regard death as merely another option'.

These comments could be regarded as the extremes of a spectrum of outlooks on death. Where we, as individuals, fit in this spectrum and, in particular, the comfort or otherwise we feel in our position will have considerable implications for both our personal well-being as nurses and the well-being of those for whom we care.

Towards the end of 1995 I was asked to give a paper at a seminar and workshop held by the Victorian branch of the Renal Society of Australasia. The theme of the program was 'Management decisions in end stage renal disease: Whose choice?' and I was asked to address the subject 'Withdrawal from active treatment —When is enough enough?'

From the outset I was impressed by the inclusion of this topic in an area usually regarded as highly technical and pragmatic. Coupled with discussions held with a wide cross-section of nursing staff at a major metropolitan teaching hospital following the circulation of the College of Nur sing Australia's discussion paper, 'Euthanasia: An issue for nurses', it made me aware that nurses are now collectively and publicly, as well as individually and privately, questioning how current healthcare decisions affect the end of life and particularly how they affect the individual whose life it is. The view so strongly and repeatedly expressed in our hospital deliberations was that 'if we were better at managing withdrawal of treatment, perhaps this (euthanasia) would not be such an issue'. It seems to me that the extent to which nurses are willing to openly question and seek for answers in this field augurs well, both for our patients and for the future of our profession.

Since the beginning of the 1960s particularly, there have been spectacular advances in the research and use of biomedical technologies, and these developments have raised hopes, some real, some false, of previously undreamt therapeutic successes. Despite their apparently miraculous nature, these technologies have also brought problems and criticism. Without wishing here to enter this complex debate, medical scientific achievement has been criticised on the grounds of its dehumanising effects on its subjects and its seeming disregard for human dignity. What set out to further liberate the individual, by offering greater choices and thereby promoting human values and interests, has, in the eyes of some, achieved just the reverse. The freedoms that we sought, in certain situations, have not made us 'more free' but rather have seemed to further enslave, by tying us to technology itself.

Certainly few would argue that, since the mid-twentieth century at least, western society has become a death-defying society. I am not suggesting that it is not a perfectly reasonable and sane desire to want to live, rather than to die, in most human circumstances. Indeed, most of us expend considerable effort over our lifetimes, and sometimes in very challenging conditions, to continue living. That natural wish to live is not what I am reflecting upon now. It is the technology-driven, one last attempt to thwart death, clutched at by patient, family or staff, that our acute care hospital nurses were talking about in relation to euthanasia. Those of us within the healthcare professions, and in particular medical researchers, must accept some responsibility for this change in community expectations of what medical technology can offer in life-threatening conditions. We have been very ready to claim media and public attention for advances or apparent 'breakthroughs'. Nonetheless, the change in community expectations has been profound. Nurses today all too often witness the total disbelief—'you mean there's nothing you can do?'—of a patient or family who is told that there are no further treatment options available.

The one-sided, or some would say selective, picture the community has of health professionals' ability to defy death brings many problems. When I was at Stanford University Hospital in 1993, I was told of a market research project done in nearby Palo Alto to ascertain the general public's knowledge of survival following cardio pulmonary resuscitation (CPR). All respondents believed that as long as resuscitation was started quickly enough, it would be totally successful in terms of both mortality and morbidity. The intensive care physician who told me of this study also introduced me to the intensive care unit. One of the patients was a young diabetic man, comatosed from severe brain damage following a fall while hypoglycaemic. The physician related that when he had finished explaining at length the serious nature of the head injury to the young man's mother, including the possibility that he may never regain consciousness, her reply was: 'But look, he hasn't got his glasses on. He'll be better if I bring his glasses in and put them on.' Perhaps 'selective' is a good word for community knowledge, or lack of it. But again I think we must take some responsibility for this, both now and in the future.

My greatest concern with what has been termed 'the medicalisation of death', and the corresponding institutionalisation, is that it isolates the dying person from the people who have been the most important in her life—her family and other loved ones. We used to know this and, as a society, respect it. When a family member was dying at home, those closest drew around, shared the burden of care and gave comfort. Those not so close, including employers, allowed and acknowledged what was happening. This acceptance gave the process of dying a dignity we most often do not accord it today. Statistics published in the *Australian Medical Journal* in 1991 showed that, in a three-month period in 1988, an astonishing 48 per cent of deaths in our Victorian population happened within a public hospital. Counting nursing homes and private hospitals, 71 per cent of all deaths in that period occurred in hospital (Clifford, Jolley & Giles, 1991). This study followed one done earlier in South Australia (1981; 1985) which looked at where patients with cancer die. Of total cancer deaths, 77 per cent were in hospital or nursing home (Roder, Bonett & Hunt, 1987). The reasons for this are of course complex, but institutionalised death is not the norm in all societies. When I worked as part of a surgical team in South Vietnam during the war in that country, we quickly learned that it was very important both for the patient and their family that they should die at home. At first, family members or local nursing staff would ask, 'should the patient be taken home now?' Soon we knew to make the suggestion ourselves, taking into the account the often slow and hazardous journeys these dying people would have to make. In the Eastern Highlands of New Guinea too, I saw the Southern Fore people caring for their family member dying of kuru, at home, with great tenderness but not forcing food or drink or attempting to prolong the death they recognised at that point as inevitable.

This home care of the dying is in stark contrast to my experience of death as a student nurse. Although I looked after many memorable patients as a junior nurse in my first ward, perhaps the patient who stands out most clearly is the first patient I saw die. This probably is not an unusual thing for a nurse to say, but this particular scenario was very different. Good talker though I have always been, I did not exchange one word with this man. He was Russian and spoke no English. He had apparently been taken off his ship at Station Pier, Port Melbourne, when he became suddenly ill. I have no idea to this day what was wrong with him, but I did know right from the start that he was very sick because the senior staff looked after him and I only ever helped with a turn or a lift. He was a big man, very pale, in retrospect perhaps slightly jaundiced. I cannot remember anything medical being done for him. He did not go to theatre although the ward was a surgical one and, worst of all, no one ever came to see him. He was probably only in hospital five or six days, but he was in a bed near the centre of the ward and I felt his big silent eyes were following me wherever I went. There seemed to be some sort of plea in those eyes. And then he died. Just like that. No fuss or noise, he just closed his eyes and was dead. I found it difficult to comprehend, and to this day have not lost my sense of sadness and perhaps guilt that he died so alone, among strangers, in so unfamiliar a place. In that first ward, and since, I have seen many physically more agonising deaths, but the feeling of aloneness attached to this one is something quite apart.

Facing up to death is essential for those who work with it, especially those as close as nurses. For many years I worked in a position that included career orientation of prospective student nurses. I used to visit parts of the hospital with them to explain how a large teaching hospital actually worked and how nursing fitted into the pattern of its work. This was very much an interactive session and I was always pleased when one of the group asked a question that meant 'how do nurses cope when one of their patients dies?' Taking time to sit down I would talk about the support offered by other nurses around them, of the truth that each of us had experienced a first time and we had survived, of the fact that with some patients it was harder than others for all sorts of reasons. But I never hid from them the fact that, despite all the supports we hope are in place and will be there to cushion us, if we are to continue in bedside nursing, we must come to grips with death for ourselves. As the individual that is us. At age 17, most of us shy away from this. I know I did and I apologise to those patients I let down by my unwillingness to share their pain, especially one beautiful young woman I have never been able to forget whose vulnerability was more than I could bear.

It was a five-year-old girl who caught up with me eventually. Her name was Mary and I was nearing the end of the second year of my training and on night duty at the Royal Children's Hospital. Mary had terminal leuk-aemia and was often awake. One night she called me over and said: 'Why am I going to die, nurse?' It was two a.m. and there was nowhere to run. With considerable trepidation I perched, rather than sat, on the edge of her bed. I wanted desperately to touch her, to hold her, to take away the hurt, but I seemed totally incapable of doing any of these. She was usually a rather silent child, unnaturally so, pale, with watching eyes that seemed too large for her tiny face. Those eyes were fixed on me now and I could do nothing but meet their gaze. Heart in mouth I asked her what made her think she was dying. 'Daddy told me', was the reply. I cannot remember what I said after this, but I do know that I could not lie or even tell half truths to this sad, serious little person who died just a few days later. And I have certainly not forgotten my own fear and feeling of total inadequacy in the face of her questioning. With hindsight I owe much to Mary, and to her father who was brave enough and honest enough to tell her she was going to die.

A quite different experience, only a few years later, shows how far I had journeyed. In the surgical ward to which I had very recently been ap-pointed charge nurse, we received a 16-year-old boy with full thickness burns to 90 per cent of his body, the result of a go-kart accident at Calder Raceway. We knew from the start that these burns were incompatible with survival. Nonetheless, both nursing and medical staff cared for Greg with all the skill and experience available to them at the time. We also cared, as best we could in the constraints of a public hospital ward, for his parents. Greg was a much loved only child and we came to love him too in the brief six days he was with us. It was the mid-1960s and peritoneal dialysis a new therapy to Melbourne. When Greg's kidneys failed, the consultant surgeon who had brought the technique back from overseas was called in and personally commenced and oversaw the dialysis. He and I were together in the single room changing the abdominal cannula when Greg died. The surgeon did not seem to have noticed, so I touched his arm gently and said 'I think he has just died'. The reaction was immediate, 'What will I do? I've never been with anyone when they've died'. I tried to reassure him that it was all right and that we had all known that death was imminent and inevitable, but he remained agitated and distressed. When I told him that Greg's mother and father were sitting in the corridor outside waiting to come in and would have to be told, he replied he couldn't possibly cope with doing that. And it was quite obvious that he could not.

My heart went out to this dedicated man I hardly knew. He had given freely of his time, knowledge and skill in an attempt to save Greg's life. Now that this therapy had proved insufficient, he seemed to have no resources on which to call. He could respond to a technical need but not to a human one. In terms of experience and professional standing, there was a large gulf between us. For this short time, in the presence of a young boy's death, we were very close. Soon, as he slipped unseen from the ward via the back stairs, I went along the corridor to break the news to Greg's parents and seek to provide some comfort for them. We kept in touch for many years thereafter.

Dying alone, or indeed facing death without support, defies what Jennifer Fitzgerald has called 'the essential interconnectedness of life' (Fitzgerald, 1995). Our society seems to have an obsession with being individual and independent, rather than social and interdependent but, as palliative care philosophy and practice has clearly realised, it does not serve the dying patient or those around them well. Uncertainty concerning our individual ability to cope with death, or the as yet unknown process of dying, produces a powerful fear for both patient and those who are closest to them. And yet, how many who have made the journey to the moment of death with a loved one have subsequently reported spending some of their most precious moments with that person during that period. I was deeply moved by hearing Joan Hurley speak on radio of her experience of 'journeying through AIDS' with her daughter. She did not gloss over the painful times, the difficult times, the anger and anguish, but, three years after her beloved Caroline's death, she was able to say, 'I am absolutely convinced that Caroline was spared much more suffering as a result of the love, care and comfort of her friends and family' (Hurley, 1996, p. 171).

When I was in the Netherlands, I was interested to learn that, although there seems to be little distinction made by doctors between euthanasia and assisted suicide, the figures show that euthanasia is requested approximately 3.5 times more often than assisted suicide (Van der Wal, 1993). (Euthanasia, in Dutch protocols, occurs when the doctor personally administers the lethal drug, and assisted suicide when the doctor supplies the drug, either directly or by prescription, and the patient self-administers.)

These figures, I think, raise some very interesting questions and ones to which I can only postulate answers, as I have been unable to track down any specific research in the area. Accepting that the patient may fear, despite the drug being specifically prescribed by a doctor to bring about death, that the assisted suicide attempt may be unsuccessful or only partially successful (leaving the patient in a worse physical situation than before) the major issues are surely:

- a fear of dying alone; or

- an unwillingness to do so and take the full responsibility for ending one's own life; or

- an ambivalence about the whole question that is eased by sharing the responsibility with another.

Any of these would be a human enough reason for requesting euthanasia rather than assisted suicide but, having both observed and heard described the cost to the Dutch medical practitioner of performing euthanasia, I feel it needs to be explored much more deeply.

If an individual wants, and reasons it is right, to maintain full control over their life until the point of death, do they also have the right to involve another in bringing about that death—particularly when that other is a professional carer rather than someone with special moral status, such as a relative or very close friend? There is certainly no compulsion on any doctor in the Netherlands to perform euthanasia. The comparatively small number who do, do so willingly and because they see it, in certain cases, 'as the final act of palliative care', 'the least worst' way out in an attempt to achieve a harmonious process of dying (Kimsma, 1994). Interestingly, both the carer and cared for also speak of the need to get to know each other more personally and to 'grow together towards death'. Nonetheless, Dr Gerrit Kimsma also told a public meeting in Melbourne that if he had to perform euthanasia more than three times a year, he 'would give up the practice of medicine'.

Perhaps there is something more to this high personal cost to practitioner and active seeking of direct help by patient than we have yet been able, or willing, to clarify. I do not think it can all be explained by the legal uncertainties in Holland where, technically at least, the practitioner does still face the danger of prosecution. Nor do I think the professional distress is only that of any caring practitioner watching their patient suffer an anguished death. After all, most doctors do not say they will give up practice if more than three of their patients die difficult deaths annually. The act of bringing about death is more than all of this, for both doctor and patient, and more also, I believe, than can be explained by the longstanding taboo in most societies against killing. It deserves further reflection.

Certainly I have no doubt that the greatest positive contribution euthanasia, or the discussion of it, has brought to Australian society has been in making us—forcing us may not be too strong an expression—face again the issue of death; to re-accept that dying is an integral, indeed sometimes welcome, part of life.

How we achieve acceptance of death will, of course, vary enormously from individual to individual. It may come as a result of age or in response to illness. It may be sought as a means to escape something perceived as worse than death or as the result of feeling that there is nothing worth living for. In these latter cases, whether we are talking about a 15-year-old, 45-year-old or 75-year-old, it is crucial that we work with the person's ambivalences about both living and dying. It is a truism that individuals do not confide in others what they perceive those others are unwilling to hear. If we do not respond to a death wish, we are denying the extent of the pain. But we should also acknowledge and affirm the pull of life, where it exists even in the face of death. As a Dutch patient said in a videotape presentation on euthanasia, 'Knowing I don't have to worry how my end will be' (i.e. knowing that he will not have to suffer beyond his own personal ability to endure) 'has freed me to live' (Hanhart, 1993). In this man's case, his life had already extended almost three years beyond that originally forecast, years that had been fulfilling for him and his family. There is a very important message here. For, in the final analysis, life is about living and whether our life span is ten years and six months or 103 years and 11 months, we only learn about life through experiencing it. This will not change, however life itself changes in the decades to come. And living must always include dying.

Not all of us will find accepting our own imminent death easy. Some of us will require help, most of us will require support. Ian Gawler has said of his considerable experience with terminally ill people, 'those who live well, die well' (Gawler, 1986). He is not making a moral judgment, since many researchers in this area also report that individuals who feel fulfilled in their lives and who have been able to achieve at least some of their life goals are more ready to accept their death than those who feel they have been cheated by, or hardly done by in, life. This is true across age groups, socio-economic groups and frequently defies objective assessment of what might constitute 'a good life' for an individual.

In her book *I heard the owl call my name*, Margaret Craven tells the story of one individual's journey along the path towards death (Craven, 1974). A young Anglican priest in Canada is diagnosed with an unnamed terminal illness, his life expectancy is less than two years. For reasons not disclosed he is not told of this, but his bishop is and decides to send him to minister in an isolated Indian village in the wilderness of British Columbia. When asked why he is sending him so far away, the bishop answers that it is where he would want to go if he was young and in his place.

Leaving aside the qualms we may experience about such paternalism, what follows is a fascinating story of Mark Brian's coming to know the Kwakutul people, through sharing their unique culture, the many physical hardships of their life and the ongoing disintegration of tribal customs and beliefs as the young go off to school and western education. I won't reveal the ultimate climax, but a Kwakutul legend relates that before anyone in the village dies, they hear the native owl call their name. One evening, at the end of his second long hard winter, Mark is trudging up the muddy path to his small home when he hears the owl call his name and suddenly understands both what has gone before and what is to come. By this time however, he has learnt enough about life and living to be ready to die.

# References

Craven, Margaret. (1974). *I heard the owl call my name*. London: Picador.

Clifford, C.A., Jolley, D.J., & Giles, G.G. (1991). Where people die in Victoria. *Medical Journal of Australia, 155* (7), 7 October, 446–456.

Fitzgerald, Jennifer. (1995, March). When 'quality of life' becomes 'quality or life', it's time to challenge the concept. *Health Issues, 42,* 19–22.

Gawler, Ian. (1986). Personal communication.

Hanhart, Frank. (1993). Videotaped interview. *In An Appointment with Death*. Toronto, Canada: WGBH Educational Foundation.

Hurley, Joan. (1996). *How far is it to London Bridge?* Sydney: Millennium Books.

Kimsma, Gerrit. (1994). Personal communication.

Roder, D., Bonett, A., Hunt, R., & Beare, M. (1987). Where patients with cancer die in South Australia. *Medical Journal of Australia, 147* (1), 6 July, 11–13.

Van der Wal, G. (1993). Personal communication.

Van der Wal, G., Van Eijk, J., Leenen, H., & Spreeuwenberg, C. (1992). Euthanasia and assisted suicide. 1. How often is it practised by family doctors in the Netherlands? *Family Practice, 9* (2), 130–134.

# 12

## Clinical, Ethical and Legal Aspects of Palliative Care and Euthanasia

### Roger Hunt

Voluntary active euthanasia and physician-assisted suicide (which will be simply referred to as euthanasia) has become a hotly debated issue in Australian society, especially since the introduction of the Northern Territory's *Rights of the Terminally Ill Act* in 1996. This chapter explores the context for the flaring of debate and considers the major arguments. Clinical cases are used to illustrate some of the ethical and legal issues.

## The changing context for end-of-life decisions

In 1850, over 90 per cent of deaths in South Australia were of people less than 40 years of age (Hunt & Maddocks, 1997). Most of these were of infants and young children who died from infections, such as gastroenteritis, cholera, diphtheria, typhoid, measles, polio, tuberculosis. The introduction of public health legislation in the latter half of the nineteenth century, and improved general living conditions, led to better nutrition and sanitation which, in turn, led to less infectious premature death. Medical advances, such as the availability of antibiotics, improved surgical techniques, and the implementation of immunisation programs, had an additional benefit mainly after World War II.

The progressive elimination of premature death resulted in expansion and ageing of the population. People now live long enough for large numbers to be affected by the degenerative diseases of the aged. The average life expectancy in Australia is now about 75 years for males and over 80 years for females, and more than 90 per cent of deaths occur in people over 65 years. The leading cause of mortality in Australia is cancer, accounting for about 26 per cent of all deaths. The average age of people who die from cancer is about 70 years of age.

Death at the end of a natural life-span from degenerative causes has become the norm—it is expected and generally accepted as an occurrence not to be resisted at all cost. Old people tend to think more about death and fear it less than young people—the death of a young person, now being quite uncommon, is seen as an 'unwelcome stranger' and especially tragic. The type of care needed at the end of a natural life-span, particularly for an illness such as progressive cancer, is palliation and a good death. Technology-intensive intervention aimed at increasing survival is much less relevant.

During the twentieth century, however, terminal care was transferred from the community and family setting to the institutional domain. This meant that death became hidden from ordinary people, which contributed to the creation of a death-denying society, and hospital professionals who had no training in care of the dying set the management agenda. Until recent decades, terminally ill patients were often not informed of their diagnosis or prognosis, and were treated as if they would get better, or were neglected out of a sense of failure. Hospital routines eclipsed more humane concerns—for example, visiting hours were restricted and family involvement was quite limited.

The rights of terminally ill persons began to be recognised and addressed in the 1960s, a time when the rights of women, racial groups, and consumers also were being considered. A 'death awareness movement' emerged to highlight the inadequacies of existing attitudes and practices, and to encourage clinicians and health care administrators to improve the cost-effectiveness of terminal care. The hospice concept offered a tangible direction for the 'death awareness' movement, and a specific alternative to conventional hospital care. The availability of hospice care meant that no longer was it routine to simply keep dying patients alive 'at all cost' or to neglect their interests and wishes. Hospice care placed greater emphasis on the value of quality of life (relative to its quantity), and open communication about the patient's agenda than did the curative mode of care in the acute hospital.

Early initiatives in the United Kingdom and North America were mainly outside the mainstream of health care, but governments have taken increasing responsibility for funding designated terminal care services. In Australia, a period of rapid hospice development occurred between 1980 and 1995, and most Australians now have access to a dedicated palliative care service. A population-based study in South Australia showed nearly two in three cancer patients who died in 1993 had involvement with a hospice service (Hunt & McCaul, 1996). In 1995, 166 services were listed in the *Directory of hospice and palliative care services in Australia*. Palliative care topics have entered many undergraduate and postgraduate curricula, and as a result the quality of care provided by generic health carers has improved. The educational enterprise has been stimulated by the appointment of five chairs in palliative care, more per capita than anywhere else in the world. Specific texts and journals are readily available, and research is expanding in many areas of palliative care.

## Hospice rhetoric and euthanasia

The slogan 'kill the pain, not the patient' epitomises the hospice movement's polarised position against euthanasia. A number of factors have contributed to the adoption of this position. The early leaders of the hospice movement, such as Dr Cicely Saunders, Dr Balfour Mount and Dr Derek Doyle, espoused a strong Christian ideology for their work, and many of the early services relied on the support of religious organisations for funds—most hospices were named to honour saints. The hospice movement was thereby encouraged to align with church and right-to-life organisations against euthanasia.

The need for the principles of hospice care to be integrated into the mainstream culture of the healthcare industry would have been more difficult to achieve if the early leaders, in addition to confronting the taboos surrounding death, embraced the controversial concept of active euthanasia. However, the desire to promote the ideal of 'a comfortable death with dignity for all' led to the oversimplification of the problems experienced by patients and their families, and to inflated claims about the effectiveness of possible solutions. This no doubt helped to generate momentum for the formative movement, but it also gave the impression that all the problems associated with a terminal illness could be adequately dealt with, making euthanasia seem unnecessary.

Palliative care workers claimed requests for euthanasia were extremely rare, and usually revoked when palliation and loving care were provided (Pollard, 1994). A sustained request was considered simply to reflect inadequate palliative care. Additionally, palliative carers witnessed the potential for reconciliation and a kind of healing that could occur during the terminal phase of life, and believed this would be undermined if euthanasia was practised. Also, research and the funding of services could suffer if euthanasia became the usual solution to terminal care problems.

## The euthanasia movement

The increasing acceptance of euthanasia by Australians is revealed by responses to the Morgan Gallop Poll question: 'If a hopelessly ill patient, in great pain with absolutely no chance of recovering, asks for a lethal dose, so as not to wake again, should a doctor be allowed to give a lethal dose, or not?' In the 1960s, less that 50 per cent said 'yes'. This proportion increased steadily. Surveys in the 1990s showed that about 75 per cent of Australians thought voluntary euthanasia should be an option for a suffering terminally ill patient, with only 15 per cent opposed. Similar results are obtained if the phrase 'unbearable suffering' is used instead of 'in great pain'. The results of Australian polls are similar to polls from other developed countries including the USA and UK.

The increase in support for voluntary euthanasia has occurred at a time of rapid hospice development. This suggests that palliative care is not a simple solution to the issue of euthanasia, and that similar forces may be driving both the hospice and euthanasia movements. These forces probably include the ageing of the population, increasing numbers of deaths from cancer, disenchantment with medical efforts to keep dying patients alive when their quality of life is poor, concern for the rights of terminally ill persons, less professional paternalism and greater patient autonomy in end-of-life decision-making.

The emphasis that palliative care places on the quality (rather than the quantity) of the remaining life of the terminally ill patients, and their autonomy, is also central to arguments favouring the availability of voluntary euthanasia. More emphasis on quality of life, and a further shift from professional paternalism to patient autonomy, is required for the acceptance of voluntary euthanasia (table 12.1).

Social change toward less traditional religious authority and greater civil liberty may also have fuelled the debate about euthanasia. It is increasingly accepted that an individual should be free to make choices about his or her life without interference from the state or church, unless other people would be be adversely affected by a certain choice. Liberty, respect for autonomy, tolerance for diversity, and the taking of responsibility for the outcomes of a choice are necessary for civilisation to flourish.

Unlike the hospice movement, which rejected the concept of euthanasia, the euthanasia movement is fully in favour of palliative care. Euthanasia advocates believe that all terminally ill patients should have access to good palliative care, and that euthanasia should be an option for those who have considered or tried palliative care and found it to be inadequate in meeting their needs. The Northern Territory's euthanasia legislation

Table 12.1   Values placed on aspects of decision-making in three modes of terminal care

| | Mode of terminal care | | |
| *Decision-making aspect* | *Curative* | *Palliative* | *Voluntary euthanasia* |
| --- | --- | --- | --- |
| Medical prescriptiveness | +++ | ++ | + |
| Patient autonomy | + | ++ | +++ |
| Quantity of life | +++ | ++ | + |
| Quality of life | + | ++ | +++ |

+ = minimum value   ++ = moderate value   +++ = maximum value stipulates that the palliative care options must be explained to patients who request euthanasia.

## The limitations of palliative care

The argument that if terminally ill patients get good palliative care they won't want euthanasia is not supported by surveys. An English survey of relatives of over 4000 people who died showed that hospice patients were in fact *more* likely to have requested euthanasia (8 to 9%) than non-hospice patients (4%). Seale and Addington-Hall (1995, p. 581) conclude that hospice care helps patients

> express their fears and exercise choice. The wish for euthanasia may then be an assertion of personal control, rather than an act of surrender . . . If this interpretation is true it intensifies the moral debate about whether one should strive to make people who desire euthanasia change their minds, or whether one should accept their wishes.

A survey of patients' spontaneously expressed statements about the duration of their dying undertaken at Daw House Hospice, a teaching unit of the Flinders University of South Australia, revealed that 77 per cent made no comment about the duration of their dying, 11 per cent wished it would hurry up, 6 per cent asked a staff member if it could be hurried up, and a further 6 per cent made a consistent and persistent request for euthanasia (Hunt et al., 1995). Interestingly, this is similar to the 7 per cent of cancer patients who have euthanasia in the Netherlands (van der Maas, van Delden, Pijnenborg, & Looman, 1991). Taken together, these figures suggest the proportion of patients dying of a terminal malignancy who are serious candidates for euthanasia is likely to be between 5 and 10 per cent, and it seems unlikely that the provision of state-of-the-art palliative care will reduce this proportion.

It is unreasonable to believe that palliative techniques can relieve all suffering. Many common symptoms associated with advanced malignancy cannot be eliminated with palliative care. For example, progressive weakness and weight loss are common, and usually cannot be reversed. Because weakness leads to a loss of function, dependence, and frequently to a loss of dignity and a diminished quality of life, it can be a reason for a patient to request euthanasia. Other symptoms, such as anorexia, difficulty breathing, nausea and vomiting, cough and confusion may be difficult or impossible to ameliorate completely. Pain can be better managed than most other symptoms and is the sole reason for a request for euthanasia in only about 5 per cent of requests (van der Maas et al., 1991).

In addition to the physical dimension, a range of psychological, social and spiritual problems arise in association with terminal illness, and cause immense suffering. Hospice advocates claim to address these aspects of suffering, but there is a paucity of systematic study to show the extent to which these problems can be relieved with various interventions. It is clear that many patients experience substantial suffering, despite the best palliative care efforts, and this sustains calls for the availability of euthanasia as an option for terminally ill patients.

## The principle of double effect

For intractable pain and suffering, the palliative repertoire of many practitioners includes resort to high doses of analgesics and sedatives to induce a state of pharmacological oblivion. This type of intervention may blot out the suffering, but it can also hasten death. It renders the patient bedbound, unable to eat and drink, to have a depressed cough reflex, and to be prone to pneumonia and other complications.

This practice is legislated under the South Australian *Consent to Medical Treatment and Palliative Care Act, 1995* which states there is no criminal or civil liability for administering a treatment with the *intention* of relieving pain or distress, even though an effect of the treatment is to hasten death, provided the treatment is with the consent of the patient, in good faith, and to appropriate standards of palliative care. This Act codifies the principle of double effect which is widely accepted by clinicians and religious groups, including the Vatican: the treatment can be justified if the primary or intended effect is the relief of suffering, and the hastening of death is regarded as an unintended or secondary effect.

However, a law based on intention can lead to ludicrous consequences. It is possible for a palliative care practitioner administering pharmacological oblivion to state that the intention is purely to relieve suffering, and he/she will receive praise. A second practitioner could state that part of the intention is to hasten the dying process in accordance with the patient's wishes, and this second practitioner could be prosecuted for murder! Two radically different outcomes for the two practitioners administering the same treatment to the same patient simply because of the different statements of intention. In this sense the law is prescribing how clinicians express what they intended to do.

Is it possible to morally distinguish between a) life-shortening palliative care and b) euthanasia?

The clinician's intention in relation to the timing of death is relevant to the morality of an act, but it is not, I believe, of absolute importance, and a number of other factors are relevant. First, the underlying motive with both a) and b) can be one of compassion. This is clearly different to the usual context of murder where the motive is sinister and the victim is violently and involuntarily killed. Some euthanasia antagonists claim that euthanasia is just another name for homicide—by ignoring the aspect of consent and the humane, indeed loving nature of euthanasia, they fall into a trap whereby they could also regard making love as just another form of rape, and a surgical incision as just another name for assault by stabbing.

Second, the hastening of death is an outcome of both practices, only it is slower with a) than with b). This suggests they differ by degree, rather than being morally distinct entities. Third, to regard a hastened death as 'secondary' and 'unintended', as the principle of double effect encourages us to do, denies that the hastening of dying may be desired by the patient and perhaps others. Furthermore, we should not downplay any serious outcome of the treatment—it is proper in clinical practice to take responsibility for a foreseen outcome of treatment, such as a hastened death, and wherever possible to discuss this with the patient and/or relevant carers prior to starting the treatment.

The principle of double effect, rather than being a valid moral principle in making life-death decisions, is a *psychological construct* which enables clinicians to palliate suffering with treatments which can hasten the demise of the patient, while at the same time áppearing to guard the sanctity of life. The more fundamental moral questions relate to the sanctity of life principle, and whether respect for the wishes of patients who are suffering and dying can justify overriding the sanctity of life principle. These will be adressed in a later section.

## Ethical questions raised by a case-study

At the age of 63, after 14 years in parliament, Gordon Bruce retired as President of the Legislative Council at the South Australian election in December 1993. He bought a campervan and looked forward to a pleasant retirement travelling with his wife, Olive. But just a few months later, in March 1994, he was diagnosed with motor neurone disease. There is no known cure for this disease which destroys the nerves which work muscles, causing progressive weakness and inevitable death.

Gordon first found he couldn't do up the buttons of his shirt with his right hand. Weakness progressively affected his legs, arms, neck (for which he was given an Oxford collar), breathing, ocular accommodation, and subsequently swallowing and speech. He was admitted to hospital because of an inability to sleep due to breathlessness and investigations showed profound diaphragm weakness, particularly in the recumbent position. Treatment with a nasal ventilator, which assists with both inspiration and expiration, enabled him to sleep well. As the disease progressed he used the ventilator for longer periods during the day, until he was using it almost continuously. The district nurse assisted with showering as his mobility and independence decreased. A domiciliary physiotherapist provided equipment and chest physiotherapy.

When I met Gordon, he made it clear he did not want his life prolonged by invasive measures such as pertracheostomy ventilation and percutaneous enterogastrostomy feeding. He wished he had a pill to carry around in his pocket so that when his life became too burdensome and difficult he could simply swallow the pill to end it all (Gordon enjoyed the humour in receiving a Christmas gift from a family member of a small box containing a peppermint which looked like a large pill). Gordon was concerned that he would be left to suffer at the end of his life, and received great comfort from my assurances that if and when his distress became overwhelmingly intolerable, I would endeavour to make him comfortable with an infusion of opioid and sedative. He was not concerned that such a treatment could shorten the duration of his life.

Gordon's photograph appeared in the *Advertiser* newspaper (Saturday, 29 October 1994) and the article quoted, 'When I am ready to go, I want to die; I do not want doctors to prolong it and save me'. He believed that eventually society would allow euthanasia. He also wrote an open letter to his former parliamentary colleagues and gave it to the local euthanasia society to use as it saw fit.

In early 1995, on my return from leave, I was told that Gordon was desperate to see me. He still had audible speech and said 'I'm past the limit of my endurance'. His breathing was extremely difficult, he was troubled by and inability to clear mucous and saliva, and had lost nearly all mobility. He said he wanted the infusion I offered as soon as possible. Gordon's wife and daughter had over recent months changed their thinking, and now believed that relief was warranted even if this involved shortening his life. I issued orders for the infusion to begin. Gordon wished to stay at home and Olive agreed with this.

I wanted to titrate the infusion of morphine and midazolam upward until the desired effect of relief and peaceful sleep was achieved. The daily doses escalated over five days, from 10 mg of morphine to 30 mg, and from 10 mg of midazolam to 60 mg. However, the desired effect was not achieved. Gordon was not sleeping well and he became quite agitated and restless at times, probably due to hypoxia. When I visited on 10 January, Gordon was restless, cyanosed and unable to communicate effectively. His wife and daughter were present—they were distressed by Gordon's distress and they felt that sedation to induce sleep was appropriate.

I gave 5 mg of midazolam intravenously which induced a peaceful sleep. But when we removed the ventilator Gordon became more cyanosed and again started to become restless. I administered a further 5 mg of midazolam with 10 mg of morphine intravenously. Following this, his colour worsened, respirations slowed, and pulse weakened. He slowly and peacefully died with his wife holding one hand, his daughter the other. They were tearful and expressed appreciation that Gordon's struggle was over, and that he died the way he wanted—'by going to sleep, rather than choking in the night'.

This case highlights three important points. First, if I were to say my intention was simply to withdraw a futile, burdensome treatment and to administer palliative medications, then officials of the church, legal and medical professions would say 'well done, you have provided appropriate, ethical medical care'. But if I said that my actions were intended to bring about Gordon's death, then I could be prosecuted for murder. Thus, I am pressured to express myself in a certain way, and perhaps to be less than honest.

Second, it may have been kinder to have left Gordon on the ventilator and to have administered a lethal injection—this would have avoided the episodes of hypoxia and agitation. The law that makes the kinder act a crime is a law that is unjust and lacking in compassion.

Third, people like Gordon can have a life-sustaining treatment removed to bring about their death, but other terminally ill people who are not receiving a life-sustaining treatment cannot have their death brought about by the withdrawal of such a treatment and are forced to live on. This constitutes a form of discrimination—some patients can have their death legally brought about as a result of a treatment decision, but others cannot get such help.

# What about utilitarian arguments against euthanasia?

Perhaps the most frequently presented argument against the legalisation of euthanasia is a utilitarian one which states that the wishes and interests of a patient who genuinely requests euthanasia must be sacrificed in order to protect the common good. This assumes that granting a person's request will inevitably lead to abuses involving other individuals and would undermine the fabric of society. This argument is often put in fear-mongering terms—that doctors will develop a lust for killing, or will conspire with governments to prey on the weak and vulnerable members of society who will be involuntarily killed. The Nazi holocaust is frequently cited in this regard, and data from the Netherlands is dubiously manipulated and used to support this position. A similar kind of argument has been put by governments that prohibit the medical prescription of opioids for cancer pain in order to prevent the widespread abuse of drugs.

However, doctors will not develop a lust for killing: they have a natural aversion to practising euthanasia, and many will opt never to be directly involved. Doctors see euthanasia only as a last resort, to be considered only after the range of palliative options has been properly tried or considered, and only when convinced it accords with the patient's wishes and interests. It is the determined and articulate patient who can 'twist the arm' of the doctor, rather than the weak and vulnerable patient, who is more likely to get his or her request met. It is certainly not clear that the harm caused by possible abuses outweighs the harm incurred by denying a terminal patient the option of euthanasia.

The moral problem with the utilitarian argument is that, whereas the suffering and the wishes of the person requesting euthanasia are very immediate and real, the claimed benefit is merely an assumed or potential benefit to as yet unknown individuals. The utilitarian approach is unjust because it treats patients who request euthanasia *not* as 'ends' in their own right, but rather as the 'means' to a presumed benefit of imagined persons. A traditional obligation in the duty of care is to treat each and every patient as an 'end', as an unique individual, and to strive to do the best for each patient. In palliative care, we must listen to each of our patients and not turn our attention away from their agenda and what is important for the satisfaction of their needs and interests.

# Is it proper for us to make decisions that affect the time of death?

Making decisions that affect the time of death is a part of the human condition. Such decisions are made at the public policy level (e.g. public health decisions, road safety, war), in medicine (e.g. surgery, prescribing medication, withholding and withdrawing life-sustaining treatments), and at the level of decisions about individual lifestyle (diet, exercise, smoking). These types of decisions are unavoidable and clearly not exclusive to God.

Given that life in itself is good, as a general rule we should act to preserve and prolong life. However, very few people adopt an absolute position on the sanctity of life. Exceptions include self-defence, martyrdom, capital punishment, war, and abortion. Right-to-life groups protest about the morality of terminations and draw analogies with euthanasia, but the two situations are morally different because the life being taken in termination of pregnancy has no say in the decision; fetal life is at the very start, as opposed to the end the life-cycle, and the fetus not necessarily experiencing suffering.

It is wrong to use medical methods to sustain a life of poor quality against the wishes of its bearer because this promotes suffering, undermines the autonomy of the individual, and wastes resources which then cannot be used for others. Most people with a terminal illness will want to keep on living as long as their quality of life is reasonable, and they will accept progressive declines in their functioning and quality of life. But some patients reach a point where further declines in quality of life, with no prospect of effective relief from progressive suffering, make life intolerable and they request help in bringing forward the time of their death. Life-shortening decisions are difficult to make, but they will inevitably be taken. In some situations, a decision to shorten life may the lesser of two evils, and may be 'right' for an individual.

## Is the law a lame duck?

Surveys of doctors indicate that despite the risk of serious criminal charges, euthanasia is being practised in Australia. Yet there have been no prosecutions of doctors. In Victoria, seven doctors stated in an open letter to the premier that they had performed euthanasia and challenged him to either change the law or to prosecute them—neither has occurred to date. The discretion of doctors and families involved in euthanasia, and the commonsense of prosecutors, seems to prevail. Nevertheless, the current situation tends to undermine respect for the law.

The current law in most jurisdictions is crude in that it does not adequately distinguish euthanasia from homicide. It lacks compassion, it is forcing doctors and nurses to be less than honest in stating their intentions about treatment, and it is unjust in not serving the interests and wishes of dying patients.

Only the most assertive, articulate and resourceful patients are likely to be able to enlist the help of a doctor in such an illegal act, which discriminates against the weaker, more vulnerable patients. Euthanasia is more possible for people who have the resources to receive terminal care in the privacy of their own home, rather than in an institutionalised setting where euthanasia practices are precluded.

Law reform would be advantageous because it would bring into the open a practice that is covert and secret. A more open approach would facilitate research and enable the development of professional guidelines to ensure proper standards of euthanasia. Many people would be reassured that they could get the help they wanted if they were dying and experiencing severe suffering. Legalisation would improve access and equity in the provision of euthanasia. Rather than acting alone, doctors would be able to seek the advice of their colleagues and be supported in the decision-making process.

However, problems are likely to accompany law reform. Some patients may fear being admitted to a facility where euthanasia is known to be practised, even though they may benefit from care there, for fear of involuntary euthanasia. The scare-mongering campaigns of euthanasia antagonists inflames this fear. Bureaucratisation is something that many doctors would rather avoid, and in the Netherlands the non-reporting of euthanasia is regarded as a problem. Also, legislation for competent patients with terminal illness does not address the problem of incompetent patients in a vegetative state (e.g. following a stroke) or those people suffering from Alzheimer's disease who had previously wished not to live under such conditions, or patients who are depressed and wish to die.

Such scenarios ensure that debate about the limits of euthanasia will continue, whatever legislative framework is introduced, and clinical challenges and dilemmas will continue to arise.

## Conclusion

The topics of terminal care, euthanasia, and death are no longer taboo, and the ageing Australian society can no longer be called death-denying. As the 'baby boom' generation enters old age, the focus on these areas is likely to intensify. The ethical and legal focus in the euthanasia debate has tended to be on the intention of the professional carers in relation to the timing of death, but deliberate decisions which can bring forward the time of death cannot be avoided. A better focus would be to ensure as far as possible that the wishes and interests of each and every patient are being met. After all, the professional carer's role is to serve the patient, rather than the patient being there simply for the good intentions of the carer.

A palliative care specialist, with an informed and wide-ranging experience in terminal illness, should be consulted to assess the nature of a request for euthanasia, whether it is congruent with the patient's character and situation or related to depression, and to ascertain if suffering could be alleviated with palliative treatments acceptable to the patient. Professional guidelines for dealing with euthanasia requests should be developed to ensure that the wishes and interests of the patient and family are best served.

## References

Hunt, R.W., Maddocks, I., Roach, D., & McLeod, A. (1995). The incidence of requests for a quicker terminal course. *Palliative Medicine, 2,* 81–82.

Hunt, R. & McCaul, K. (1996). A population-based study of the coverage of cancer patients by hospice services. *Palliative Medicine, 10,* 5–12.

Hunt, R. & Maddocks, I. (in press). Terminal care in South Australia: Historical aspects and equity issues. In Clark et al. (eds.), New themes in palliative care. Buckingham: Open University Press.

Pollard, B. (1994). *The challenge of euthanasia.* Sydney: Little Hills Press.

Seale, C. & Addington-Hall, J. (1995). Euthanasia: the role of good care. *Social Science & Medicine, 40* (5), 581–587.

van der Maas, P., van Delden, J., Pijnenborg, L., & Looman, C. (1991). Euthanasia and other medical decisions concerning the end of life. *Lancet, 338,* 669–674.

# 13

## Palliative Care within the Euthanasia Debate

### Margaret O'Connor and Marguerite Menon

During the first six months of 1995 the daily debate in the Australian newspapers about euthanasia as a result of the 'right to die' bill in the Northern Territory became significantly polarised and acrimonious (Brown & Pinkney, 1995; Buchanan, 1995; Davies, 1995a, 1995b; Gawler, 1995; Oderberg, 1995; O'Sullivan, 1995; Singer, 1995; Uren, 1995; Woodruff, 1995). The replication of the Kuhse and Singer (1992) study of euthanasia attitudes among Victorian nurses was presented and discussed among palliative care nurses (Aranda & O'Connor, 1995). The Royal College of Nursing Australia published a discussion paper on euthanasia intended to stimulate debate and increase knowledge about the issue among nurses (Hamilton, 1995).

Much of what appears in the popular media about euthanasia is biased towards the sensational and the extreme. A cursory examination of the press would lead most to think that people frequently die alone and unsupported in extremes of pain and suffering (AAP, 1995; Perron, 1995; Allingham, 1995; Kelly, 1995). Attempts by nurses to redress this with more balanced reporting have been generally unsuccessful because the media seem largely uninterested in the ordinary day-to-day stories of caring for loved ones in their final days. Nurses' views are mostly ignored by the press and television.

The legalisation of euthanasia in the Northern Territory (1995) catapulted Australia into addressing this issue 'ready or not'. The Australian community generally seems ill-equipped to deal with the implications of such legislation, often deriving their attitudes to euthanasia from heartrending TV stories and the popular press. Of particular concern is the overuse of the extreme example drawn from the individual 'worst case' scenario to argue for a change in the law (Alcorn, 1996). The consequence is a vehement demand for the 'right to die' based on the needs of a single individual with an argument that the law must change for everyone.

Against this background of daily discussion in the papers, on radio and on television, a series of four focus groups were held in Melbourne to identify and clarify palliative care nurses' perspectives and meanings about euthanasia (Menon, 1996). Qualitative data gathered consisted of dense descriptive explanations clarified by anecdotal practitioner experiences detailing the contextually located perspectives of euthanasia.

These palliative care nurses voiced strong views that the euthanasia debate was: confused as to the practical realities of euthanasia; simplistic in scope; based on an emotive view of suffering without real knowledge of dying people's needs; ignorant of the real experiences and treatment of dying people; and disrespectful of dying people's rights for comfort and simple human caring.

In this and previous studies (Aranda & O'Connor, 1995; McInerney & Seibold, 1995), nurses qualified their responses to questions about euthanasia in a contextual manner, telling stories and anecdotes about their experiences, rather than simply commenting or providing an opinion either for or against euthanasia. Responses were not in simple black and white terms; rather they depended on the circumstances of the family situation, the stage of the illness and the manner of the discussion surrounding the request. This chapter explores some of the issues nurses raised that contribute to the overall debate on euthanasia.

# What constitutes euthanasia?

Research and media reports suggest that there is confusion within the healthcare professions about what constitutes an act of euthanasia (Aranda & O'Connor, 1995; McInerney & Seibold, 1995; Menon, 1996) reflecting the recognised confusion that exists at all levels of society. This confusion is in part due to the terms used to define an act of euthanasia.

## *Definitional issues*

Nurses in both the Menon (1996) and Aranda and O'Connor (1995) studies identified the confusion that exists in definitions of euthanasia. The terms 'active', 'passive', 'voluntary' and 'involuntary' were perceived as misleading the debate and leading to confusion of the withdrawal of medical treatment with the deliberate ending of a person's life. The question to ask, therefore, is whether discussion of legislation to allow euthanasia is appropriately conducted within a situation of confused understandings.

Palliative care nurses identify euthanasia as a deliberate act to cause the death of a dying person on the grounds of compassion. 'Euthanasia is the deliberate action by a physician (or another individual) to kill a patient at the patient's request' (Coyle, 1992, p. 42). The cessation of medical treatment is not euthanasia; turning off life-sustaining treatment is not euthanasia, and respecting a person's wishes to refuse active medical treatment is not euthanasia. Instead, the dying person's desire to legally refuse treatment, together with a focus on relief of distressing symptoms, is good palliative care. Palliative care is directed towards relieving the symptoms of suffering in order to maximise the quality of life and living when a person is dying.

The term 'passive euthanasia' is misleading since it implies that refusal to continue with 'active' medical treatment is tantamount to euthanasia. This confusion is perhaps related to the portrayal of euthanasia as a 'good death' or 'dying with dignity', when palliative care is defined and thought of in similar terms. Nurses regard the clarification of these terms as crucial to upholding the rights of the terminally ill to refuse burdensome treatments and to be better provided with palliative care services.

## Intention

Relieving suffering created by pain is seen by palliative care nurses as good care. Symptom control is clearly aimed at providing a pain-free existence. The intention of comfort is the crucial motivation. Where the intention is comfort and pain relief, that is good palliative care even if the levels of analgesics provided may inadvertently shorten life. Palliative care motivated by the intention to provide relief of symptoms should never be confused with or equated to actions taken to deliberately end a life.

The argument that the end point for all these patients is death and consequently the actions in both cases are a form of euthanasia regardless of motivation (consequentialism) denies the reality of palliative care practice. This reasoning inevitably leads proponents to say that euthanasia is just a clarification of what is already happening and therefore it should be legalised. This argument undervalues palliative care, and nurses who work with the dying regard it as fallacious. They point out that in the Netherlands where euthanasia has been supported by this reasoning, there is a disgraceful lack of adequate palliative care available for terminally ill people who are therefore unable to gain effective relief of their pain and suffering.

Nurses should be very clear about their motivations when giving large doses of analgesia to relieve extreme pain for terminally ill people. A simple check may be employed to establish intention. If the end result has not been achieved by the administration of the drug, what does the practitioner do? If the intention was to end the person's life and they have not died, then the action would be to continue administration of the drug until the death has occurred. If, however, the intention was to relieve the pain, the drug would be administered only until this goal has been achieved.

# Why people request euthanasia
## *Suffering*

Nurses feel that most requests for euthanasia occur in situations of inadequate alleviation of suffering. An holistic understanding of the complexity of suffering must involve a range of health professionals from different disciplines. Because the experience of suffering is so subjective, one needs to be open to hearing the individual's experience and be able to respond appropriately. Suffering will not always involve physical pain; indeed, alleviation of the spiritual and psychological suffering at the end of life is often most difficult. In fact many nurses feel that the circumstances and medical history of each dying person is so complex that it is difficult to accept simplistic debates about euthanasia (Menon, 1996; Aranda & O'Connor, 1995).

The cry for euthanasia seems to come often from fear of dying, fear of the unknown, fear of loss of control and fear of helplessness (Saunders, 1992). People are demanding to be cared for at home more and more. Suffering is seen in a much more positive light when people find meaning in their lives and quality of living in their relationships.

Coyle (1992) notes the importance of the subjective context for nurses, pointing out that it is the nurse who must cope with the patient whose symptoms are out of control, and with the family's distress (p. 45). In seeking to promote the best quality of life for the patient, this can only

> be ascertained by the individual and communicated by the individual concerned and may be fluid in nature, being influenced by physical, psychological and spiritual factors (p. 42).

## *Depression*

Depression too plays a part in decision-making at the end of life. Research (Chochinov, Wilson, & Enns, 1995; Hooper, Vaughan, Tennant, & Perz, 1996) into the mental state of those who seek an active end to life found that depression influenced these requests in a majority of cases. Depression is a normal reaction and an expected state of mind when a person is facing the end of life, particularly if the end is earlier than expected by the individual; much hinges on the treatment and supports provided for a person in such a vulnerable mental state. Perhaps because of the acceptance of the 'normality' of depressive states in terminal illness, diagnosis and treatment are less actively sought. Some studies report that non-psychiatrically trained personnel miss diagnosing up to half of those people with a medical illness who present with a major depression (Nielson & Williams, 1980; Clarke & Smith, 1995). In palliative care, the link between depression and requests to die is only recently being given credence within the multidisciplinary team.

## Uncontrolled symptoms

Palliative care nurses identify that some people ask for help to die when they are distressed because: they fear death; fear severe pain; fear extreme unrelieved vomiting, diarrhoea, dyspnoea, depression and so on; and feel they cannot cope any longer with such a burden of suffering. These nurses have evidence derived from personal practice experience that people who have relief of these distressing symptoms and who feel effectively supported became involved in living their lives again and no longer request assistance to end their lives (Menon, 1996).

People who think their brain is likely to be affected fear the loss of the mental capacity to be a rational human being, fear losing their personal dignity, fear being a burden on the family, fear being unable to cope with pain, and fear dying without support. The fear that living will be an unbearable burden on others contributes to the desire to 'end it all'. People hate being helpless, dependent and lacking in dignity. Palliative care nurses identify that these people, despite the fears, still do not want to die. When the symptoms causing fear, loss of control and the unbearable suffering are alleviated, often so is the desire to seek suicide and death. Nurses know that palliative care can make this difference for people (Menon, 1996).

The elderly dependent patient in a nursing home is in a totally different situation to the one dying with terminal cancer in a hospice. But this is the kind of patient of whom some say: 'Poor old dear. She just sits there with no quality of life. We should put them out of their misery' (Kennett, 1995). The reality is, however, that very few wish to end their existence and cling to the spark of life they have. Few people in the general population seem to realise that the Northern Territory euthanasia legislation excluded these dependent older people who require full-time care. Nurses have expressed a concern that the debate about euthanasia could very easily shift from people with a terminally ill condition to those who are simply old and frail, have debilitating depressions, require full-time health care, or simply have a miserable existence in the eyes of those who are concerned about the costs associated with their care, or even those who hate to see a loved one suffer. Families may request euthanasia to lessen their own suffering.

Many ill-informed health professionals and people in the community mistakenly think that high doses of narcotics of themselves will kill people. Palliative care nurses have seen that giving high doses of morphine can support a quality of life that enables people to live their lives as effectively as possible. Outside the practice of palliative care, these nurses feel there is little understanding of the effective use and dosage of morphine required to adequately relieve distressing symptoms such as pain or dyspnoea in patients with advanced cancer. Relief of symptoms is the aim in palliation and a balance between the relief of suffering and the complications of high dose medication needs to be achieved. People do not die of large doses of narcotics properly titrated to relieve pain, but this does not appear to be common knowledge. Many health professionals, including nurses and medical practitioners who did not have the constant experience of symptom management for terminal patients, have misconceptions also (Aranda & O'Connor, 1995). An understanding of the complex pharmacology of morphine and of narcotic tolerance when it is used for pain relief is crucial to providing effective analgesia in advanced cancer.

## A death-denying society

Nurses see the dilemmas faced by health professionals as reflective of the death-denying attitude held in our society. If death is regarded as a medical defeat rather than a natural conclusion to a life lived, those who care for the dying will receive little peer support, and perhaps develop a skewed view of their work as being inferior. Nurses recognise the need for education of health professionals and the general community to clarify what is euthanasia and what is palliative care.

Palliative care appears to be one of those areas of work that the community really does not want to know about until it is needed, and thus community views about death and dying are distorted. The community desires to be reassured in some covert way that someone, somewhere, is supporting the dying, but does not want to know the details. Thus hospice workers are expected to carry a burden of silent and undervalued care on behalf of the community.

> We leave it to the workers at the coal face to deal with the myriad of possibilities for life and death as best they can. Health care workers therefore get little guidance from the community they serve. The community to a great extent leaves the health care professional to deal with what is put into the too hard basket. (Morieson, 1993, p. 31)

With the community's implicit collusion with medicine's reliance on increasing technological possibilities at the end of life and the consequent acceptance that death occurs in hospital surrounded by professionals, heroic intervention and machines, families are disempowered in the roles they could provide to support the death of a loved one in a more domestic setting. Death is a natural part of the human life-cycle, and as much as possible ought to be returned to its rightful place within the family unit and the community of supporting friends. However, our community needs assistance from knowledgeable health professionals to manage such care effectively.

# What does palliative care offer?

Palliative care involves an overt shift of power over care from professionals to the sick person and the family, enabling the transfer of decision-making about the directions of medical treatment. This transfer may not be popular with everyone in our community, since people may not have confidence in their skills to manage death in the home setting. They often feel the burden of social taboos about death strongly and prefer not to expose their difficulties and vulnerability to neighbours.

Caregiving, once a normal family task at home, has become a professional career. Palliative care seeks to return home caregiving options to those who wish to participate in the care of family and friends. Palliative care is a complex intimate sharing of physical, emotional and spiritual experiences and meanings derived from the mystery and uncertainties of dying and death.

Palliative care nurses report that decisions about treatment interventions for dying people are too often based on having the medical capacity to provide them. Such treatments have been applied without adequate consideration given to: the real desires of the patient and their family; the effectiveness of the real life outcomes for the patient during or after the intervention; and/or an inadequate exploration of alternative treatments available. Palliative care nurses believe that they need to speak up on behalf of dying people to advocate for good palliative medicine, and to request the cessation of treatments that create an intolerable burden of suffering.

> In a climate where the pressure to produce seemingly overrules the duty to care, the increasing isolation of the sick and elderly in many ways and the frequently indifferent or negative attitudes towards the increasing numbers of elderly—I wonder whether euthanasia would remain voluntary for long . . . I have concern that any legalised 'right to die' may translate for many vulnerable people as a subtle 'duty to die'. (O'Connor, 1993)

Expert care of the dying has become the domain of the medical specialist and anecdotes appear in the media telling of unnecessary sufferings of people denied access to the desired specialist care.

> It is a bitter paradox that euthanasia is being promoted, primarily because of poor medical care, at a time when we know better than ever before, how to care well for the dying. The medical profession has in its hands the best social answer to the call for euthanasia. It is at once the partial cause of the problem and the best hope for the effective remedy. (Pollard, 1989, p. 132)

Arguably, the palliative care approach to symptom management for the outcomes of the best quality of life is well within the general expertise of any health professional. When working with dying people who have severe pain, however, experience is recognised as essential for effective outcomes. Most cancer pain and other distressing symptoms can be well controlled by palliative care methods when experienced, specialist advice and support is available. Yet there seems to be a reticence to embrace basic rules of good palliative care when dying is inevitable. Nurses refuse to give what to them appear to be overlarge doses of prescribed analgesic, for fear of 'killing' the patient, thus supporting some of the misconceptions about the actions of commonly used medications (Aranda & O'Connor, 1995).

The complex and holistic nature of palliative care requires care to be delivered by a multidisciplinary team. Such a team has developed a uniquely interconnected and collaborative decision-making process which recognises and uses the specialised skills of each member of the team. The team includes representatives from medical specialties and general practice, as well non-medical health professionals. To achieve teamwork of this complexity requires time dedicated to the team process and well-informed respect by all team members for the practice expertise of other professionals and practitioners, and the full involvement of patients and families in the decision-making process. In the modern practice of acute curative medicine, the pressures of time and technology mitigate against such multi-layered consensus methods of decision-making.

Additionally, an air of professional arrogance can still be observed among some health professionals; this arrogance creates tensions in the multidisciplinary team, preventing effective decision-making processes. Doctors can still feel that only they know what is best for the patient, and may disregard the opinions and knowledge of other professionals involved in palliative care. Nurses can undervalue the contribution of professionals who do not provide 24-hour care for people because they have traditionally provided everything when others have been absent from the bedside.

Palliative care fosters an approach to care that does not tolerate the sense of *power over* knowledge. Health professionals in palliative care operate from a model of having 'fuzzy boundaries' with those with whom they work. So the pastoral care worker is not threatened by the nurse who provides spiritual support while showering the patient, nor is the social worker concerned when the nurse uses counselling skills to resolve an issue which arises with the family.

Past traditions operate from the background of the generalised social denial of death and need for a belief in the ultimate curative power of science and medical knowledge. The skills of palliative care are still not well recognised or utilised, particularly in the acute settings of care where the emphasis is on seeking a cure. There is evidence of a subtle denial of death in the healthcare system which results in reticence to refer people to palliative care at the early stage of a probably terminal illness. Palliative care is seen by some as a challenge to orthodox medicine (Woodruff, 1992, p. 4). Woodruff argues that palliative care ought to be available alongside 'active' treatments and that the role of palliative care increases as the needs of the person and the family alter towards the goals of quality of life and acceptance of dying (p. 4).

> The principles and practice of palliative care should be initiated at such time as the patient with cancer has been shown to have an incurable disease, and should never be withheld until such time as all modalities of anti-cancer treatment have been exhausted. The intervention required will vary; . . . but the groundwork for the future involvement of the palliative care service can be laid. (Woodruff, 1992, p. 10)

## Palliative care nurses as advocates for the dying

In the eyes of many nurses, a law such as that passed in the Northern Territory does not set up a system that protects those people who are most vulnerable—those people who are facing the imminent end of life. Anecdotal reports describe terminally ill patients as already feeling a subtle pressure to devalue their remaining life in response to what they read in the media. Patients who are not able to express their wishes directly and are not free to make decisions about care need the reassurance that ongoing care will be provided.

Palliative care nurses believe that nursing should develop a clear public position which supports those they care for to make informed decisions about their life when they are dying. Nurses have a trust relationship with the community. They must advocate for access to good palliative care services and for improved quality of life for people with terminal conditions. Palliative care nurses believe that nursing should publicly identify euthanasia as irrelevant to good nursing practice. The real nursing focus should be on the work of caring for people no matter what their condition, context or beliefs. The community recognises that nurses can be effective advocates for people in the healthcare system and, as a result, nursing cannot support euthanasia without damaging this trust relationship.

> It seems to me that in life the possibility of suffering is inevitable. Only the misery is optional. Rather than bowing to the potential of misery and seeking to kill it, we need the understanding, training and support to seek the deeper meaning of suffering and to transcend it. (Gawler, 1995)

Palliative care can give people and their families the capacity to live and die supported, loved and empowered in the context of inevitable death. It provides support for people to complete the unfinished business of their life. Palliative care nurses believe that the debate about euthanasia needs to be refocused to advocate for palliative care, community resources and community-based services which provide that care effectively.

If the Australian community is to examine the options for termination of life, then surely there must be adequate research into the way people die. Many questions remain unaddressed and unanswered in the current debate—how are people in Australia dying at present?; what inadequacies are they experiencing?; how can care at the end of life be improved? Only by having a full picture of the experience of dying in Australia currently can we gain a proper understanding of needs and of the appropriate responses to requests for assistance to end life.

## Conclusion

The three qualitative studies discussed in this chapter identify the perspectives held by palliative care nurses about euthanasia and provide much food for thought (Aranda & O'Connor, 1995; McInerney & Seibold, 1995; Menon, 1996). They show the rich multidimensional complexity of the context, circumstances, medical/nursing variables and the consequent meanings surrounding the oversimplified debate about euthanasia. Euthanasia in this context is identified as potentially disastrous in relation to clarifying the resource needs for the care of those with terminal conditions in our society (Hockley, 1993; Maison, 1994).

Palliative care nurses recognise and support the need for adequate resources for further research, for professional education for those providing palliative care, for the dissemination of information to the community, and for improved financial support for multidisciplinary palliative care teams in the community. The experience of palliative care nurses is that money spent on these services will ultimately control and manage the needs of older people in such a way that it reduces the need for costly curative medical technology when it is really inappropriate. The debate about euthanasia urgently needs to be shifted from unproductive arguments about legalisation, which derive from the emotive concerns of a few articulate people, to an informed discussion about the practical allocation of resources for those with terminal conditions who need compassion and effective relief of their suffering and distress.

## References

AAP. (1995, 26 May). Wife's death key to M.P.'s deciding vote. *Herald-Sun* (Melbourne), p. 4.

Alcorn, G. (1996, 17 April). Why a nurse wants to choose her time to die. *Age* (Melbourne), p. 1.

Allingham, R. (1995, 4 April). Reflections on one year in the life of the dying. *Age* (Melbourne), p. 14.

Aranda, S. & O'Connor, M. (1995). Euthanasia, nursing and care of the dying: Rethinking Kuhse and Singer. *Australian Nurses Journal, 3* (2), 18–21.

170   Death and Caring for the Dying

Brown, T. & Pinkney, M. (1995, 26 May). Mercy law wins praise. *Herald-Sun* (Melbourne), p. 1.

Buchanan, R. (1995, 27 March). Charge euthanasia doctors, says right to life. *Age* (Melbourne), pp. 1, 2.

Chochinov, H.M., Wilson, K.G., & Enns, M. et al. (1995). Desire for death in the terminally ill. *American Journal of Psychiatry, 152,* 1185–1191.

Clarke, D.M. & Smith, G.C. (1995). Consultation psychiatry in general medical units. *Australian New Zealand Journal of Psychiatry, 29,* 424–432.

Coyle, Nessa (1992). The euthanasia and physician assisted suicide debate: issues for nursing. *ONF, 19* (7) (Supplement), 41–46.

Davies, N. (1995a, 25 March). Helping patients to die. *Age* (Melbourne), pp. 6, 23.

Davies, N. (1995b, 25 March). A matter of life and death. *Age* (Melbourne), feature in Saturday Extra.

Gawler, I. (1995, 29 May). Letter to the Editor. *Age* (Melbourne), p. 14.

Hamilton, H. (1995). *Euthanasia: An issue for nurses,* Discussion paper no. 1. Deakin, ACT: Royal College of Nursing Australia.

Hockley, J. (1993). The concept of hope and the will to live. *Palliative Medicine, 7,* 181–186.

Hooper, Stuart C., Vaughan, Kevin J., Tennant, Christopher C., & Perz, Jannette M. (1996). Major depression and refusal of life sustaining medical treatment in the elderly. *Medical Journal of Australia, 165,* 416–419.

Kelly, David (1995, 7 April). A balancing of harm on the scales of justice. *Age* (Melbourne), p. 9.

Kennett, J. (1995, 26 May). Head to head: Yes, to euthanasia. *Herald-Sun* (Melbourne), p. 12.

Kuhse, H. & Singer, P. (1992). Euthanasia: A survey of nurses' attitudes and practices. *Australian Nurses Journal, 21* (8), 21–22.

Maison, Michel Sarrazin (1994). Position on euthanasia. *Journal of Palliative Care, 10* (4), 23–26.

McInerney, F. & Seibold, C. (1995). Nurses' definitions of and attitudes towards euthanasia. *Journal of Advanced Nursing, 22,* 171–182.

Menon, M. (1996). Palliative care nurses' perspectives on euthanasia in 1995. Unpublished research report.

Morieson, B. (1993). A nursing perspective on euthanasia. *Conference Proceedings* from Active voluntary euthanasia: The current issues. Melbourne: Monash Centre for Human Bioethics.

Nielson, C. & Williams, T.A. (1980). Depression in ambulatory medical patients: Prevalence by self-report questionnaire and recognition by non-psychiatric physicians. *Arch Gen Psychiatry, 37,* 999–1004.

Oderberg, D. (1995, 22 March). Dying with dignity ignores the basic good of living. *Australian Financial Review,* p. 3.

O'Connor, M. (1992). A better way: palliative care nurses and their experiences of home based care of the dying. Unpublished MN thesis, RMIT, Melbourne.

O'Connor, M. (1993). Weighing up the arguments on euthanasia and palliative care—a nurse's perspective. *Conference Proceedings* from Active voluntary euthanasia: The current issues conference. Melbourne: Monash Medical Centre.

O'Sullivan, K. (1995, 30 April). Dignity in death. *Herald-Sun* (Melbourne), p. 6.

Perron, Marshall (1995, 26 May). Wrong to ignore the pain. *Age* (Melbourne), p. 12.

Place, Michael (1993). Why we should not legalise euthanasia. *Health Progress,* March, 39–70.

Pollard, Brian (1989). *Euthanasia: Why kill the dying?* Sydney: Little Hills Press.

Singer, P. (1995, 30 March). Letter to the editor: A challenge to the AMA on euthanasia. *Age* (Melbourne), p. 12.

Saunders, C. (1992). Voluntary euthanasia. *Palliative Medicine, 6*, 1–5.

Uren, K. (1995, 18 April). The euthanasia debate: Warning on abuse. *Progress Press* (Melbourne), p. 3.

World Health Organization (WHO) (1987). *Declaration on euthanasia*, 39th World Medical Assembly. Madrid: WHO.

Woodruff, R.K.W. (1992). *Palliative medicine*. Melbourne: Asperula.

Woodruff, R. (1995, 30 March). Letter to the editor: Facts needed to balance doctors' euthanasia push. *Age* (Melbourne), p. 12.

# 14

# Breaking the Silence: Palliation for People with Dementia

## Jennifer Abbey

## The long death of dementia

The life expectancy for people with dementia is increasing, as is our knowledge of how to inject some quality of life into the day-to-day care of those who suffer from diseases that cause the condition. The care of people who exhibited behaviour that was irrational, abnormal or outside social norms has depended on the prevailing social and economic conditions of the time. In recent history people who were demented were incarcerated in mental institutions and labelled 'mad'. Scanning the histories of the treatment of those perceived as insane (Foucault, 1967; Barton, 1976; Bates, 1977; Porter, 1987) reveals what seems in retrospect barbaric institutional practices and individual cruelty based on ignorance, superstition and insensitivity.

Advocates from the disciplines of philosophy, social policy, medicine and nursing challenged the thinking and practices of earlier times, and today, in the main, people with late-stage dementia are cared for in nursing homes where standards are well controlled by government regulations. Institutional practices are based on a policy that recognises an individual's rights to freedom and dignity. Care is guided by a philosophy of choice based on the principle of the least restrictive alternative in an environment that values the social role people have in society. That progress has been made is undeniable. However, knowledge of the historical perspective reminds us of the need to see ourselves as the next era will see us.

Within the rapidly changing contemporary environment, any discussion of whether to make palliative care available to people with dementia, or what form that care would take in clinical terms, may be discouraged or ignored because of the cultural and ethical difficulties our community has with the concept of death as a managed process. If and when these curtains of silence are raised, usually by force of circumstance, polarised positions develop quickly. Palliative care discussed in this context may well be labelled as a covert form of euthanasia. Such labelling is rare when palliative care is being discussed in relation to cancer and other conditions, reminding us that the general assumptions and the patterns of care provided in acute settings do not adequately encompass the experience and needs of the person with dementia.

In a hospice unit, for example, the philosophy has been spelt out: the role of the unit is to assist people to a peaceful, pain-free and dignified death. But most people with dementia die in nursing homes. For people with dementia who are dying, and for those who care for them, an atmosphere of ambiguity, both in the community and in aged-care facilities, leads to confused and unplanned care. Nurses are under moral and professional pressure 'to protect the vulnerable against carrying a disproportionate burden of suffering in health care contexts' (Johnstone, 1996, p. 124) but are not provided with conceptual frameworks or established decision-making procedures that allow them to weigh this pressure against the habits of established practice in an appropriate way. This leaves people in the terminal stages of a dementing illness, and those who care for them, in a most vulnerable position. Nursing home residents appear to suffer greatly and many families indicate that 'they would not have chosen to stay alive like this'. The ambiguous atmosphere that exists is worsening as the euthanasia debate is sensationalised in the media. Despite, or because of this, nurses' choices are most often limited to safe, life-extending care.

## The issues

This chapter will explore only a few of the difficult issues regarding the death and dying of people with dementia. I argue that early discussion is needed of the likely course of the disease and an opportunity must be given to the person who has been diagnosed with dementia to register preferences concerning treatment in the late stages. I point to the consequences of the failure of present-day policy to encourage the development of a structured process that enables nurses, doctors and relatives to consult together to make a number of decisions about questions which the course of the illness will almost inevitably reveal. Some criticism is then offered of the part that the philosophy and practices of normalisation play in suppressing discussion of and preparation for the death trajectory associated with dementia. A discussion of the ambiguities inherent in current concepts of advocacy serves to highlight some of the obstacles that a shift towards palliation would meet, especially since so much of our thinking about palliation and treatment options derives from acute settings very different from nursing homes.

Some of these issues hover at the fringe of consciousness for the public and health professionals alike. If they are not drawn out and dealt with in a constructive manner, everyone can suffer. In the process of addressing this suffering in the next decade, a new role for nurses who care for residents in aged-care facilities is likely to emerge. This new role will involve reconceptualising duty-of-care relationships with people who suffer from late stage dementia. Case conferences, with a defined agenda and an openness and sensitivity to different paradigms of care, are pro- posed as worthwhile innovations.

An essential base from which to explore this new territory is an under- standing of the condition of dementia.

## Dying and dementia

Dementia, in the main, is a disease of the old, affecting one in four people over 80 years of age. Of people in nursing homes 80 per cent suffer from some form of dementing illness. The first sign of dementia is usually that forgetfulness increases to the point where it interferes with normal management of life, and either the affected person or their family or friends seek medical advice. The dementia syndrome is characterised by the triad of memory impairment, intellectual deterioration and per- sonality change.

Alzheimer's disease (AD) and multi-infarct dementia (MID) (Schmitt & Sano, 1994) are responsible for most cases of dementia and neither is susceptible to well-recognised treatments or any cure. In either form, cognitive and behavioural malfunctions of a person will flow from and depend on the parts of the brain that are damaged, but differences in the way the disease progresses tend to alter the nature of the death and may have other implications for care in the later stages. In elderly people the condition of dementia is often labelled 'Senile Dementia of the Alzheimer's Type' (SDAT) as multiple factors may affect the cognitive impairment.

There is no reason why choices about end-stage care cannot be carefully raised and discussed with the person who has dementia as the disease progresses. Experts argue that a person in the early stages of dementia, after a definitive diagnosis has been made, can retain their testamentary capacity for some time, and are therefore legally competent and able to sign an advanced directive (Peisah & Brodaty, 1994). For palliative care to be introduced effectively in the late stages of SDAT it is important that both the person with dementia and the family have explored issues about treatment and management of the progressive decline that is inevitable. Yet, there is little point in undergoing this process if requests and views will be discounted, as often happens, during final stage care.

During the early and middle stages, the family dynamics that will influence the care provided to the person with dementia begin to emerge, and differences of opinion as to the course care should take are likely to cause strains within the family and, sometimes, between family members and health professionals. It seems fair to conclude that these strains are often exacerbated by the absence of a clearly recognised framework for discussing the issues that arise and the choices that are available.

## Late stage dementia

A description of the late stage of the disease is not found in the literature about dementia but its symptoms will be familiar to most gerontic nurses. A person may lose the ability to recognise family or friends, not know themselves and spit out food, fluid and medications. He or she may be highly aggressive, belligerent, sobbing or screaming; or strikingly passive and quiet, immobile and non-verbal; and, sometimes, each by turns. In the late stage of dementia, people are inevitably incontinent of urine and faeces; and they may be in pain but have difficulties in expressing this. The development of contractures, skin tears and peripheral shutdown occurs as body breakdown slowly progresses. This stage may last for months or, sometimes, years.

## Decision-making

The long dying process characterised by physical and cognitive decline can be complicated by conflicting personal and professional obligations which mark the perceptions and conduct of those family members and health professionals who play a part in directing the course and character of terminal care.

For example, family members may be quite insistent that the person with dementia who has lost most cognitive ability would not have wanted to stay alive in that condition, and they will request no active treatment, wanting him or her to be left to die peacefully. A nurse described the decision-making process when Mr C became acutely ill. He was suffering from SDAT, emphysema and congestive cardiac failure. She sets out the doctor's report of a conversation he had with relatives:

> What do you want us to do? [the doctor said] . . . do you want us to be active in our treatment or should we be conservative and let nature take its course? I can give him an injection of Lasix and it will ease it off but other than that he has to go down to the hospital and have this, this and this done. Now how do you want us to go?'

The nurse notes the family's acceptance of the inevitability of death and their preference for comfort measures only. She goes on to comment, supportively: 'I mean, he had emphysema and obviously it really wasn't going to help him that much. So he had his injection of Lasix and stayed with us and he'd gone in a couple of days' (Abbey, 1996).

Here, where all the parties were of like mind, leaving the choice of the decision-making mechanism to the doctor was unproblematic; but in other cases, the views of the doctor, the nurses and the family may be at odds with one another.

This situation is illustrated by these extracts from a meeting held to discuss care options for Mrs M, a nursing home resident with late stage dementia who had a gangrenous foot. The relatives and most of the nurses believed that Mrs M was in great pain. The concerned relative visited every day and had done so for the entire time that Mrs M had been in the nursing home. When nurses passed on the relative's request for an increase in the dose of morphine, the general practitioner expressed the opinion that, taking into account Mrs M's history and previous agitated behaviour, her screams arose from apprehension, not pain, and his opinion was that the

> family want to bump her off—it is illegal, it does not matter how compassionate we want to be. The only reason for morphine will be pain . . . apprehension is *not pain* [speaker's emphasis]. Apprehension and fear is to be dealt with by Haloperidol not Morphine. (Abbey, 1996)

The various replies from nurses to this comment reflect their own value positions. They said:

> 'we know she is dying. So she must go with dignity. Does it matter if it is pain and/or agitation?';
> 'I would hate to err on the side that it is her dementia not pain—she used to say I will scream if you do that to me';
> 'Give her the benefit of the doubt—I would want cover—I hope there is someone advocating for me';
> 'She's on a lower dose today and just as comfortable';
> 'That leg is horrendous. If you cannot increase their life expectancy then surely we should make her comfortable'. (Abbey, 1996)

As a result of the meeting, no changes were made to the morphine dose; the doctor's views prevailed.

In both cases death was imminent, and yet, the judgments of the participants were heavily and unpredictably influenced by factors other than the demented person's behaviour and apparent condition. The interactions between doctors, nurses and relatives demonstrate not only a diversity of opinion, but also a striking absence of any orderly way of bringing the various bodies of knowledge, opinion and belief to bear on the choices that will inevitably be made, whether deliberately or by inactivity.

# The nature of the dying and the dilemmas attached

Particular patterns of case management emerge from these two examples, and specific lines of criticism can be raised about how each situation was handled. In the first case, sections of Australian society would be likely to see an instance of immorality constituted by neglect of the patient's best interests and an unacceptable level of arrogance; other sections of society will see those same attributes in the very different handling of the second case.

It is understandable that, among this confusion, nurses too hold diverse opinions about whether limits to treatment and the giving of narcotics constitute palliative care or passive euthanasia. Because of the lack of clear guidelines about their role as advocate, or their duty-of-care responsibilities, nurses are often prepared to leave the negotiation about the progress to death of people with dementia to the treating doctor, in spite of the fact that most of the care that keeps people alive is performed by nurses. Rarely are palliative care experts contacted in relation to residents with dementia who are close to death. One study found that palliative care consultation was sought for some nursing home residents but never for residents with dementia (Maddocks, Abbey, Pickaver, Parker, Beck, & DeBellis, 1996). When the general practitioner is known to have a firm position on such issues, nurses are unlikely to put forward conflicting views.

Nurses' clinical reasoning is hampered by the nature of aged care policy which is based on the normalisation and social role valorisation (SRV) principles as outlined by Wolf Wolfensberger (1932; 1975; 1981). Wolfensberger's insistence that 'the best strategy for disadvantaged people to avoid further devaluation is for them to achieve positive social roles' (Bleasdale, 1996, p. 4) has led to the conception that the optimal care in nursing homes will be one where the best quality 'home-like' environment exists. In recent years, Wolfensberger has added further moral overtones by insisting that any discussion of care other than that which supports the maintenance of life 'even if one lives in physical pain and misery' (Wolfensberger, 1994, p. 410) is tantamount to death-making behaviour.

In nursing homes this 'normalisation' philosophy, based on social values not practical realities, has infiltrated so far into the aged-care psyche that there is little questioning that the 'right thing' to do with frail old bodies is to get them out of bed, dress them in clothes, and sit them in a chair. If a person develops a rattle in their chest or a urinary tract infection is suspected, the doctor is often asked to prescribe antibiotics, even when the tablets are spat out. Also, hours are spent trying to encourage the shell of the person who is left to take mouthfuls of softened food, or, when this fails, to drink dietary supplements.

For some relatives, this is important and the treatment they desire. An extract from one carer's story tells of her mother's last days.

> Mum is no longer able to tolerate solid foods so her diet is liquids and very soft foods. She is given Ensure which I am told has all the necessary vitamins that she needs. She was enjoying an egg flip when I called in on her this morning and the staff are very kind in trying to give her various things to encourage her to eat. Even with all the tender loving care Mum has still gone down very quickly in the last few weeks, some days even the liquids are too much for her to tolerate. I have said my last goodbyes on several occasions lately and thought I would cope with this sad time when it did eventuate but I am finding it very difficult. Just to see Mum fading away not able to take fluids of any sort, it is very hard to put my feelings into words. Mum appears to know we were there, when we spoke she answered by blinking her eyes but she was just so very tired. Her breathing was very heavy and it seemed to take all her energy just to get her breath. (Abbey, 1996, appendix 7)

For another carer, this kind of waiting was too stressful. Bill and Violet had been happily married for 60 years. Bill had cared for Violet through the early and middle stages of her dementing illness but was now finally facing the realisation that their shared life was at an end and that she would have to be cared for by others in her last months. In a way, at this point, Violet was no longer alive for Bill. Her personhood had slipped away. Watching her body break down, waiting and wishing for her physical death was suffering of the worst kind for him. Bill's comment was 'I hope Mum does not last too long in a way—the girls look after her and all that but that is no good for my position' (Abbey, 1996, p. 177).

The nurses and carers were aware of Bill's views and struggled with the choices of feeding and turning Violet and dressing her wounds. Although morphine was given before turns or dressings, it seemed clear that both Violet and Bill suffered agonies in the last few weeks of Violet's life. The nurses, in spite of their commitment to providing palliative care for Violet, had great difficulties in changing their learned role as clinicians. Their only way to express their love and devotion to both Bill and Violet was to make Violet look as 'normal' as possible. She was showered, even when the pressure of the shower water tore the skin off her legs, dressed, perfumed and fed until the day she died. These actions were all performed with the utmost in tender care. Alternatives were discussed, even the fact that fasting can produce a state of comfort and, at times even mild euphoria, but the idea of what seemed like 'doing nothing' was so at odds with the care paradigm in nurses' minds that they felt unable to change their normal practice. The entrenched hierarchical relationship of doctor and nurse combined with the constraints of policy and practice produced unwanted and fruitless suffering in spite of the very best of intentions of all those involved.

How, then, can these dilemmas be made to come to the surface, to emerge in everyday practice, to be presented in an orderly and consistent way; how can discussion that draws on all the available kinds of knowledge held by the different participants encompass all the possible choices and lead to a resolution that delivers the dignity owed to any person approaching death? Should someone be nominated to make the choice? If so, who should it be in the case of a person who has left no advance directive? Is relief of suffering to be the final arbiter? Unfortunately, the relief of suffering is a problematic mandate (McCullough & Wilson, 1995) because the concept of suffering itself can be understood only in relation to our own unique understanding of ourselves in the world; and in the case of advanced dementias, the person with the principal interest is no longer able to contribute or give instructions when the questions can no longer be avoided. Until such questions are addressed, nursing staff will often find themselves unsure of what their professional responsibilities require of them.

## Facing the future

The future reality the gerontic nurse is going to have to deal with is that nursing homes will house many aged people with late stage dementia who will be suffering from a gradual overall systemic breakdown. These people will no longer be able to give or withhold consent for treatment, though some may have left advanced directives.

For many nursing home residents, no close relatives visit and therefore the nurse feels a responsibility to act as an advocate on behalf of the person with dementia. An advocate is defined as 'person who acts as a mouthpiece for another, for example, with officials or institutional staff' (Creyke, 1995, p. xxix). There are two models of advocacy, either one of which might be adopted, depending partly on the advocate's philosophy and partly on the context. Advocates can act either 'in the best interests of a person', in which case the advocate uses his or her judgment as to what is best for the person being represented. Or 'substitute judgment' can be exercised (Creyke, 1995, p. xxix–xxxii); this requires a 'substitute decision maker' to attempt to do what a now-incompetent person would have done in the same situation. The availability of these alternative guiding principles contributes to the complexity in acting as an advocate for people who have lost the capacity to make decisions for themselves. Advocating is difficult enough in areas such as finance and accommodation; advocating for people's right to die with dignity is even more difficult.

It is not only the person with dementia who may need support. Nurses, either in the community or in residential settings, may also feel obliged to play an advocate role for relatives. When relatives wish to choose palliative care, the nurse may be caught up in a difficult situation where it is the carer who needs an advocate. Burdekin cites evidence showing the services that exist for people with dementia and their carers all a 'bureaucratic nightmare' and 'a hotch-potch . . . without a thought for a strategy' (Human Rights & Equal Opportunities Commission, 1993). This lack of a legislative or cultural paradigm for dealing with such cases leaves the community nurse or case manager caught in the middle of what may all too easily become a dialogue of the deaf.

The ideal place for a gerontic nurse to play an advocacy role in defining palliative care for an individual with dementia is as part of a case conference team. But the first task will be to press for institutional philosophies and clear frameworks of care, so that death decisions are not made by default or by the overbearing combination of accepted wisdom, the medical model of care and the rigid assumptions of current public policy.

Competencies, developed and used by the profession, indicate that an advocacy role is part of a nurse's responsibilities (Australian Nursing Council, 1993). However, this area of activity is intricate and complex and needs an open approach with a good measure of lateral thinking. Suppression of deeply ingrained habits acquired during professional socialisation may be needed. It appears that a significant proportion of health professionals are more inclined to make judgments for people rather than to assist them to make their own choices. Evidence suggests that the professionals much prefer to 'take over', and tend to judge both 'best interest' and 'substituted judgment' from their own perspectives (McCullough & Wilson, 1995).

In purely legal terms, the Commonwealth publication, *Who can decide? Legal decision making for others* (Creyke, 1995), outlines the principles that are to be followed in proxy decision-making in Australia. *The International Covenant on Civil and Political Rights* and the *United Nations Declaration of the Rights of Disabled Persons* outline overriding ethical standards. Article 10 of the *International Covenant on Civil and Political Rights* states that all people of the world have the right to be free from 'cruel, inhumane or degrading treatment or punishment' (Human Rights & Equal Opportunities Commission, 1993, p. 22). Australia does not have a bill of rights but has agreed to abide by these covenants and standards. It is questionable if these endowed rights are available to all people with dementias, especially those in the late stage of the disease.

Guidance in the matter of advocacy for case managers and nursing home staff may be summed up as follows:

- If no indication of preference has been left in any form of advanced directive, then the best interest of the person should prevail.

- If any form of living will or documentation that cites a preference for care is available, and considered to be valid, then a substituted judgment approach would be appropriate.

But this guidance is given with caution.

## Care issues and dilemmas

History, habit, fear, lack of debate and the ambiguous position nurses find themselves in will make it very difficult for them to change to being independent clinical activists and advocates. It will be hard to switch from automatically calling a doctor when a person's temperature rises rather than commencing tepid sponging, even if the relatives and the doctor have tacitly agreed that only palliative care measures are to be implemented. But this change will be demanded by consumers and by people with dementia themselves who have left advanced directions about their wishes. In meeting this demand, discretion must be applied before this change can, or should, occur.

One of the difficulties in making a change to what some consider 'suffering-making' nursing care is the increasing risk of litigation. An accepted cure-oriented clinical route feels safer than the notion of exploring creative and personal options for people with late stage dementia.

The nurse acting as an advocate or changing 'curing' practice to palliative care can be in a difficult position. In the present context, the practical effect of aged-care policy forces a philosophy of body maintenance on staff. Brans warns that nurses may be exposing themselves to a situation where their relationship with the resident is challenged when they act as a patient advocate in order to benefit, or to represent the patient's 'best interests' (Brans, 1995, p. 14).

In introducing palliative care for people with dementia, questions of medications, mobilisation and nutrition are intertwined and cross the boundaries between professional responsibilities. Take the instance when a nurse detects that a person with dementia is having difficulty with their swallowing reflex. A bedside decision could be taken by the nurse to cease feeding. More commonly, however, the nurse will call the treating doctor who will order that an opinion from a speech therapist be sought; and then it is almost inevitable that high-calorie food supplements will be ordered. The nurse is then obliged to carry through that order. We see a chain of habit, hierarchy and obligation lead to the continuation of nursing care based on body maintenance. Johnstone (1994) indicates that this structure of control over nurses' work is still very real and enforceable in law.

Palliative care for people with late stage dementia will only be successfully introduced when efforts have been made first, to reduce or eliminate the taken-for-granted status of normalisation and, second, to find a structured way to feed the intimate and specialised knowledge that nurses have of people with dementia into organised death-care planning. A nurse is at risk in taking on an advocacy role without these two issues being resolved.

## Conclusion

A major change in culture and policy is required. The first step must be to lift the veil of silence. This can be done by discussing and making overt the suffering that people with late stage dementia exhibit. Nurses would do well to demand individual case conferences for people with dementia who are judged to require palliative care. Support can, and should, be obtained from people who are experts in palliative care.

Present-day policy in aged care shows us to be a society that marginalises our most vulnerable group, the elderly with dementia. If our society continues to accept inaction and passivity as adequate responses to the dilemmas of care that surround suffering in the period shortly before these people meet their death, it will be falling short of the standards it would like to claim for itself. Nurses have the major role, and incur the greatest legal risk, in meeting humane and professional obligations to all those who suffer with SDAT, the living death. As the 'right to die with dignity' movement grows stronger, it will be nurses who carry the brunt of the blame if their advocacy and clinical role in the relief of suffering becomes confused in the public mind with euthanasia.

Only by breaking the silence that hides the choices associated with planning the care of the elderly person with late stage dementia can the ethical differences between keeping people alive and letting them fade away in peace and dignity be made explicit. Until this happens, nursing care plans, which are suitable for use in everyday practice, which allow nurses to draw on the knowledge and views held by different participants, and which deliver the dignity owed to us all as we approach death, will develop only slowly and with difficulty.

## References

Abbey, J. (1996). Death and late-stage dementia in Institutions: a cultural analysis. Unpublished PhD thesis. Deakin University, Victoria.
Australian Nursing Council (1993). *National competencies for the registered and enrolled nurse in recommended domains.* Melbourne: ANC.
Barton, R. (1976). *Institutional neurosis*, 3rd edn. Bristol: John Wright and Sons.
Bates, E. (1977). *Models of madness.* St Lucia, Qld: University of Queensland Press.
Bleasdale, P. (1996). Evaluating values—a critique of value theory in social role valorisation. *Australian Disability Review*, 1, 3–22.
Brans, L. (1995). Patient advocacy: Is it in the patient's best interests or the nurses?

*Conference Abstracts.* Impossible Demands: Ethical and Legal Quandaries for Nurses Conference, 13 October. Melbourne: Monash University.

Creyke, R. (1995). *Who can decide? Legal decision-making for others.* Canberra: AGPS.

Foucault, M. (1967). *Madness and civilization: A history of insanity in the age of reason.* London: Tavistock Publications.

Human Rights & Equal Opportunities Commission (1993). *Human rights and mental illness: Report of the National Inquiry into the Human Rights of People with Mental Illness,* vol. 2 (Brian Burdekin, Chairperson). Canberra: AGPS.

Johnstone, M. (1994). *Nursing and the injustices of the law.* Sydney: Harcourt Brace & Company.

Johnstone, M. (Ed.) (1996). *The politics of euthanasia: A nursing response.* Melbourne: The Royal College of Nursing.

Maddocks, I., Abbey, J., Pickhaver, A., Parker, D., Beck, K., & DeBellis, A. (1996). *Palliative care in nursing homes, Report to the Commonwealth Department of Health and Family Services.* Adelaide: Palliative Care Unit, Flinders University of South Australia.

McCullough, L. & Wilson, N. (1995). *Long-term care decisions, ethical and conceptual dimensions.* Baltimore: The John Hopkins University Press.

Peisah, C. & Brodaty, H. (1994). Dementia and the will-making process: The role of the medical practitioner. *Medical Journal of Australia, 161* (6), 381–384.

Porter, R. (1987). *A social history of madness: Stories of the insane.* London: Weidenfeld and Nicolson.

Schmitt, F. & Sano, M. (1994). Neuropsychological approaches to the study of dementia. In Morris, J. (Ed.), *Handbook of dementing illnesses.* New York: Dekker.

Wolfensberger, W. (1932). *The principles of normalisation in human service.* Toronto: National Institute of Mental Retardation.

Wolfensberger, W. (1975). *The origin and nature of our institutional models.* New York: Human Policy.

Wolfensberger, W. (1981). Social role valorization: A proposed new term for the principles of normalization. *Mental Retardation, 19* (1), 1–7.

Wolfensberger, W. (1994). The growing threat to the lives of handicapped people in the context of modernistic values. *Disability and Society, 9* (3), 95–413.

# Part III
# CHALLENGES IN CONTEXT

# 15

# Negotiating New Goals and Care Options in the Presence of Irreversible Disease

## Ruth Redpath

> The definitional context in which the awareness of terminal illness initially begins for the cancer patient is the treatment situation. There is no facile boundary between the end of mainstream 'treatment' and the beginning of 'dying' in many instances: dying will begin in the larger context of an illness calendar already in existence, often in treatment centres the public mandate of which is 'cure'. (Schou, 1993)

This chapter examines the notion of the 'facile boundary' noted by Schou (1993) that exists at the turning point between the end of treatment and the beginning of terminal care. The very imprecise nature of this boundary points to the need for expert negotiation of decision-making to ensure the best outcomes for the patient. This chapter discusses situations in which such a turning point is reached and suggests ways in which a satisfactory transition can be negotiated. Barriers to the successful negotiation of this transition will be explored and strategies for improving care at the turning point will be suggested.

## A critical turning point

The point at which it is acknowledged that active medical intervention will do little or nothing to halt or reverse the downward course of a person's illness is likely to be a time of distress and adjustment. The realisation of the terminal nature of illness will occur at different times for those involved but is unlikely to be instantaneous, occurring instead as the result of processing information from a variety of sources.

There are many possible clinical scenarios in which such turning points from acute to palliative care occur. Each different context will affect the way both the medical practitioners and the person and their family approach the transition. People come to the turning point having been:

- incurable from diagnosis with no active treatment offered;
- incurable following one or more periods of remission; or,
- incurable as their disease becomes increasingly unresponsive to treatment.

The lack of a precise boundary between active and palliative treatment has been compounded by an increasing ability to achieve periods of relatively stable disease with non-curative treatment. Thus some people with incurable disease may follow a chronic disease trajectory over many months or even years of non-curative treatment.

Recognition that cure or control of disease is no longer possible is often first discussed within the doctor–patient consultation process without involvement of staff of other disciplines. If the disease is incurable from the time of diagnosis, few other professionals may have been previously involved in the patient's care, but this is not usually the case. Frequently, the person has undergone a period of intensive treatment with involvement of a multidisciplinary team and the potential exists for a more holistic approach to the negotiation of goal changes at the turning point.

## Barriers to negotiation of the turning point

Reports and experience indicate that communication and dialogue at this time of new direction may be handled in ways that leave the person confused and bewildered, with a sense of isolation from help (Anon. 1983). While it would be foolish to expect that the pain of such crises in the individual's life is totally avoidable if only the healthcare team did the job well enough, it is important to acknowledge and address potential barriers to the negotiation of this communication that may relate to the health system, health professionals and the patient and family.

### The healthcare system

Structural constraints within the healthcare setting may mitigate against successful negotiation of the transition to palliative care. Factors such as non-integrated medical records, lack of team accessibility, limited or no access to interview rooms, and pressures to reduce patient stays and reduce clinic visits all work against effective communication about goal change. Delivery of information by junior medical staff in busy outpatient clinics also affects the quality of the interaction.

## Medical practitioners

Medical training tends to focus on the pathophysiology of disease and the technology of its investigation and treatment. This biomedical approach may also prevail in practice, especially within the acute hospital setting. Doctors may concentrate on the task of disease reversal, with deterioration and death being seen as a failure, and consequently be unwilling to face reality. This is compounded by a lack of universality of response to different treatments.

The doctor also faces definitional problems, 'determining when treatment for cancer should become "palliative" rather than "radical", deciding/revising definitions of prognostic likelihood and determining when an individual becomes expressly "terminal" as opposed to "incurably ill" or as having advanced disease' (Schou, 1993). This ambiguity may lead to discomfort in speaking with the individual patient who may find the uncertainty difficult to accept.

In addition, the doctor may have known the patient and family a long time and invested much emotional energy and technical expertise in their life and survival, making it difficult to admit that there are no more treatment options.

Cancer treatment, associated complications of illness and treatment and other associated medical conditions may necessitate the attention of multiple specialists. Obtaining an agreed approach to care which takes account of the whole clinical picture, let alone the person's wishes, may prove difficult. In some instances, it may be hard to distinguish between a side-effect of treatment, reversible with intervention, and the ongoing disease process. The general practitioner who may be an important source of support to the patient and family may be left out of the decision-making and communication processes around goal change.

Apparent indifference on the part of doctors and others may relate to poor communication skills. While the problems are many and varied, of particular importance is the use of distancing. Maguire (1985) reported fear of personal emotional overload or of difficult questions or the unleashing of strong emotions by patient or family as common reasons for distancing by doctors and nurses. Staff must be trained so that they feel more confident in the appropriate interviewing and counselling skills to cope with these fears as well as there being mechanisms, formal or informal, for staff support in such work.

Significant time within medical students' curriculum is now given to the teaching of communication skills and, in palliative care courses in particular, to providing the prospective doctors with some insight into some of the more personal factors that can influence communication in emotionally demanding situations. However, the learning demands on new practitioners make the utilisation of these skills difficult. While communication is a key issue in the negotiation of goal change, it is not within the scope of this paper to address it specifically.

## Team involvement

The point at which it is acknowledged that the patient is no longer responding to treatment is not reached by all team members simultaneously. It is not uncommon for doctors and other staff, particularly nurses, to be in disagreement over the point at which to recommend withdrawal of curative or remission based treatment. Prescott and Bowen (1985) indicate that the commonest cause of doctor–nurse disagreement is the general plan of care, with specific areas of tension being the extent of treatment, its degree of invasiveness and the timing of its withdrawal. However, these authors also suggest such disagreement acts as an important catalyst for the exercise of the complementary role of the two disciplines and their varied insights into care.

Nurses may view investigations and treatments as sources of suffering more readily than doctors (Dudgeon, 1992). The nurse may also have developed an understanding of the patient's expectations through daily physical care that may offer important insights into the patient's readiness to accept treatment withdrawal. As Fincannon (1995) identified, in the oncology service it is the nurses who are the most consistent observers of the patient's emotional responses. Night nurses may have a particular contribution to make that needs to be incorporated (Hanson, 1994).

Similarly, medical social workers, pastoral care workers and other allied health professionals may have valuable insights into the patient and family's perspective. There must be collaboration in sharing of goals, planning, problem-solving, decision-making, responsibility (Kertstetter, 1990), with recognition and acceptance of separate and combined spheres of activity. Building such confidence between members of the team does not occur overnight; a slow and sometimes painful process may be required to achieve this.

The implication of this approach is that the multidisciplinary team may move to an agreed position about the need to change direction and address the new reality gradually, not always abruptly. From there due consideration can be given to the best way of sharing these understandings with the patient. Such communications should not be seen as an event, happening only when it becomes clear that the patient is terminally ill, but part of an ongoing exchange of health-related information throughout the course of the person's illness.

## Patient/family/others

Pre-existing factors may also influence the way that a person and his/her family/friends receive the news of the change in direction of care. Some factors that may influence the communication process are:

- age and family status;
- life experience;
- family history of illness, treatment and bereavement;
- spirituality and worldview;
- cultural and language barriers;
- family dynamics;
- presence of pain and other symptoms;
- depression and mental status;
- weakness;
- poor concentration.

While it is common for the patient to want to continue treatment despite mounting evidence that it is not effective, it is also not rare for a patient to ask for treatment to be stopped or to refuse a new program of treatment. Such requests need to be carefully considered by the treatment team. The person may be depressed when making such a request, or be under duress by feeling themselves a burden to others. The request may be presented as a weariness with, or intolerance of, the treatment and its side-effects. Treatment may be perceived as diminishing their quality of life and the patient may want to use their remaining time in other ways.

While it is not surprising or unreasonable that the medical team should seek to dissuade the person from choosing the option of withdrawal from treatment, the benefits of treatment should be carefully considered. A willingness of the treatment team to re-examine both the treatment plan and the person's understanding of it will help to ensure that the best decisions are made for the individual patient. The patient and family need full scope to express the reasons for their request and to receive clarification of the present state of the disease and its prognosis with, and without, treatment.

Again, involvement of the whole staff team in this process is vital, creating an atmosphere in which the person is respected and can feel free to discuss the decision with any member of the team. It may be appropriate for an assessment as to whether treatable depression is present, and helpful to offer the support of a spiritual adviser or counsellor, if they are not already involved, as such a turning point is contemplated.

## Successful negotiation of the turning point

Most commonly the critical encounter with the patient will take place within the acute hospital environment, be it an in-patient ward, a day ward, or an ambulatory care clinic, less commonly in the specialist's consulting rooms and occasionally in the general practitioner's rooms. Rarely, the encounter may occur in the patient's home.

Attention to the setting of the encounter is important, especially when the patient is not in their own environment. Issues such as privacy, freedom from interruption, presence of a support person, time for clarification and questions, and the involvement of another health professional are important (Faulkner, Maguire & Regnard, 1994). Additionally, a time for follow-up is also paramount. Later, further questions can be articulated, information repeated to check accuracy of understanding, and a more considered careplan discussed.

For the doctor, the complexities of offering the right information with clarity and empathy in individual circumstances, in such a way that the person feels that they have been an active participant in the process, call for much skill and sensitivity based on continuing clinical experience and education programs. Involvement of other professionals, with whom the patient and family have communicated well, may be appropriate.

As well as the patient/family needing support, it should be recognised that the doctor who has had the task of confronting this difficult interaction probably needs to debrief, at least informally. The encounter with the patient and family may include strong emotional responses and anger which stretch the doctor's tolerance. It may be difficult for a doctor to admit to colleagues that he/she needs to talk about a stressful meeting of this kind. But the work culture should encourage this within the team context and within confidential boundaries, even by the formation of staff support groups (Maguire, 1985).

It is important that all team members are familiar with the change in direction. This may be conveyed through a regular staff meeting, though notifying everyone is not always easy—as Kerstetter (1990) says, the novice to the oncology unit is struck by the sheer number of people involved in cancer care. Attempts to do so must be pursued rigorously, with detailed documentation in the patient's medical record. Failure can result in mixed messages and fragmentation of care. There may not always be full agreement with the decision that has been taken, but it is important that the patient does not get confusing information from other members of the team.

Sometimes, the patient relates closely to a staff member other than the one who discussed the change in direction with them. This person often then acts as an advocate for the patient in seeking more information or revisiting the care plan which has been agreed. This possibility should be acknowledged by the team and such interventions on the patient's behalf should be handled in a suitably professional manner without personal antagonisms.

## Adjusting to the changed direction

The adjustment to the information that the focus of care has now shifted to one of maximising quality of life and symptom control is highly individual.

Developing an appropriate care plan at a time of transition is not easy, especially if the disease is progressing rapidly. In addition, the person is often a hospital in-patient when this turning point is reached, but may be discharged home at the very time when they are most vulnerable emotionally. Members of the family or other carers must also adjust to the changed goals of care. Even though they may long have known that treatment had been for prolongation of life or remission rather than cure, a shift in thinking has to occur when no more treatment is being recommended. As they come to terms with the fact that the person is dying, fears and questions may arise. Preparation for discharge and referral on to appropriate services are therefore paramount.

The sick person may not discuss these details; rather their spoken concerns may relate more to not wanting to be a burden to those at home and the feeling of apparent abandonment by the hospital team/specialist to whom they have become emotionally attached over a period of illness. Alternatively, they may not yet be ready to accept their terminal diagnosis and may behave as though no change of direction has yet occurred.

## Referral to palliative care

In Australia palliative care teams have been established in acute care hospitals. There is a strong case to be made for the visible and practical integration of the palliative care team into an oncology centre's staff to facilitate the change of focus from treatment of disease to symptom control and attention to the multiple factors that cause distress as the end of life approaches, even if death may still be months away (Kramer & Dwyer, 1989).

Similarly, for the care of patients in other parts of the acute hospital, an identifiable team should mean that eligible patients have the opportunity of referral, and should smooth the transition from the active treatment mode to a palliative approach for both staff and patients. Too often, palliative care practitioners are seen as being in opposition to the medical team whose main focus has been on disease reversal. Indeed, in their attitudes and their statements, palliative care workers sometimes give the impression that they are the ones who care for the person while everyone else is caught up in curing.

These attitudes, however they arise, can lead to misunderstanding and may deny the person who is ill another option for this stage of their care. Burucoa (1993) has identified several misconceptions about palliative care that may hinder referral, including a preoccupation with death, the removal of hope, limitation of further treatment and loss of control by the referring team.

Referral to palliative care also underlines the terminality of illness and necessitates open communication which may be difficult for the treating team. Resistance to making patients aware of palliative care services may be symptomatic of the problem staff can have in adjusting the focus of care for a particular person. If the role of a palliative care team is not understood and the referral is not made, direct discussion of the turning point may not occur and the person may be sent home with no more than a discharge letter to the family practitioner, without support mechanisms, and with poor understanding of the future. Referral should occur early, without the pressure of imminent discharge, allowing for a full assessment and appropriate ongoing referral to non-acute services.

The way in which the possibility of referral is raised with the person is often problematic because of the misconceptions that the practitioner or the patient may have about its implications. The referring doctor may give a very vague explanation of why this is recommended and give the person little choice or understanding of their options (Aranda, 1994; Turley, 1994). Open discussion with the patient about the positive aspects of involvement of palliative care practitioners is more likely to result in a smooth transition (Hyman & Bulkin, 1990). Rejection of palliative care referral is also a possibility and the challenge then is to ensure that the patient has access to appropriate support later if they should require it.

# Discharge planning

## *Assessment*

At the time of referral, a comprehensive assessment needs to be made so that the best options for future care can be determined and an appropriate plan developed. Questions which might form the basis of the assessment include:

- What understanding of the illness does the person and their family have? Have they been given adequate information?
- What symptom complexes are present and to what extent are they controlled by current measures? Does the medical information available explain them adequately or does more investigation need to be done?
- How rapidly is the situation changing? Are there issues that can be predicted to occur that should be considered now for care planning?
- What other elements of distress are present—emotional, social, spiritual? To what extent are these part of the normal adjustment process? Do any particular interventions need to be initiated or continued after discharge?

- What are the person's and the family's perceptions of their needs? What are their resources, practical, emotional, social, spiritual? Who is family? Who is at home during the day and at night?
- Is there a significant past history of abnormal grief or a psychiatric history in the person or in the family?
- How do the family communicate and share information?
- What additional resources should be offered?

This assessment may take considerable time, especially if the family is to be involved. Family meetings are often helpful to identify concerns, to clarify misconceptions and to negotiate jointly the care plan. The assessment process should take place in the context of the person's own cultural background, using appropriate interpreter services if needed.

If possible, there should be active participation in care planning by staff who have known the person over the course of the illness to ease the fear of abandonment, to act as a resource with further information, to be advocates for them in their new relationships with professionals and to facilitate acute readmission should this be required.

## Development of care plan

A critical focus will be on the location of future care, whether the person is to be discharged from an acute care setting to home, to an in-patient palliative care unit or hospice, or to another in-patient setting such as nursing home or local hospital. Factors involved in such a decision include:

- patient and family wishes;
- availability of potential carers;
- local community resources;
- proximity of in-patient facilities for visitors;
- expected prognosis;
- particular physical care needs;
- availability of professional support.

Many patients, but not all, express the wish to be in their own homes to the end of their lives, if they can be assured of the right assistance. Some will be relatively mobile and physically independent in most respects, and home would be the recommended option. If no carer is available, supervised accommodation with community monitoring by healthcare workers could be feasible. In-patient care may sometimes be the only alternative. Regardless of the decision made, planning should be flexible so that the patient and family are reassured that alternatives exist if care becomes too burdensome.

In some centres where there is not an established palliative care team, social workers have played a major role in discharge planning. They may understand the concepts of holistic palliative care and have detailed knowledge of resources, but are often hampered by a lack of understanding of the disease process, expected symptoms and prognosis (Weissman & Griffie, 1994). This limitation can lead to lack of clarity in management and planning goals, and it is always advisable for a full clinical assessment by experienced staff to be performed.

Healthcare workers always endeavour to ensure that the person is fully informed about what options are available and is able to decide on that basis. However, the speed with which some of these decisions need to be made may not allow for someone who is severely distressed to make necessary emotional adjustments and decisions before being discharged. In these circumstances, the need for continuing nursing supervision of the person's care may be used as a means of ensuring that the person is not sent home entirely unsupported, even if they do not yet acknowledge more multidimensional needs which a palliative care service could address. A nursing focus may be seen to provide a legitimate link to the care the person has received in hospital (Aranda, 1994). Community services called into the home may find that the person and the family seem unprepared for this transition (Aranda, 1994), increasing the importance of good liaison between all those involved in the patient's care.

## Preparing for discharge

While the medical and nursing members of the team develop the assessment, other team members, including occupational therapists, physiotherapists, dietitians, financial counsellors will begin to organise their services. These team members will be able to provide aids for daily living, education about care provision and financial counselling if required. While such interventions may require delays to discharge, the risk of acute readmission is reduced if the necessary support mechanisms are in place prior to discharge.

It is important for the hospital medical officer and/or palliative care team to make phone and written contact with the general practitioner and the community palliative care service to communicate the relevant immediate information which makes for a smooth transition of care.

## Continuity of care

In most cases, the transition from an active interventionist mode of treatment to a palliative approach, with focus on quality of life and symptom control, will involve a move from a hospital bed to care at another site or to care at home master-minded by the general practitioner and the community palliative care program.

Reassurance of the person/family at this time is particularly important to prevent a feeling of abandonment from a team of people they have come to trust. Various practical measures assist this, including having a member of the community palliative care program visit them before discharge if they are going home, arranging a visit to the hospice by the person and family prior to transfer, providing names and contact phone numbers of relevant care co-ordinators, and supplying brochures about the program or in-patient unit to which they have been referred.

It must be recognised that there may later need to be moves within the continuum of care, in any direction between the person's present place of residence, the acute hospital and the in-patient palliative care unit or hospice. As the person's illness continues, their needs and those of their family may be difficult to predict, and flexibility is needed to advise which options are in their best interests at a particular time. For these options to be accessible at short notice, up-to-date knowledge of the person's situation is required by members of the care network. Access to the acute hospital may be required for complications such as pleural effusion, fracture, or hypercalcaemia. There may also need to be a transfer from home to an in-patient palliative care unit or hospice for symptom control, for respite care, or for the last days of life.

Depending on the frequency of referrals from a particular hospital unit to a community palliative care service, a brief weekly report sheet on all the mutual patients may be exchanged with supplementary phone calls for more immediate changes. But many services rely on personal contact by phone because of the strong network which develops, particularly between the community and hospital nurses. It can be very reassuring to the person and the family to know that these interactions occur and that their specialist is kept well-informed and available for advice even if they are not actually seeing him.

It is similarly educative for the referring team members to receive feedback that their discharge planning has been effective or otherwise (Armitage, Kavanagh & Hayes, 1995) as well as encouraging for them to feel some contact with the person who is now out of their immediate care. Of great importance is the communication to all involved of the patient's death. While time-consuming, such communication helps to ensure appropriate contact with the family and allows long-term carers to acknowledge any sense of loss they may feel.

## Conclusion

Negotiation of the turning point between acute treatment and palliative care for the dying is a challenging task. Perhaps at the centre of this challenge is the necessity for good communication with the patient, family and all involved in the provision of care. The technological orientation of today's acute hospital and the funding formulae for healthcare services make it difficult to provide staffing levels to support such an approach. However, it is rewarding professionally when a team can recognise their contribution to meeting the needs of each individual patient and family.

# References

Anonymous (1983). Personal paper—Cancer care: the relative's view. *The Lancet*, 19 November.

Aranda, S. (1994). On the receiving end. *Journal of the University of Melbourne Medical Society*, 3 (3), 10–12.

Armitage, S.K., Kavanagh, K.M., & Hayes, L. (1995). An analysis of continuing care at the interface of hospital and community nursing services. *Study report*. Sydney: Faculty of Nursing, University of Sydney.

Burucoa, B. (1993). The pitfalls of palliative care. *Journal of Palliative Care, 9* (2), 29–32.

Dudgeon, D. (1992). Quality of life: a bridge between the biomedical and illness models of medicine and nursing? *Journal of Palliative Care, 8* (3), 14–17.

Faulkner, A., Maguire, P., & Regnard, C. (1994). Breaking bad news—A flow diagram. *Palliative Medicine, 8*, 145–151.

Fincannon, J.L. (1995). Analysis of psychiatric referrals and interventions in an oncology population. *Oncology Nursing Forum, 22* (1), 87–92.

Hanson, E. (1994). Psychological support at night. *Cancer Nursing, 17* (5), 379–384.

Hyman, R.B. & Bulkin, W. (1990). Physician reported incentives and disincentives for referring patients to hospice. *The Hospice Journal, 6* (4), 39–57.

Kerstetter, N.C. (1990). A stepwise approach to developing and maintaining an oncology multidisciplinary conference. *Cancer Nursing, 13* (4), 216–220.

Kramer, J.A. & Dwyer, B.E. (1989). Palliative care in the teaching hospital. *Cancer Forum, 13* (1), 4–7.

Maguire, P. (1985). Barriers to psychological care of the dying. *British Medical Journal, 291*, 1711–1713.

Prescott, P. & Bowen, S. (1985). Physician nurse relationship. *Annals of Internal Medicine, 103*, 127–133.

Schou, K.C. (1993). Dying in the cancer treatment setting. In Clark D. (ed.), The sociology of death: Theory, culture and practice (pp. 246–247). Oxford: Blackwell.

Turley, A. (1994). Managing continuity of care for clients. Unpublished M.Bus. thesis, School of Management, Swinburne University.

Weissman, D.E. & Griffie, J. (1994). The palliative care consultation service of the Medical College of Wisconsin. *Journal of Pain & Symptom Management, 9* (7), 474–479.

# 16

## Referral Issues

*Anne Turley*

The process of delivering palliative care to clients begins at referral. As Ruth Redpath (see chapter 15) has pointed out, the transition or referral to hospice palliative care is often described as shifting gears or changing the direction of care. Rarely do clients request a referral to hospice palliative care on their own initiative; most referrals are initiated by the care provider (Beresford, 1993), hopefully after thorough consultation with the client. Client need should be the basis of referral to palliative care.

In 1978, Cicely Saunders outlined three desirable attributes of palliative care; they were:

- continuity of care;
- continued liaison with clients' former doctors;
- a clear route back to the curative care system.

Achieving a smooth transition for clients between care settings, and facilitating continuity of care for clients across service providers form the essence of 'best referral practice' in palliative care.

In its 1996 report, the Victorian Department of Human Services suggests that in order to achieve continuity of care for clients, a triangle of care service model should be adopted. The triangle would include: community-based palliative care (provided in clients' own homes), an in-patient hospice palliative care unit, and acute hospital palliative care. Clients should, the department suggests, be able to move freely between these three settings according to their clinical and support needs (DHS, 1996).

Most referrals for palliative care in Australia come from acute hospitals. Ensuring continuity of care and holistic care provision for clients as they move from hospital to the community is an ongoing difficulty in palliative care. Therefore, this chapter seeks to explore the referral challenges confronting providers if continuity of care for clients and holistic care is to be achieved. It draws on comments made by clients and referral sources in two studies conducted by a community-based palliative care organisa-

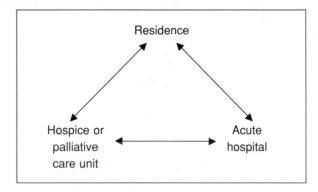

**Figure 16.1    Triangle of care service model**

tion. One study explored whether clients perceived that the care they received aligned with the philosophy of care espoused by the agency. The other study explored client and referral source understanding of the service, and whether clients knew their prognosis and the continuing nature of their care. It also asked clients and referral sources whether clients had been involved in the referral decision.

This chapter:

- draws attention to how the continuing tensions between two paradigms of service delivery affect client care;
- looks at problems surrounding prognosis-based admission and late referral;
- explores clients' perceptions of fragmented care and the ways that continuity of care is undermined;
- illustrates how a lack of collaborative teamwork can negatively affect client care;
- suggests some ways forward.

It acknowledges that all of us, whether health professional, patient or family member, view situations and frame our world in uniquely personal ways, influenced by our own life experience, cultural background, spiritual beliefs, relationships and formational training. This chapter too needs to be viewed as a personal, not a definitive way of seeing!

## Challenges in facilitating referrals

### Tensions between models of care

The whole person focus of palliative care stands in strong contrast to the biomedical or disease model of care for terminally ill people. While the biomedical model has been fundamental to the great strides made in understanding, categorising and treating disease, problems arise when it is used in clinical practice to the exclusion of humanistic considerations (Dugeon, 1992). The biomedical model leaves little or no room for the psychosocial and spiritual dimensions of illness. It encourages illness to be viewed in linear, cause-and-effect, concrete terms. It also encourages physicians to believe that disease pathology is more important than the illness the person is experiencing (Kleinman, 1988). The traditional medical paradigm of care for terminally ill people centres on curing the patient. Patients are most commonly cared for in the acute setting, separated from their significant others. Active treatment is frequently pursued up until death. Patients are given little information about what is happening to them and choices about care are predominantly made by the health professional.

The following client statement illustrates the tensions that exist between these two paradigms of care: 'You're just a number there (in the acute hospital) . . . not a person with a family or dreams or nothing, . . . they're not interested in all that sort of stuff' (Turley, 1994). The client perceived that caregivers in the acute setting were not interested in them in any way other than as a number or case to be treated. This comment unfortunately is not an isolated one. In recent studies carried out by Melbourne Citymission Hospice Service, clients often spoke of feeling powerless and frustrated within a system that viewed them as a case to be dealt with. They talked of the 'system' taking over and suddenly everyone else knew what was best for them. One woman, whose husband died, said

> it was hard to formulate the right questions to ask the health professionals . . . Formulation of questions . . . takes time and assumes knowlege of the right language . . . It requires people to be assertive in an environment that many find intimidating . . . I found it intimidating . . . I remained silent because I didn't want to take their valuable time, and in any case I didn't know how to put words to my questions.

Tensions between the biomedical disease model of care of terminally ill persons and the hospice model have been contrasted by Bortnowska (1991), who talks of the ethos of cure and the ethos of care. The ethos of cure encompasses military values like endurance, and not giving up. The ethos of care sees illness in the context of the person's spiritual, cultural and social realities. In curing, the physician is 'General', making most of the decisions regarding ongoing treatment, site of care, etc. In caring, the patient is 'sovereign', making their own choices about their ongoing care. The hospice paradigm shifts the power and control balance of care decisions to the client—away from the health professional. It radically changes the way care is delivered and how decisions are made. Whereas in the past, control of treatment and choices about care have predominantly been made by health professionals (Beckhard & Rubin, 1979)—with some clients handing over their independence and rights of self-determination to health professionals—the hospice palliative care paradigm requires that health professionals see the client as a whole person, within the context of their spiritual and cultural environment. It requires that clients be given information, the time to consider their options, and make choices about their future care and if possible the site of that care. Both studies referred to in this chapter found that clients had been provided with minimal information about the palliative care service they had been referred to (often having been told only that someone would visit them). Many felt that they had not been involved in the referral decision—they had been told what would happen. As a consequence, on admission to a palliative care service, many clients often appeared to be unaware of their prognosis, the nature of their continuing care, or the holistic multidisciplinary focus of the care team they had been referred to.

## *Prognosis-based referral*

Most palliative care services operate with a six-month prognosis criteria for referral and admission. In reality, most referrals are made much later than this. (Clients in the service referred to in this chapter had an average length of stay of 77 days.) Referral sources canvassed in recent studies (Hockley, 1991; Turley, 1994) indicated that clients had been told of their prognosis and the continuing focus for their care. They indicated that they were unsure, however, about what the clients had actually heard, as some clients appeared to comprehend only part of the message. Others appeared to reframe the information to make it more palatable, or manageable, and others denied they were told. A number of referral sources indicated that they found it extremely difficult to convey the news of terminal illness to clients in ways that did not shatter hope. Special attention needs to be paid to timing, the choice of language and how this information is communicated. Knowledge should not be forced inappropriately on the client just because they are leaving hospital or because of perceived needs on the part of service providers. Clients should be allowed the time and space to come to an awareness of their dying in their own time and way.

> I didn't even know he was going to die. I didn't know he was terminally ill . . . nobody said anything to me. I don't know whether they told him. He was a very private person and I think if we had had long to get used to it we would have talked about all this, in fact I know we would have . . . but we didn't really get to the stage of getting over the shock of it before he died. (Aranda, 1993)

This client indicated her wish that she and her husband had had more time to talk, to plan, to set their affairs in order, and to arrange for the well-being of family members. One can only guess at the reasons behind why this couple came to an awareness of his dying so late. This woman was obviously dissatisfied with the way communication of the situation was handled. Frequently, as with the couple above, clients are admitted for care in the last weeks of their or their loved one's life. The realisation of the terminal nature of the illness brings, for some, increased feelings of loss and grief and of being in crisis. In a limited time span, and with depleted emotional, spiritual and physical resources, clients often work against the clock to 'get their heads around' this new reality. For some, like this couple, the news or realistion came too late and the discussion never took place. Is there a better way to facilitate information dissemination and manage referral processes?

## Needs-based referral

A needs-based, rather than a prognosis-based referral may more appropriately meet the needs of all. For instance, at the time of diagnosis of a potentially terminal illness, the notion of palliative care and its philosophy could be introduced to clients along with other care options and treatments. As a result, clients would become aware of the full range of services available and the choices open to them. The services of the multidisciplinary palliative care team could be available earlier, assisting clients with the many spiritual, psychological and social adjustments they are confronted with as they assimilate news of a potentially terminal illness.

## Some ways in which continuity of care is undermined

'I'm really frightened, I felt safe in hospital. What will happen here if a I fall or mix up my pills . . .' (Turley, 1994)

Clients often feel uncertain and confused about how their continuing care needs will be met outside of the hospital. They may see discharge from hospital as desertion by health professionals they have trusted. Going home or to another care facility is like stepping into a frightening void. High levels of anxiety, distress and despair among these clients is reported. They need reassurance that they have not been discharged into a void and that their care will be facilitated across service providers through collaborative teamwork (Gomas, 1993; Doyle, 1993). Unfortunately, the only information many community-based palliative care services are given about clients at referral is their name, address, phone number, age and diagnosis. With these details comes a request to contact the client, and advice that the client has been or is about to be discharged. Such inadequate information and lack of discharge planning affects clients negatively, particularly those who are highly anxious. Community-based palliative care organisations then have no option but to start gathering information about the client's medical and social history from the beginning. This completely undermines the notion of continuity of care for clients across service settings.

Fortunately, the establishment of palliative care units within some acute hospitals has facilitated a smoother transition of palliative care clients across service settings.

In cases where a smooth transition has occurred, discharge planning has been done well.

- The continuing care needs of the client have been discussed with them.
- Information has been provided, options explored and decisions have been made about future care.
- The client is aware of the change in focus of care and what the community-based organisation or hospice palliative care unit can provide.
- Referral has been done well in advance of discharge from hospital and a full medical and social history has been received by the agency responsible for ongoing care.
- Appropriate communication links between the services have been established, and the client is aware of the links and how they work.

Twycross (1991) suggests that continuity of care cannot be done by individuals, only by individuals and/or agencies working together as a team. The composition of the team may vary, but includes the patient, the immediate family, friends, doctor(s), nurses, chaplain, counsellors, social workers and other allied health staff.

## *Barriers to collaborative teamwork*

'I'm confused, so many people have told me things, I don't remember half of it . . . I have no idea who you are or what you do . . . perhaps you can tell me.'(Turley, 1994)

By the time a client is referred to hospice palliative care, they will have been exposed to a wide variety of health professionals and multiple service providers. Hobbs (1993) describes one of his clients who had been seen by twenty health professionals from at least three healthcare services in the last episode of his care. His client, he said, was having difficulty understanding the interconnectedness (if any) of all of these services and activities. Too often, the professional thinks in terms of 'my patient', rather than 'our client'. Competition and boundary disputes undermine cohesive care for clients (O'Shannessy & Medenthorp, 1993). The notion of collaborative multidisciplinary teamwork within and across service settings grew out of a recognition that fragmented care does not meet the medical, social and psychosocial needs of individual clients. A collaborative multidisciplinary approach, using various professional disciplines each with their expertise, can more effectively meet the wide-ranging needs of clients than can any one discipline (Ducanis & Golin, 1978). A real advantage of collaborative practice, say Bloom and Parad (1976), is that it appears to enhance service effectiveness in general and continuity of care to patients in particular.

However, individuals trained in different disciplines do not become a team merely by calling themselves one. A system to effect collaboration must be specifically set up. If the basic format and structure is not clear to all members of the team, effective interaction and communication will not occur. Collaboration involves the sharing of goals, planning, problem-solving, decision-making and responsibility. Time to build an effective team must be allocated if collaborative teamwork, a sophisticated method of interaction that results in joint formulation of client care plans, is to work.

While the establishment of palliative care units in acute settings has eased some of the difficulties surrounding the transition of clients to other service settings, much more needs to be done if continuity of care is to be achieved for all clients.

## Some possible ways forward

### Appointment of liaison staff

Funding for and introduction of a liaison person from other palliative care settings into the acute palliative care setting when discharge and referral are being discussed may facilitate referrals of clients across service settings. The presence of both the referral source and the home-based care team members could help reassure clients that their continuity of care will be met. Liaison staff may also be able to meet clients in the general practitioner's rooms as a way of establishing clear links between the GP, client and the community-based palliative care service.

### Better teamwork

Expanding our understanding of 'team' to be inclusive of all participants in care provision may enhance collaboration across service providers for the benefit of clients. An awareness of how other disciplines and organisations work would need to be fostered over time. Opportunities for case-study reflection, educational seminars, joint project and research work, staff placement and exchanges, and social events could lay a helpful foundation for this process.

## Establishment of integrated care networks

Integrated or organised care delivery systems, which have been widely promoted recently, are organisations that provide, or arrange to provide, a co-ordinated continuum of services across service settings to a defined population of clients. The focus is client health and well-being, not illness. In order for integrated care networks to develop, a common vision and culture across various care settings and agencies must be established, and supersede local agency and institutional directions. Factors that promote integrated care across service settings are:

- a common vision of integrated service delivery and activities based on the goal of improving care delivered to patients and families;
- visionary leadership and the establishment of creative partnerships between clinicians, administrators, and funding bodies;
- team-building, opportunities that facilitate multidisciplinary team communication and understanding of other disciplines' expertise across service settings.

Integrated care networks are known to improve co-ordination of care and care outcomes, facilitate better communication among care providers, and provide increased patient and caregiver satisfaction (Porter et al., 1996).

## Conclusion

The establishment of palliative care units within acute settings has facilitated referrals of palliative care clients across service settings in recent years. However, if continuity of care is to be achieved for all clients, much more needs to be done. We need to advocate for clients, especially when the biomedical disease model of care overrides their holistic palliative care needs. Taking a more proactive approach when a potentially life-threatening illness is diagnosed and adopting a needs-based referral process may assist clients to feel more in control of their lives.

Understanding the unique expertise of other disciplines and organisations, and choosing a more inclusive approach within and between organisations may facilitate client care and best use of scarce resources. Finally, our referral practices and care provision must respond to the uniquely individual whole person needs of our clients. Our aim should be to provide our clients with cohesive care that facilitates their sense of dignity, right to self-determination and physical, spiritual, emotional and social well-being.

## References

Aranda, S. (1993). *What is the relationship between palliative care philosophy and care received by dying patients and their primary caregiver? A qualitative evaluation of the Melbourne Citymission Hospice Service.* Melbourne: Citymission Inc.

Beckhard, R. & Rubin, I.M. (1972). Factors influencing effectiveness of health teams. *Millbank Quarterly*, July.

Beresford, L. (1993). *The hospice handbook: A complete guide*. Boston: Little, Brown and Company.

Bloom, B.L. & Parad, H.J. (1976). Interdisciplinary training and interdisciplinary functioning: A survey of attitudes and practices in community mental health. *American Journal of Orthopsychiatry*, 46 (4), 669–675.

Bortnowska, H. (1991). Why palliative medicine? *Henry Ford Hospital Medical Journal*, 39.

Department of Human Services, Victoria (DHS) (1996). *Palliative care: The way forward*. Melbourne: DHS.

Doyle, D. (1993). *Oxford textbook of palliative medicine*. Oxford: Oxford University Press.

Ducanis, A.J. & Golin, A.K. (1979). *The interdisciplinary health care team*. Germantown, MD: University of Pittsburgh, Aspen Systems Corp.

Dugeon, D. (1992). Quality of life: A bridge between the biomedical and illness model of medicine and nursing. *Journal of Palliative Care*, 8, 14–17.

Gomas, J.M. (1993). Palliative care at home: A reality of mission impossible. *Palliative Medicine*, 7, 45–49.

Hobbs, R.N. (1993). Walk with me: Physician and patient stories and their role in palliative care education. *Journal of Palliative Care*, 9 (2), 41–46.

Hockley, J. (1991). *Role of the hospital support team*. Edinburgh: University of Edinburgh.

Kleinman, A. (1988). *The illness narrative: Suffering, healing and the human condition*. New York: Basic Books.

O'Shannessy, D. & Medenthorp, J. (1993). C.O.P.D. and hospice: Collaboration or conflict. *American Journal of Hospice and Palliative Care*, Nov./Dec.

Porter, A.L., Van Cleave, B.L., Milobowski, L.A., Conlon, P.F., & Mambourg, P.D. (1996). Clinical integration. *Nursing Administration Quarterly*, 20 (2), 65–73.

Saunders, C. (1978). Hospice care. *American Journal of Medicine*, 65, 726–728.

Turley, A. (1994). *Managing continuity of care for clients across service providers*. Melbourne: Melbourne Citymission Inc.

Twycross, R. (1991). Why palliative medicine? *Henry Ford Hospital Medical Journal*, 39.

# 17

# Expertise in Palliative Care Nursing: A Nursing View of the Generalist/Specialist Debate

## Susan Lee

Palliative care and the hospice movement were born out of the realisation that the care of dying patients in an increasingly technological and 'cure' centred environment was inadequate. In 1980, Wald, Foster and Wald cautioned that for the philosophy of hospice to survive in healthcare, a balance needed to be maintained between the ideals of palliative care and the economic realities of the system. In the past, the debate between models of palliative care has centred on whether the generalist or the specialist model can better fulfil the ideal of palliative care practice. Of course, this issue is entirely 'academic' if the model cannot be funded. The debate about palliative care should more appropriately question how the ideals of palliative care are promulgated in a range of environments and should also question the development of the science of palliative care.

This chapter explores the background to the palliative care practice model debate. It discusses some insights into the development of specialisation in nursing and the development of palliative care as a discipline.

## The ideals of hospice and palliative care

In the early 1980s when the development of palliative care in Australia was in its infancy, a medical colleague suggested during an open discussion that there was no need for a palliative care movement; that if 'we did our jobs properly' (in the education of health practitioners), dying patients would be well cared for. Intuitively, most healthcare practitioners might agree with the doctor who stated this. We would reasonably expect every caring health professional to uphold the principles of palliative care. These principles are underpinned by standards for treating patients' psychological and spiritual as well as physical needs; for offering family-centred care; for encouraging involvement in decision-making; for fostering autonomy and standards for relief when cure is not possible. These are standards for holistic care that ought to be a part of good practice in any setting and by any healthcare practitioner.

There is a clear danger in oversimplifying the issue of specialisation by shifting the responsibility of the provision of quality palliative care onto all healthcare practitioners, who already struggle to cope with the information explosion in healthcare. To suggest that palliative care simply requires caring healthcare professionals who are able to frame their care holistically, with sensitivity to the human condition and without a focus on curing illness, is problematic on at least two counts. First, this suggestion assumes that prior to the introduction of palliative care organisations, the problems regarding care, as experienced by people who were dying, were due primarily to a lack of education about holistic care. Since the concept of holism has been featured in nursing literature over the past 20 years, this is clearly not the case. Second, it ignores the complexity of the problems that people and their families face at the end of life. Though it would not be unreasonable to demand that all healthcare professionals care sensitively and holistically for the needs of the dying, clients are likely to require quite unusual interventions and resources. Since specialisation is a reality of modern healthcare, the demand that all healthcare practitioners be experts in palliative care is unrealistic.

## The great 'best practice model' debate

Historically, community palliative care in Australia developed to meet a need. People in the community who were dying needed to be cared for with more sensitivity than the healthcare service provided. The type of organisation that developed in a particular community depended on many factors, such as the population and geographical area, current healthcare service interest and commitment to palliative care, available expertise and funding. Communities aimed to develop services that would most effectively meet the unique needs of their area. In-patient palliative care service is currently developing in a similar way, evidenced by the multiple models of practice.

Nursing services in community palliative care organisations can be provided in two major ways, depending on many of these developmental factors. Palliative care nursing services can be provided by generalist nurses who work with many patients, some of whom are palliative care patients. Alternatively, palliative care nursing services can be provided by nurses who work only with palliative care patients. In either situation, the nurses have varying degrees of expertise in palliative care and ideally ought to be supervised by an expert palliative care nurse. Such supervision occurs in most organisations and recognises the need for the maintenance of palliative care standards as identified by the Australian Association for Hospice and Palliative Care (1984).

Each model has particular difficulty in providing palliative care of a high standard (Wade & Moyer, 1989). The rivalry between those who advocate the generalist model and those who advocate the specialist model can often be traced to the way an individual palliative care service has developed. Some generalist community nurses complain that the specialist services have ignored their long history of dealing with dying patients in the community and have taken over some of their most satisfying work. They have expressed concern about the ability of specialist services to provide adequate 24-hour services, and about how expensive specialist services are. Specialist services complain about the lack of expert symptom control available in generalist services and about the lack of multidisciplinary support and communication.

Whether a particular model continues to meet the needs of its clients and community must be rationally and deliberately evaluated, not supposed, or cursorily rejected on the basis of superficial comparison. Comparing one model to another could result in very narrow conclusions based on standards of practice and economic measures. Such conclusions may lead to a choice of one model over another while failing to recognise that both models have advantages in education and in practice. An oversimplified comparison of models will do little to foster the development of excellence in palliative care practice, particularly in nursing.

## The need for specialisation in palliative care

In palliative care, the care of clients (patients and families) is based on their needs. One argument for specialisation in palliative care is that it is in the interests of clients. According to the Naylor and Brooten (1993), the benefits of clinical nurse specialists on patient and family outcomes, in a range of clinical practice areas, included reduced hospitalisation times and improved family abilities in self-care. Naylor and Brooten also report on a 1989 study by McCorkle, which investigated the use of oncological clinical nurse specialists in home care services (though not in palliative care) and noted that 'the group that received home care by an oncological CNS [clinical nurse specialists] had fewer hospital admissions for symptoms and complications associated with malignancy' (Naylor & Brooten, 1993, p. 76). A palliative care nurse specialist ought to provide specialised knowledge of symptom control and support to families and, as it is specialised, that care should result in similar advantages in an improved ability to manage symptoms and in the choice to stay at home.

However, an underlying assumption here is that specialisation in palliative care is equivalent to or synonymous with expertise in palliative care, and that expert care can be provided only in a specialist environment. In generalist organisations, the clinical nurse specialists would provide consultation on cases within their sphere of expertise. Naylor and Brooten also note the clinical nurse specialist's skills in teaching, in assisting novice or inexperienced nurses develop, in research and evaluation, and stress the 'ability of the CNS to build teams, influence changes in the system and monitor practices and outcomes' (Naylor & Brooten, 1993, p. 74). As the nurse specialist's role develops and leadership expands, he or she is less likely to provide direct care.

If we were to agree that palliative care nursing involves maximising the autonomy of a person who is dying, and agree that this can be achieved by: the ability to recognise and provide care for a range of the physical and non-physical needs of patients and families; providing vigilant, accurate and superior symptom control; communicating with openness, sensitivity and honesty; and working as an effective member of a multidisciplinary team; then we might come some way in being able to describe an expert in palliative care nursing. But the expert palliative care nurse is not simply a palliative care nurse who manages care of dying patients and their families well. In all care environments, expert palliative care nurses would surely be expected to be able to teach others the skills of palliative care nursing, or to use Patricia Benner's term, to 'coach' (Benner, 1984, p. 46) those less expert in the art of palliative care. Such an expert should also be active in the development of policy and direction in palliative care by monitoring and evaluating palliative care practice. In short, an expert palliative care nurse has expertise in the provision of palliative care and must also be able to provide the same sort of leadership in palliative care nursing that would be expected of a palliative care clinical nurse specialist. Whether the organisational context is generalist or specialist is irrelevant to the expectation of palliative care expertise and leadership from nurses who are expert in palliative care.

The assertion thus far is that specialisation and expertise in palliative care are forms of excellence in palliative care, and that patients benefit from expert palliative care nursing. My interest is not only in how nurses develop that expertise, but also in the development of palliative care as a discipline of excellence.

## The development of palliative care practice

Palliative care as a discipline of nursing will develop as a result of critical reflection on practice, and as a result of education and research.

Reflection on practice is a technique now fostered in education as a valuable method of learning that has been used for generations of nurses as a way of understanding and improving the work of nursing (Benner, 1984). The process of critical reflection can be an internal inclination to review a significant practice event in the mind, analysing the players, their motivations, actions and the outcomes and also attempting to review possible alternative actions and outcomes. Critical reflection can be enhanced by externalising the review in writing, particularly in journalling. Once the experience is written down, often with the passion that accompanied it, the writer can examine the event with a little more distance and reflection can be a richer exploration of the possibilities.

Reflecting on practice is also enhanced by discussing experiences with others. The 'tea room' and 'handover' are common times when this type of reflection occurs. It is informal and involves telling the story of the significant event and the outcomes. In sharing the event, the story-teller expresses their concerns and the other offers support and their own experiences. In this way, there is an opportunity for informal mentorship and support whereby learning occurs through the exploration of each others' experiences.

Reflecting on practice is a valuable learning tool and can be fostered by organisations as part of staff development. In palliative care such reflection can be encouraged in team meetings. What can be learned from these episodes of reflection is enhanced by the presence of nurses with varying levels of expertise who can share their insights into the situation being explored and test their understanding by the knowledge of others. Such reflection often leads to the sharing of literature and the resources of other members of the team. Gaps in the development of the discipline of palliative care can be identified as areas for further research. In this way, reflecting on practice develops practice in the workplace and links practice to education and research.

## Education

Education in palliative care is also essential in the development of expertise in the specialty. Many leaders in palliative care, particularly in the United Kingdom, have researched and written on educational curricula for palliative care workers (Jeffery, 1994; Copp, 1994). Some of their suggestions are for education in symptom control; bereavement care; communication and team skills; complementary therapies; social, cultural and spiritual aspects of care; and care for particular groups of patients such as children. Gina Copp (1994) has reviewed research on death education for nurses and concluded that reflection on practice as a method of education is a powerful factor in nurses learning about their own practice. She cites two studies that demonstrated that 'the use of didactic methods of teaching were less effective than experiential approaches' (Copp, 1994, p. 554).

As an educator, I have found that relating practice experiences to the theory that I wish students to grasp creates a dynamic learning environment. Students begin to examine their own practice experiences and analyse their actual and potential actions in the light of new knowledge and past experiences. Clinical learning environments become a focus of learning in nursing, a forum for the students to gather experiences from observing expert nurses in practice and also from their own patient contact.

## Research

The body of knowledge of a discipline of nursing has been described by Carper (1978) as consisting of four patterns of knowing: ethical knowledge, aesthetics, personal knowledge and empirical knowledge. In palliative care, nursing practice has, to date, developed through the exploration of ethical and personal knowledge and aesthetics, but not through empirical knowledge. Nursing practices have developed in palliative care based on an attempt to understand and value the lived experience of dying as an aesthetic value, to foster a more just healthcare environment that advocates for patient choices and builds on the experience of nurses in a range of healthcare environments. The body of knowledge developed in palliative care is incomplete and distorted without a scientific basis for practice, without a testing of the empirical evidence of excellence in nursing care (Kristjanson, 1996).

Expert specialty practice also develops through research. Through research, theories may be tested and new practices formulated. In palliative care, the research road has been slow to develop. There are many possible reasons for this. In nursing, much of the palliative care that we do is extremely difficult to articulate—for example, the work related to 'being with' a patient. With the development of higher education programs for palliative care nurses in Australia and with greater federal and community funding, empirical research in palliative care is a new commitment. Because some palliative care nurses have developed their research skills in academic programs and because palliative care organisations need to be able to justify the funding they receive through program evaluation, there are new opportunities for research.

For research in palliative care to contribute to excellence in practice though, the research questions in palliative care must be developed through and as a result of palliative care practice, including patient care. The research must therefore involve palliative care practitioners as more than just participants in research—they must also be the generators of research. It is palliative care nurses who, through their reflections on nursing care, will identify the significant gaps in practice knowledge that need to be researched. As in education, research is linked to the practice environment.

## Environmental conditions for the development of excellence

In order to encourage the development of palliative care, there are certain conditions in the patient care environment that organisations need to foster.

Since expert nurses function in part to assist the development of inexperienced or novice nurses, organisations which provide palliative care ought to be committed to the employment of expert palliative care nurses who function in this role. Each member of a successful healthcare team brings particular skills to the group. Skill in clinical leadership—as well as financial management—are necessary in a healthcare team, and nurses who can provide that clinical leadership are essential. The organisation must ensure that clinical leadership is expected of these nurses, by describing and funding their jobs appropriately. The palliative care standards as developed by the Australian Association for Hospice and Palliative Care (1984, especially standards 5 and 7) highlight the significance of the community education and research role of palliative care organisations. Palliative care nurses, therefore, have a collective responsibility for the development of the specialty and a duty to share their expertise with novices, participate in palliative care educational programs, and actively engage in and foster research programs in palliative care nursing.

Because education and research are interwoven in practice issues, models of practice cannot be ignored in a discussion about the environmental conditions for palliative care excellence. Involvement of specialist nurses improves patient care outcomes, which supports the employment of these specialists, but this is a message not only for organisations working in the generalist model. All organisations are tempted to reduce expertise in lean financial times. Nevertheless, it must be recognised that, for a specialty to survive and develop in a generalist organisation, a commitment to it must be fostered despite competing interests from other specialties.

Organisations must also acknowledge that specialist development will also occur with greater ease and more quickly in a focused, single specialty work environment. After all, during any period, a nurse working in a specialist environment will see more patients who are dying than one in a generalist environment. A larger volume of cases will enable the nurse to 'work through' the process of reflection and change over a shorter period. The recognition of patterns of practice that leads to the generation of research questions is more likely to emerge when people are working within a specialist framework.

By collaborating on the development of palliative care specialisation, the specialist organisation should become a resource for the generalist service both for the education of staff and for the dissemination of new knowledge. As a component of educational programs, generalist nurses who wish to develop palliative care expertise ought to be able to attend a specialist service and work alongside specialists to develop skills and observe 'best practice' examples. Specialist nurses within generalist organisations ought to be able to seek professional support and advice through the formal special interest groups as well as through informal support networking involving specialist and generalist services. Through participation in these education initiatives, specialist services gain insight into further educational needs in the nursing profession and into research questions. The practice in the generalist service is improved by the new understandings and successes in care being shared and by knowledge about skilled palliative care being passed on to other generalist nurses in the organisation.

If only specialist palliative care organisations are maintained or if they are isolated from a region's general services, the propagation of the ideals of palliative care into mainstream healthcare may be seriously jeopardised. This danger was recognised by Layzell and McCarthy (1993), who found that specialist HIV/AIDS teams in the United Kingdom acted in some areas as a disincentive to general nurses becoming involved with the care of these clients. The overall level of competence in the care of patients with these special needs will not improve if nurses are only required to refer to another service rather than seeking knowledge to provide the care under some sort of specialist guidance. Similarly, in the United States, Sloan (1992) expressed concern about the lack of diffusion of the hospice concept through urban areas where specialist hospice services operated. The generalist model for palliative care provision, with specialist support, provides an environment for the dissemination of the ideals of palliative care through a population of nurses who might otherwise not have sought such knowledge. In engaging in palliative care practice while supported by specialists, generalists are challenged by the questions left unanswered and buoyed by their successes. From this pool of enlightened and curious nurses, future palliative care specialists are drawn, attracted by their experiences in a generalist environment.

While specialist palliative care service may showcase palliative care for the development of the discipline, generalist services may be the only way palliative care can be provided to all the citizens who require it. One of the concerns noted earlier was about the best way of meeting patient need: if a generalist service will meet more needs and quality can be assured through the support of palliative care specialists, then this must be examined as a viable model. A generalist organisation cannot provide for the development of excellence in specialist practice in isolation; in order to maintain and develop quality palliative care practice, it will need to collaborate with specialist services.

## Conclusion

The clear message from this discussion about models of practice in palliative care is that the development of excellence in palliative care nursing will be fostered by a commitment to the practice of palliative care. The question of whether one model or another can provide better patient care has not been addressed here, for pursuing it is of doubtful value. Specialist and generalist organisations should not be competitors in a race to provide better service to clients. Specialist organisations have the capacity to drive palliative care evolution in specific skill development and research. Correspondingly, if committed to the development of excellence in palliative care, an organisation that provides service through generalist nurses reaches a greater number of clients and has the capacity to inspire and advance the cause of palliative care to a large proportion of the nursing population. While specialist services are critical for the development of palliative care through education and research, generalist services are the tools by which we can spread that knowledge through the profession. By collaborating with specialist organisations, generalist organisations may utilise that focused environment to develop their own staff, and thus together they will increase the pool of knowledge and foster excellence in palliative care in a variety of care environments.

## References

Australian Association for Hospice and Palliative Care Inc. (1984). *Standards for hospice and palliative care provision*. Perth, WA.

Benner, P. (1984). *From novice to expert: Excellence and power in clinical nursing*. Menlo Park, California: Addison-Wesley.

Carper, B.A. (1978). Fundamental patterns of knowing in nursing. *Advanced Nursing Science, 1*, 13–23.

Copp, G. (1994). Palliative care nursing education: A review of research findings. *Journal of Advanced Nursing, 19*, 552–557.

Jeffery, D. (1994). Education in palliative care: A qualitative evaluation of the present state and the needs of general practitioners and community nurses. *European Journal of Cancer Care, 3*, 67–74.

Kristjanson, L. (1996). Research in palliative care seminar. Unpublished. Monash University, Melbourne.

Layzell, S. & McCarthy, M. (1993). Specialist or generic community nursing care for HIV/AIDS patients. *Journal of Advanced Nursing, 18*, 531–537.

Naylor, M. & Brooten, D. (1993). The roles and functions of clinical nurse specialists. *IMAGE: Journal of Nursing Scholarship, 25* (1) (Spring), 73–78.

Sloan, S. (1992). The hospice movement: A study in the diffusion of innovative care. *American Journal of Hospice and Palliative Care*, May/June, 24–29.

Wade, B. & Moyer, A. (1989). An evaluation of clinical nurse specialists: Implications for education and organisation of care. *Senior Nurse, 19* (9) (October), 11–16.

Wald, F., Foster, Z., & Wald, H. (1980). The hospice movement as a healthcare reform. *Nursing Outlook*, March, 173–178.

# 18

## The Role of the Nurse Consultant in the Acute Hospital Setting

### Kate White

> It is now very important we guard against a viewpoint which sees
> the hospices as the sole repository of good practice in terminal care.
> Learning and skills have been disseminated from the hospices into
> wider settings and there are indications of palliative care being
> taken more seriously in general hospitals and in the community.
> It is this triad of services that should be the focus of
> attention . . . (Clarke, 1993, p. 176)

Little is written about palliative care in the acute hospital setting, and even less on the role of the palliative care nurse consultant (PCNC) in this arena. This is not surprising given the emphasis placed on community and hospice settings as the ideal environments for the palliative care patient. Is there a need, as suggested in Clarke's (1993) quote, for palliative care in the acute hospital? Can hospitals provide good palliative care? This chapter will describe the role of the PCNC in the acute setting.

## Reasons for palliative care services in the hospital setting

Hospital-based palliative care nurse consultant positions developed through a recognition that the acute hospital is a frequent site of death, that palliative care is not restricted to cancer care and that most palliative care is initiated in the acute setting.

Despite the growth of home and in-patient hospice services, patients continue to die in acute hospitals. In Australia 60 per cent of deaths due to breast cancer (Coates, Day, McCredie & Taylor, 1992), 100 per cent of deaths due to leukaemia (Maddocks, Bentley & Sheedy, 1994) and 58 per cent of deaths due to colorectal cancer (Woo, Mann, Stewart, Dent, Chapus & Bokey, 1991) occur in an acute hospital. These patients require the same skilled care and symptom control provided by palliative care services in other settings.

218

The focus of palliative care services has primarily been patients with cancer, yet patients with other incurable and progressive illnesses can benefit from these services (O'Neal, 1989). Patients who die of diseases other than cancer are more likely to be cared for in the acute hospital setting and provide a challenge for the nurse trained to provide care aimed at cure. Difficulties in predicting prognosis in these diseases may preclude admission to home-based palliative care or hospices. Additionally, the needs of the terminally ill geriatric population in relation to symptom control and prolonged palliative care have been identified (Wilson, Lawson & Smith, 1987; Blackburn, 1989), and these patients are often not considered candidates for hospice care (O'Neal, 1989).

Integration of palliative care into mainstream services facilitates earlier access to appropriate support services, and optimal symptom control. The model for integration adopted by the World Health Organization (WHO) (1990) encourages palliative care services to be seen as a continuum of care that can be implemented at any stage in the patient's illness, not just in the terminal phase. This not only facilitates improved access to symptom control, but also gives the patient a sense of continuity in the ongoing management of their disease and related symptoms (Dunlop & Hockley, 1990; Expert Panel on Palliative Care, 1991; MacDonald, 1992). Services therefore need to be located at the acute hospital where the patient receives their primary treatment. Experienced palliative care nurses are essential to the provision of palliative care in the hospital setting.

## Key functions of the role

While the PCNC role can be developed in a number of ways, certain functions are common to all. The clinical nurse consultant has been described as an 'expert practitioner who provides a . . . consultancy service to health care providers', which includes acting as a resource person, providing a clinical service, education, and research in the area of speciality (Wentworth Area Health Service, 1993). Each of these aspects is an essential component of being an agent of change and in challenging the belief that palliative care can only be provided in specialised units to people at the end of life. The key aspects of the role are described below, with some brief journal excerpts that help to illustrate the daily practice of the PCNC in the acute hospital. Most aspects of the role are premised on the PCNC's symptom management and interpersonal communication skills and knowledge.

## Being a resource to others

Unlike nurses with direct care roles, the PCNC achieves patient goals through others and thus support and education of unit staff is a major focus. The support and education of staff occurs formally and informally, and relies significantly on the relationships that have been fostered in role development. It is important that the PCNC does not undermine the skill and knowledge of other nurses while developing this specialist role within the hospital.

At times it is important that the PCNC function as an independent practitioner. This independence underpins a professional role that is focused on the palliative care needs of the patient and is outside of usual ward dynamics. Specifically, independence helps the PCNC to undertake a role as advocate for ward nurses in improving the palliative care of the patients in their care, as illustrated in this excerpt from the reflective journal kept by a hospital PCNC:

> Today I was approached by nursing staff who expressed concern about planned investigations for a patient on the ward who is unconscious and appears to be imminently dying. Their requests to cancel the procedure to junior medical staff have been unsuccessful. The nursing staff were angry, frustrated and distressed, believing it highly likely the patient would die during the investigation. I reviewed the patient and agreed that the patient was close to death. Then I reviewed the case notes, and contacted the registrar, but despite a lengthy discussion, the registrar did not believe he had the authority to cancel the investigation. I contacted the medical consultant, explained the situation, the concerns of the nursing staff, and requested clinical review of the patient prior to investigation. The investigation was cancelled by the consultant after this review. This incident was followed by a discussion between nursing unit manager, medical consultant and nursing staff where concerns about communication were discussed. This situation was resolved without further conflict, the medical consultant being sensitive to the nurses' concerns both about the patient and the lack of clinical review. I discussed with the staff avenues that are open to them to help resolve conflict over treatment. The patient died peacefully five hours later.

The PCNC helps staff to explore the issues that cause them distress. Informal support through one-on-one contact with nurses appears to be very effective; therefore, location within the hospital and a high level of visibility on the wards are both essential. Conversations are most likely to occur in a relaxed atmosphere—staff need to feel that they are safe, listened to with appropriate responses, and that their concerns will be treated confidentially. It is important for the PCNC to be perceived as both knowledgeable and approachable. The PCNC should be a resource person to provide support, guidance and education, not seen simply as someone who has come in to take over the care.

Calls for support can come at inopportune times and from areas not traditionally associated with palliative care, offering exciting opportunities to extend palliative care skills. To meet these calls for support, the

PCNC needs to be flexible and prepared for a working day that lacks predictability.

> During lunch I am paged by a nurse from the intensive care unit. These calls always fill me with dread as there is no way of knowing what to expect. Today the nursing staff are concerned about the decision to withdraw treatment from a patient. This 34-year-old woman has been with them for several weeks, is conscious but unable to survive without life support, and has a rapidly progressive incurable neurological condition. The decision to withdraw treatment has been made by the patient and family, but the nursing staff are finding it very difficult. I arrange to visit the unit during handover to talk with the staff. I always feel very out of place in the ICU, all those alarms and machines. The meeting with the staff is but a prelude to what will be several meetings, as they grapple with their concerns about the morality and ethics of the decision that has been made, and the unusual experience of caring for a conscious patient, whom they have come to know and who is close to them in age. An intensive care unit is perhaps seen as a strange place for a palliative care nurse, but after initially helping the nurses with some difficult cases of 'constipation', and giving in-service lectures on acute grief and bereavement, I have received increasing requests for involvement and support. . . . [While these requests] may not fit the picture of mainstream palliative care, it is rare that I am unable to use the skills I gained as a palliative care nurse to help.

## Counselling

Referrals are not always made because of physical symptoms and as palliative care becomes accepted, referrals to provide emotional support or to assist in the care of 'difficult or stressful' patients increase. Early rather than late referrals are more common when the PCNC role is accepted and leads to increasing involvement in family conferences, particularly around the delivery of bad news.

> Today an immunology consultant asks me to see a new patient and get to know the family as things are 'starting to look like they are not going well'. I also arrange and attend a family conference for another patient with the medical team as there was a lack of understanding about the aim of treatment and likely outcome.

A considerable amount of time may be spent with the patient and family listening, clarifying and answering questions regarding treatment and disease. Various studies indicate that communication with patients is a major area of deficit (Audit Commission, 1993; Buckman, 1987; Glasser & Struass, 1965; Maguire, 1985; Wilkinson, 1991); therefore the PCNC must have excellent communications skills in order to model these for other hospital staff.

## Specialist knowledge

The PCNC must have expert knowledge and skills to be able to care effectively for the palliative care patient, and to provide both informal and formal education to staff in the acute hospital. Acceptance of the PCNC's role is strongly linked with having credibility and a presence within the hospital that is recognised by a wide range of professionals. Time is a major factor in establishing a presence; however, confidence in the nurse's knowledge and skills plays a significant role. Expertise includes the use of effective communications skills, which facilitate liaison with different disciplines and speciality areas, and leads to an increased ability to be a troubleshooter. The complexity of daily practice is illustrated by these journal excerpts.

> During the round my page goes off on three occasions: a community nurse with concerns about a patient discharged two weeks ago, who may require readmission; a nursing unit manager with a query about a patient's morphine dose as the patient is having a procedure and is nil by mouth (despite documentation in patient's notes and order on drug chart for morphine to be given)—this query is answered with detailed explanation; and the third is a request for review of patient on haematology ward due to increasing pain.
>
> After completing the ward round I review the patient in the haematology unit. Then, after discussion with the patient, a new pain management plan is determined and discussed with medical and nursing staff. An arrangement is made for me to review the patient in the afternoon. I meet with the nursing unit manager in the main oncology ward to discuss concerns nursing staff have in relation to several patients in this unit.
>
> Next, I contact community nurses to arrange a patient's discharge in a few days. I arrange home oxygen, and contact the patient's GP. I meet with the patient's wife to go over discharge requirements and support services she may require. I explain the patient's medications with both the patient and his wife. She remains reluctant to allow community nurses from the local hospice to become involved, but has agreed to let the generalist community nurses visit.

## Discharge planning

A major role of the PCNC is the assessment and streamlining of the palliative care patient's discharge. The addition to the team of a PCNC can significantly increase the number of patients discharged home. Medical staff may be less likely to encourage home discharge, unaware of resources available, and concerned that practical care could not be delivered outside the institutional environment. Discharge planning requires skill and knowledge of community resources, and education for the patient and carer. While this can be a time-consuming and complicated task, when it achieves the patient's goal it is rewarding.

# Education

There is considerable evidence that nurses feel inadequately prepared to care for patients who are dying (Benoleil, 1985; Hamric, 1977; Lev, 1986; Rutman & Parke,1991). Nurses who infrequently care for dying patients are more likely to experience feelings of inadequacy, as they have had little opportunity to gain confidence and knowledge in this important clinical area. The PCNC helps provide education to the patient and family, and staff, gradually increasing confidence and transferring more of the direct care role to the ward nurse.

Staff education is achieved in a variety of ways, including role modelling, mentoring, and formal and informal education. Regular in-service lectures on specific topics provides education and an opportunity for staff to raise issues of concern. Developing expertise at ward level has the distinct advantage of providing improved care, and extra resources for other staff. It is extremely rewarding when ward nurses elect to continue their education in this area by undertaking formal studies in palliative care.

> Following lunch, I give an in-service lecture on pain management to staff on a surgical ward. There is much discussion about nurses' concerns about patients being under-medicated in relation to pain. Ways to overcome nursing and medical reluctance to administer appropriate analgesics are discussed. At these sessions, it is important to move the focus away from solely blaming the medical staff, and explore with the nurses their own hesitancy to administer opioid medications, reasons for this, and other methods they can use to help alleviate pain and distress. Encouraging nurses to move away from a model that is dependent solely on pharmaceutical approaches remains a challenge.

Pain and symptom management is crucial in ensuring patient comfort. While nurses frequently berate medical staff for their lack of knowledge, research has shown nurses may also lack knowledge and skills (Donavon & Dillon, 1987; Hamilton & Edgar, 1992; McCaffery, Ferrell, O'Neil-Page, Lester & Ferrell, 1990; Myers, 1985; O'Brien, Dalton, Konsler & Carlson, 1996; Rankin & Snyder, 1984). The importance of the educative role of the acute hospital PCNC in this area cannot be underestimated (Hockley, 1988; Whedon, Shedd & Summers, 1992).

# Research

An area of increasing importance in the PCNC's role is research. For many nurses, limited time and lack of research experience makes this a difficult endeavour. As experience in undertaking research in the area of palliative care increases and more nurses attain research degrees, the volume and quality of research will increase. With the development of tertiary-based courses in palliative care nursing the opportunities for collaborative research with academics has grown. This provides an avenue for cross-fertilisation of ideas and skills, with benefits to both the clinical and the academic nurse, and to patient outcomes.

## Developing the role

The PCNC role develops over time with success linked to both the skills of the individual nurse and the effort taken to integrate the role within the hospital. The new PCNC may arrive full of enthusiasm and commitment, only to experience frustration when few referrals are received and hospital staff appear hostile. Change often occurs slowly within the healthcare system and avenues for gradually establishing the position and creating a profile need to be explored.

The role development occurs within the context of the palliative care team. Team structure will be determined in part by the setting and the nature of the client group. In large metropolitan hospitals, the nurse will be part of a small palliative care team, perhaps consisting only of the PCNC, a consultant PC physician and a trainee registrar. Regardless of the team structure, good communication helps to present the service as an integrated whole to the hospital, thus ensuring the success of the service. Detailed team meetings and daily informal discussion determine the patient visits, which team members are to attend ward rounds in key clinical areas and so on. Team members also conduct in-service education and attend local palliative care meetings. This regular communication ensures that everyone is up to date with patient progress and can therefore respond appropriately when the need arises.

The first step in role development is to gain acceptance by clinical units. Acceptance facilitates early referral and the involvement of the palliative care team in patient management. Ward rounds are an important aspect of this and a common setting for referrals. The round also provides an opportunity to review current care with the care team, discuss issues related to treatment plans and what is happening for the patient, to plan discharge arrangements and raise other areas of concern. This process helps create a collegial and collaborative approach to patient care, with mutual respect for the skills and expertise that different disciplines and specialities provide.

Collaboration between speciality areas and disciplines has a direct benefit for the patient and family by streamlining care and ensuring optimal symptom control. It also helps to establish and facilitate acceptance of the PCNC. A further advantage is that education in relation to palliative care occurs informally during the round, with advice and suggestions regarding patient management being made without formal referral.

Involving ward nurses in the decisions made about patient care, ensuring they have a clear understanding of treatments to be implemented and the rationale for these, is not only vital for patient care and an important approach to teaching, but ensures a team approach to the patient's care. For acceptance of the PCNC to be complete, she/he must be perceived by the ward nurses as a member of the ward nursing team, with shared goals.

## Issues affecting the role

Acceptance of the role of the PCNC is necessary to the effective functioning of this position. This acceptance requires consistent administrative commitment, integration within the hospital structure, resolution of role conflict and territorialism, and acceptance of the concept of 'nurse to nurse' referrals.

Without formal and continuing support from hospital administration, there is the potential for many problems, including a yearly battle to maintain funding. There is a possible perception that palliative care patients are more likely to have prolonged hospital stays, could be transferred to a hospice, and that palliative care is a 'frill' the hospital can no longer afford.

Commitment is essential not only for funding of clinical positions, but also for resourcing these positions adequately with office space, located close to ward areas, secretarial support, computer equipment, and a fund to purchase specialised equipment such as special mattresses.

A key to the success of any service is integration within existing hospital services. If the palliative care service is perceived to be in competition with existing services or departments, then there is the potential for conflict and role confusion. The World Health Organization (1990) argues for a model where the palliative care service is an integrated component of any cancer centre, and there are advantages for this approach. Not every hospital will have a cancer centre, however, and the PCNC will provide care for patients with other diseases. Of greatest importance is acceptance of the PCNC as part of the hospital staff, with a commitment to the institution and to its staff and patients.

## *Maintaining the role*

The experience of being in a consultative position provides opportunities, challenges and frustration. If moving from a direct clinical position the nurse may experience role transition difficulties in the initial period. In making the move to this style of nursing practice, the nurse needs to be familiar with the consultative role, and be prepared for the frustrations that can occasionally develop when unable to intervene or provide direct care for the patient.

The PCNC role can be isolating and emotionally draining. The heavy demands to support nursing staff, patients and families highlight the need for PCNCs to develop and maintain healthy support mechanisms. Some nurses will have established support mechanisms in a network of collegial support. If the PCNC is part of a small team, then this group can be supportive. Professional supervision can provide a mechanism for both support and professional development and is worth considering.

## Preparation for the role

Traditionally PCNCs were nurses experienced in palliative care, often with a background in cancer care. While experience remains critical, educational preparation for such consultancy roles is receiving increased emphasis. Tertiary qualifications in palliative care are increasingly required and should include some preparation in research and evaluation as more emphasis is placed on evidence-based practice in nursing. Ideally, preparation for the PCNC role should be at the Masters degree level.

## Role conflict and territorialism

Overcoming role conflict and territorialism are important to PCNC role development. Role conflict can be experienced if clear objectives for the PCNC's role are not established at the outset. Before addressing possible areas of overlap, the PCNC must be very clear and confident in what the role entails but must also respect the expertise of other staff. Working closely with colleagues and maintaining good communication between disciplines go a long way in preventing conflict.

Territorialism, where staff are reluctant to refer or have the PCNC involved, may stem from a lack of understanding of the role. There may be either a perception that the involvement of the PCNC is a criticism of the nursing care being provided, or a general reluctance to have other health professionals involved in the patient's care. Open communication, explanation of the PCNC's role, and gentle perseverance will overcome this problem, as will some early success in symptom management or other aspects of patient care.

## Conclusion

As is evidenced in the journal extracts of the nurse's day, palliative care can be practised and implemented in the acute hospital environment. The nurse who works in this role must be an expert practitioner, with skills in all areas of palliative care. The PCNC in the acute hospital can make a difference for the patient, family and staff by providing support and clinical expertise to relieve symptoms and improve quality of life. It is also timely to recall that Dame Cicely Saunders' initial intent was that 'hospices needed to move out of the NHS [hospital system] so that attitudes and knowledge could move back in'. It was never the intent that the knowledge, skills and practice remain exclusive to these institutions.

# References

Audit Commission (1993). *What seems to be the matter: Communication between hospitals and patients*. National Health Service Report Number 12.

Benoliel, J.Q. (1985). Loss and terminal illness. *Nursing Clinics of North America, 20* (2), 439–448.

Blackburn, A.M. (1989). Problems of terminal care in elderly patients. *Palliative Medicine, 3*, 203–206.

Buckman, R. (1984). Breaking bad news: Why is it so difficult? *British Medical Journal, 288*, 1597–1599.

Clark, D. (Ed.) (1993). *The future for palliative care: Issues of policy and practice*. Buckingham: Open University Press.

Coates, M., Day, D., McCredie, M., & Taylor, R. (1995). *Cancer in New South Wales: Incidence and mortality 1992*. Sydney: NSW Cancer Council.

Donovan, M. & Dillon, P. (1987). Incidence and characteristics of pain in a sample of hospitalised cancer patients. *Cancer Nursing, 10* (2), 85–92.

Dunlop, R.J. & Hockley, J.M. (1990). *Terminal care support teams: The hospital–hospice interface*. Oxford: Oxford University Press.

Expert Panel on Palliative Care (1991). *Report to Cancer 2000 Task Force*. Toronto.

Glasser, B.G. & Strauss, A.L. (1965). *Awareness of dying*. Chicago: Aldine.

Hamilton, J. & Edgar, L. (1992). A survey examining nurses' knowledge of pain control. *Journal of Pain and Symptom Management, 7* (1), 18–26.

Hamric, A. (1977). Deterrents to therapeutic care of the dying person: a nurse's perspective. In Barton, D. (Ed.), *Dying and death: A clinical guide to caregivers* (pp. 183–199). Baltimore: Williams and Wilkinson.

Hockley, J. (1988). Setting standards for pain control. *Professional Nurse*, May, 310–313.

Lev, E. (1986). Teaching humane care for dying patients. *Nursing Outlook, 34* (5), 241–243.

MacDonald, N. (1992). Cancer centres—Their role in palliative care. *Journal of Palliative Care, 8* (1), 38–42.

Maddocks, I., Bentley, L., & Sheedy, J. (1994). Quality of life issues in patients dying from haematological diseases. *Annals Academy of Medicine, 23* (2), 244–248.

Maguire, P. (1985). Barriers to psychological care of the dying. *British Medical Journal, 291*, 1711–1713.

McCaffery, M., Ferrell. B., O'Neil-Page, E., Lester, M., & Ferrell, B. (1990). Nurses' knowledge of opioid analgesic drugs and psychological dependence. *Cancer Nursing, 13* (1), 21–27.

Myers, J. (1985). Cancer pain: Assessment of nurses' knowledge and attitude. *Oncology Nursing Forum, 12* (4), 62–66.

O'Brien, S., Dalton, J., Konsler, G., & Carlson, J. (1996). The knowledge and attitudes of experienced oncology nurses regarding the management of cancer-related pain. *Oncology Nursing Forum, 33* (3), 515–520.

O'Neal, P. (1989). Services for the dying. *Nursing Times, 85* (9), 36–37.

Rankin, M. & Snyder, B. (1984). Nurses' perception of cancer patients' pain. *Cancer Nursing*, April, 149–155.

Wentworth Area Health Service (1993). *The standard for work practice for clinical nurse consultancies*. Sydney: Wentworth Area Health Service.

Whedon, M., Shedd, P., & Summers, B. (1992). The role of the advanced practice oncology nurse in pain relief. *Oncology Nursing Forum, 19* (7), Supplement, 12–19.

Wilkinson, S. (1991). Factors which influence how nurses communicate with cancer patients. *Journal of Advanced Nursing, 16,* 677–668.

Wilson, J.A., Lawson, P.M., & Smith, R.G. (1987). The treatment of terminally ill geriatric patients. *Palliative Medicine, 1,* 149–153.

Woo, H.H., Mann, L.J., Stewart, P.J., Dent, O.F., Chapus, P.H., & Bokey, L. (1991). Frequency of intermediate admissions and place of death of patients with advanced colorectal cancer. *Australian and New Zealand Journal of Surgery, 61,* 603–607.

World Health Organization (1990). *Cancer pain relief and palliative care: Report of a WHO expert committee.* Technical report series 804. Geneva: World Health Organization.

# 19

# Children with
# a Life-threatening Illness

## Margaret Noone

To speak of dying and death in the context of children is to go against what is, in our society anyway, considered the natural order of things. Parents have a worldview that they will die before their children just as grandparents believe they will die before the parents of their grandchildren. Therefore, to speak of palliative care in the context of children with a life-threatening illness is to step into an area of social discomfort. While it is often difficult for people to come to terms with the impending death of any person close to them, this may be even more difficult in the case of a child.

Many children with life-threatening and terminal illnesses never receive palliative care, as acceptance of palliative care implies acceptance of the child's impending death. The reasons for this are complex and at least in part relate to this difficulty of accepting death as inevitable in one so young. I recall the night a father pleaded with the doctor to do anything just to keep his child alive even if only for another half hour. His child was 17 months old, had never gone past her birth weight, had had surgery and was lying in a coma. The mother was asking that the child be left in peace and allowed to die. In such a case the doctor is caught in an impossible situation.

The imperative to keep treating, perhaps working from the principle that where there is life there is hope, is a much more common scenario in the care of dying children than is early referral to palliative care services. We must remember doctors are trained to 'make people better' and can see death of one so young as a failure. I find the language so often used by doctors interesting, 'I lost a patient' being almost a denial of the word death.

The media is full of news about extraordinary advances in medical science with many illnesses and medical conditions once considered incurable and fatal, now treatable and curable. We need only to look at childhood cancer to see the great advances in the survival rate over the past 20 years, where now more than 60 per cent of those diagnosed will be 'cured'. Such advances lead to the modern perspective that death can be delayed and this belief applies very much with childhood illnesses. Thus it is extremely difficult for everyone, the parents, doctors and all who have a vested interest in the child, to face the fact that in some cases active treatment of the disease is of no further benefit. To discontinue treatment is viewed by some as failure, giving in, and giving up hope. To stop treatment is an acknowledgment that the child no longer responds to treatment and will soon die. The result is that some children are treated aggressively right up to the day of their death. These children, and their families, are often denied palliative care, minimising their access to pain and symptom control that may enhance the quality of remaining life. The efforts of the care team need to be focused on helping parents and others come to acknowledge the child's impending death so that appropriate palliative care services can be instigated.

## The child in the context of the family

The most important social context within which the child exists is the family; thus the care of dying children must be family centred. Care efforts cannot focus on the child to the exclusion of the family, as anything that affects the child has direct ramifications for and on each person in that family. All children with a life-threatening or terminal illness and their families have special needs that can be understood only in the specific family context and it is through this knowledge that the care team is able to plan care that will enhance the quality of life for the dying child and their family. The family may feel alone and not understood by relatives and friends or may not know how to ask for or receive help from those willing to offer support. The family needs assistance to prevent the continual build up of the all too reasonable feelings and emotions each member is trying to grapple with each day.

### Parents

How difficult it is for parents to care for themselves in a holistic way during the weeks, months and sometimes years of the child's illness. The sense of guilt is often very strong, with parents believing something they did or did not do caused their child's illness. It seems to be an instinct to stop everything else in life and to dedicate oneself completely to the sick child. It is often only when everyone in the family is exhausted both physically and emotionally that a family will reach out and accept help from others. That cry for help is natural and must be heard. In most cases, it is the mother who is left to do most of the nurturing and care of the sick child, which leaves little time for siblings, husband and herself. She is lost in a sea of doing and she herself is lost. The father may want to be more involved but the imperative to keep working to support the family is especially strong when the burdens of long-term care have eroded the family's financial resources.

## Siblings

A major issue facing many parents of sick children is how to provide suitable parenting to a sick child and to the other children in the family. Normal parenting practices, such as disciplining a child who is dying, often seem out of place, and yet the family must continue to function in 'normal' ways for the remaining children. So often the sick child is the 'special child' in the family, with a level of specialness the siblings feel they would never reach and indeed may resent. This may lead the siblings to think that their parents really wouldn't care if they were dying or even to wish they were the one who was sick. Some siblings defend the sick child, while others are embarrassed by the sick child's physical appearance. Guilt may also be an aspect of the siblings' experience. Young children, in particular, tend to have an inflated view of their power and may believe a past wish for their sibling to die or go away has become reality. Behavioural problems among siblings at home and school are not unusual. Their performance at school may become disruptive and their study habits may deteriorate. Siblings may be confused as to what is happening to the family or sense a real feeling of neglect, and their self-worth may diminish. During the child's illness, the siblings may not have as much contact with the parents as before, as the parents' time is completely taken up with the physical and emotional care of the one who is to die. Separation of the family is also a reality as the sick child may need to go to a distant centre for treatment.

While the sick child is being cared for so intensely, the other children often miss out and at times are left to their own devices. The sick child may sense the apparent neglect of their brothers and sisters and also feel a sense of guilt. Children are aware of the traumatic impact their illness has on the whole family and feel responsible for the extremely painful emotions displayed by different members of the family. While parents express fear, despair, anger and disbelief, the siblings may regress or mature beyond their years. Immense strain is put on marriages as partners cope and react differently at different times. Some families are resilient and grow stronger through this experience, while others are torn apart.

## Grandparents

For the grandparents there is a double sorrow when a grandchild has a life-threatening illness or is dying. Grandparents often question the early death of a child who has their whole life in front of them and question why it is not they who are dying when they have lived their life. Grandparents also suffer for their own child who is the parent of the one who is so ill. Many grandparents are extremely helpful to the family during the time of the child's illness, while others may be unable to assist because of distance or their own physical condition. Some just don't know how to help and walk away from the situation. Alternatively, grandparents may be excluded through efforts not to worry 'the old people', which only creates more suffering and pain. We can't shield people from pain and we haven't a right to do so.

Recently, I was asked to have lunch with a group of grandparents, some of whom had a grandchild with a life-threatening illness and others who had had a grandchild die. We sat around a table, introduced ourselves to each other and I was beginning to wonder what the next move might be. It didn't take long before the room was full of voices, soft gentle voices, as people began to tell the story of their grandchild to the person next to them. Someone was brave enough to say they nearly didn't come as they were not sure they wanted to be there. Another sat quietly wondering if anyone really wanted to hear her story. Suddenly, it seemed a safe place to talk about their grandchild. No one was there to judge them. There was a real feeling of unconditional love. Each accepted the other as they were all experiencing similar feelings and emotions.

After we had eaten a hearty meal and enjoyed a glass of wine, the expectation was for me to share some of my experiences with families. I assured them that in no way could I begin to imagine how each was feeling, as I didn't have children or grandchildren of my own and it would be presumptuous on my part to say 'I know how you feel'. How often do we hear people say this, failing to acknowledge the uniqueness of human experience. Each person's relationship to the child is unique, as are the feelings and emotions generated by the experience of watching a child die. What is important is that we own our feelings and acknowledge them and have them acknowledged by others as valid and important.

Grandparents may feel they need to be strong for their own children and other grandchildren. Grandparents have a lifetime of experiences behind them which may be of help to their family but they must remember they themselves need time out to face their own grief. By the end of the meal, there appeared to be a good feeling that they were not alone and it was okay to be concerned for their children and grandchildren, but they still needed to have time away just for themselves. They also needed to allow their children to do the same. There are times when families need to grieve together and there are times for personal grief.

One grandfather asked, 'why were you not around 11 years ago when our grandchild died?'. How many times have I heard that over the years. A concern of mine that kept coming up that day, as it has so often come up with parents, is the apparent hesitation of some doctors to be honest and forthright about the child's condition in a caring, sensitive way. How essential it is for families to be fully informed and well prepared for the death of the child. For one who came in as a stranger to the group, I left feeling we were the better and wiser for having met. At critical times in our lives we all need a safe environment where we can be heard without being judged.

## Palliative care for the dying child

Palliative care is for the whole family, not just the sick person. It involves total care of the sick person's physical needs as well as the psychological, social and spiritual requirements. Their pain and symptoms should be managed to achieve the greatest possible level of comfort, while addressing the possibilities of quality of life for the whole family. The modern hospice movement began in the late 1970s in Australia but has been largely centred on the care of terminally ill adults; the concept that it is necessary for children is still inconceivable to many. It is now 14 years since the first children's hospice was built in the United Kingdom. Helen House in Oxford was built because Sister Francis Dominica recognised the needs of families caring for a child with a limited life owing to a progressive, life-threatening illness. While the number of children needing palliative care is very small compared to adults, their illnesses and needs are often very different.

Paediatric wards in hospitals are for the acutely ill and are often inappropriately set up for any child requiring palliative care. It is difficult to reconcile the care of children who are dying alongside the intensive efforts to cure those who are not terminally ill. Home is by far the better place for the child so long as the family can manage and have ready access to skilled back-up if and when required. While home is possibly the best place for the care of dying children, this is not always possible, especially when the care demands are burdensome. Many hesitate to have their child in hospital, even for short-term respite, as they lose much of the control over the type of care given to their child, but for many, hospital is the only option. The community is only now beginning to recognise that children do die and they have few choices of where they can receive the type of care they require. The first children's hospice in Australia, Very Special Kids' House, opened in Melbourne in 1996 and will cater for children and the families needing palliative care and provide respite for those with a life-threatening illness. It will also provide a focal point for the development of expertise in the care of dying children and their families that will help to improve the ongoing care of dying children in all contexts.

## The child's awareness of death

Children are very articulate and thought provoking about many things in life and yet, when it comes to subjects like death and dying, adults suddenly begin treating them as if they are unaware of their condition. Children are aware of their physical state of health long before anyone is willing to talk to them and discuss this with them. Children like honesty and respect those who are truthful with them and treat them with the respect they deserve. If a sick child asks questions concerning their illness, it is always advisable to check out with them exactly what they are asking and not presume we know the intent of their questions. The old story of the little boy who asked his father where he came from exemplifies the difficulty of making assumptions about children's questions. The boy's father gave him a thorough explanation of procreation and birth, after which his son turned to him and said, 'it's just that Jimmy comes from Melbourne and I was wondering where I came from'.

Children often carry unnecessary burdens because adults lack the courage to discuss and tell them the truth. Children know when they are dying even if they are unable to articulate the words. Their drawings express what they know and understand. Elisabeth Kübler-Ross (1974) has written at length of her experiences with children who were sick and dying. Earl Grollman (1990) is another authority on this subject. Kushner (1982) had first-hand experience during his own son's protracted illness and early death.

My first experience of listening to, and trying to come to terms with the amount of pain and suffering adults expose children to when these questions go unanswered was in Tiburon, California, when I worked at the Center for Attitudinal Healing with Dr Jerry Jampolsky. At this centre, children found that the company of other children in a group allowed them to be authentic about what was happening to them. They seemed to accept my presence in the group, perhaps recognising that I was not going to deny this open discussion about the most important thing to them, their life and their death.

Volumes have been written about children's need to talk about their life and their death. I have been amazed how even very young children know about their approaching death. Elisabeth Kübler-Ross has always said that even the very youngest child knows when they are dying. It was only after first-hand experience with very young babies that I could accept that they did know.

## Preparing for a child's death

Being told their child may not reach adulthood is a devastating experience for parents. Life can never be the same for them without that child, although in time, they learn to live with the pain and hurt, and hope one day the pain will lessen. As one mother commented after the death of her child, 'I just ached all over and now after many years, I keep that ache in one place, close to my heart'.

Children sense the sorrow and pain they are causing their parents and they will often try to protect them. One three-year-old turned to her mother and said, 'mummy, I will try very hard not to die for you'. Another child said to her parents, 'I am so tired I can't try any more'.

I remember parents who had been preparing for their child to die for nearly four years and felt they had equipped themselves to cope after their daughter's death. Some years later they admitted to me that they had no idea how devastating the death would be for them. The father to this day admits that his daughter taught him what it was to love. This frail little child would often talk about dying to the nurses in her ward during the small hours of the night when she was unable to sleep. These children have so much to teach us if we only allow them.

Each family deals with a child's death in their own way. One mother spoke of the number of requests her son had which were quite out of the ordinary on the morning of his death but added, 'he didn't know he was dying because we never told him'. What a hard secret that little boy carried over the last weeks of his life at home alone with his parents.

The father of a beautiful teenage daughter was afraid to talk to his daughter about death in case she gave up trying. While it must be the most difficult and terrifying experience for a parent to talk to a child about their death, imagine the isolation of the child when the parents are unable to openly acknowledge what is happening. Some parents excuse themselves by saying, 'we didn't have to tell our child, they knew but we never talked about it'. Is it our fear of death? Our fear of seeing the child upset? Our inability to deal with the whole range of emotions that the child may express? How must a child feel when no one cries with them, no one tells them how much they are loved and how they will be missed in the family? Or when no one talks to them about what would they really like to do and who would they wish to say goodbye to before they die? They may wish to plan for their own funeral. There may be relations, friends, classmates to whom they wish to say goodbye. Elisabeth Kübler-Ross so often speaks of 'unfinished business'. Children may like to make a will and give their favourite toys and precious belongings to particular people.

The meaning of death differs for each child depending on their age and experience within their own family. It is a subject so often not spoken about when children are around but one they are often fascinated with very early in life. Very young children don't see death as something permanent because they have no sense of time or finality and may ask when the person who has died will visit again. Young children may express their fear of going somewhere without their parents. They may express fear of the unknown. Many speak about heaven as being a happy place where there is no more pain. Families need to be able to work through many of these issues of separation. If the family is receiving good palliative care, and the child has good symptom and pain control, the family has more opportunities of facing some of these issues together in a homely and more familiar atmosphere.

The death of a child is always viewed as a tragedy as it leaves a trail of suffering behind. One feeling which lingers is anger, along with questions like 'why my child?', 'why our family?'. Not only immediate family but all who come in contact with the child experience some pain and even regrets. The ripple effect can spread far, making it difficult to celebrate the life of the child and to recognise just how much good has come from knowing that particular child and family. The one thing which stands out is the courage and patience of the child and how forgiving they are when subjected to painful procedures. I believe they have an innate understanding of and belief in an afterlife. Many families sense an urgency about the sick child's activity. The father of an eight-year-old daughter who had a short time to live commented that she did more living than her three brothers put together.

## Grief and bereavement

The whole area of anticipatory grief relates to the painful experience of watching a child deteriorate day by day. The two-year-old diagnosed with spinal muscular atrophy which causes spinal nerve cell deterioration and muscle wastage, with no cure and no treatment, leaves parents feeling numb and powerless. This alert, intelligent little boy busy doing what all two-year-olds love doing now finds things he did six months ago impossible. When he falls, he can no longer get up without assistance. He is adorable, which makes it all the more difficult and painful to know he will die very young.

One of the problems is that we all grieve differently, and these differences often set up barriers to support. Grief does not follow any pattern and one person's experience of grief may seem alien to a partner, family, friends and certainly to the wider community. If we reflect on the Azaria Chamberlain case in Australia, no matter what that mother did or said she was judged.

At the time of death, religious rituals are important for many people. In our modern society, many of these rituals have been eliminated or shortened to fit into the ever increasing pace of life. Within a few weeks of the death, it seems to be taken for granted that all is right with the world and one needs to get on with life. This is possibly the time when the reality of the death and the terrible emptiness and absence of the person begins to set in, yet everyone is expecting it to be over and put behind them. It is very difficult to allow people to grieve in their own ways and to resist the temptation to try to alleviate their pain. We must allow each person to grieve when and how it is appropriate for them.

Sometimes grief is delayed, which can prove to be more difficult and prolonged. I recently met a 60-year-old man whose twin brother had died at the age of six. His dead brother's name was never mentioned within the family after his death. The man had photos of the two of them when they were very young but over the years he often wondered if perhaps his brother had not died but had been adopted. Last year this man returned to his native country and checked the death register and found his twin's death was recorded. He felt he could have been spared a lot of unnecessary grief, if his brother's death had been treated differently.

The large amount of care required by a terminally ill child can also mean a large void exists in the family following the death. After years of regular visits to the hospital and of focusing the family routine around the needs of the sick child, a return to 'normal' family life may be more difficult than many realise or expect. Families often find this a time of high anxiety which may be exacerbated by reduced or no access to the care team who had been supporting them during the child's illness. Recognition of this important time of transition helps to ensure that ongoing support is available as the family learns to adjust to their changed circumstances.

## Conclusion

The dying and death of children brings forth many human emotions and is a difficult time for all involved in the child's care and support. The families of these children are our future and should receive every possible help to enable them to live full and productive lives both during and following their child's death. Many times these families are left hurt and wounded with nowhere to turn for support. The death of a child need not be only a time of sadness and pain as the dying child has much to give. The families need the opportunity to look back with joy on what their child brought to their lives and in time to recognise the strength, gifts and talents within the family which may never have been discovered without the painful experience of their child's death.

## References

Grollman, Earl A. (1990). *Talking about grief*. Boston: Beacon Press.
Kübler-Ross, Elisabeth. (1974). *Talking to dying children*. New York: Macmillan.
Krushner, Harold S. (1982). *When bad things happen to good people*. London: Pan Books.

# 20

# The Interface of Palliative Care and Technology in Critical Care

## Elizabeth Manias

This chapter examines the tensions between technology and palliative care in the critical care environment. A profession whose central tenet relates to commitment to care, nursing is continually constrained and shaped by the predominant technocratic tendency influencing the structure and delivery of this care. The conflicts confronted by the nurse involving the provision of palliative care are nowhere more apparent than in the micro-culture of the critical care environment. Here, the dominance of technology often renders attempts towards palliative care invisible and nullified.

The micro-culture of critical care will be examined and related to the discourses of technology and palliative care. Medical and scientific discourses are the dominant ways of talking and thinking about reality in the critical care environment, often to the sublimation of other types of knowledges. In critical care, the knowledges that are pertinent to palliative care include: an acknowledgment of the shared human condition that the patient manifests; patient and family vulnerability to the ordinary; and the often unpredictable responses to this vulnerability. These knowledges are appropriated and subjugated to the level of other, as they do not fit into what constitutes legitimate knowledge.

## Theoretical underpinnings

Central to the analysis of the interface between palliative care and technology in critical care are the concepts of power, knowledge, discourse and subjectivity. The work of Michel Foucault provides an insightful framework of these concepts, and of the metaphors and assumptions in an environment where the focus is on saving lives. This form of critique will open up spaces, creating new opportunities for palliative care in the critical care environment.

Foucault considers power a force relation, with ceaseless struggles, confrontations, contradictions, inequalities, and the integration of these force relations (1990, p. 92). Although radical ruptures and revolutions are possible, the usual impacts on power struggles are 'mobile and transitory points of resistance' (Foucault, 1990, p. 96). Furthermore, resistance, like power, is heterogenous in that it is distributed in an 'irregular fashion'.

While technology and scientific knowledge may be associated with dominant forms of knowledge, Foucault's reference to the '*insurrection of subjugated knowledges*' (Foucault, 1980, p. 81, italics in original) is an appropriate description of other types of knowledges pertinent to palliative care. They may include the knowledges relating to spiritual guidance provided during the terminal stage of a patient's life, or the need to have debriefing meetings which focus on nurses' emotions and general nursing care of a terminally ill patient, rather than the rationales underlying the use of various medical interventions.

One common view sees power as domination or imposition by constraint which can be exposed through truth or knowledge (Keenan, 1987). Foucault's alternative notion of mutually interdependent power-knowledge 'challenges assumptions that ideology can be demystified and, hence, that undistorted truth can be attained' (Diamond & Quinby, 1988, p. xi).

Discourses are ways of constituting knowledge, together with the social practices, power relations, and individual consciousness which occur in such knowledges and the relationships between them (Weedon, 1992). Experts of dominant discourses analyse and recognise the truth by specific questions and answers. This allows claims to particular forms of knowledge and therefore truth. On the basis of this ownership to discourse, experts can make claims to power.

For discourses to be effectively used, they need to be activated through an agency of individual subjects. In the traditional, humanist view, the subject (or individual) is understood to be unified, rational and autonomous. In other words, the power of human nature is able to solve problems through self-realisation and reason. Foucault has argued that this humanistic conception of the subject is insufficient to deal with the forces involving power relationships in society. This argument is particularly relevant to nursing's confrontation with technology in the critical care environment. Instead of believing in the subject as the cause and solution of experiences, a Foucauldian understanding enables examination of the historical conditions that make different and specific subject positions possible, and how these subject positions are constituted through resistance to the dominating effects of technology. At the same time, subjectivity also refers to the conscious and unconscious thoughts and emotions of individuals, and their ways of understanding how their sense of themselves relate to society (Weedon, 1992).

## Discourses of technology and palliative care within the critical care environment

In the context of critical care, technology is associated with the medications, equipment, medical procedures, and the supportive organisations and systems underlying patient management. In critical care, not only is the context defined and appropriated by technology, but palliative care experiences are also rendered invisible. The relationship between nursing in the critical care environment and technology has been described as one involving conflicting, irreconcilable forces (Cooper, 1993; Sandelowski, 1988). Indeed, Sandelowski (1988) argues that this relationship concerns the dominating effects of technology: 'nurses for the most part neither invent nor control but rather apply medical technology, [and] are insufficiently aware of the conceptual systems they accept when they uncritically integrate medical technology into their practice' (pp. 35–36). She further contends that attempts to extend nursing's sphere of influence and to humanise machine-orientated health care may prove futile. Undoubtedly, technology has saved the lives of many patients who would have otherwise died. Indeed some of these patients are able to go home and enjoy an improved quality of life (Ashworth, 1990; Pearson, 1993). Critical care is dominated by the delivery of technology-orientated model of care, while nursing struggles in its attempt to address humanising aspects of caring. The challenge for nursing has been therefore, to incorporate the complex technology with care, and to deliver quality patient care.

Palliative care has been described as a holistic approach, encompassing the interacting, physical, intellectual, emotional, social, and spiritual aspects of the patient and family during the terminal stages of illness when curative treatment is no longer effective. Emphasis is placed on the professional skills of the multidisciplinary team, whose aim is to improve the patient's quality of life or prevent deterioration where cure or remission is considered unlikely (Buchanan, 1989; Coates, 1982; James, Gebski, & Gunz, 1985). As caring occurs within a relationship of reciprocity (Marck, 1990) and empathy (Olsen, 1991), palliative care recognises that a sharing of the human condition between individuals makes them vulnerable to ordinary experiences of suffering, joy, hope, pain and despair. On the other hand, McGilly and Haines (1995) view palliation as active, total care of patients whose disease process no longer responds to curative intervention. Blues (1984) is concerned with the definition of palliative care applying to an incurable patient as it is difficult to determine incurability with absolute certainty. Palliative care is often associated with the use of comfort care measures of a terminally ill or dying patient. Faber-Langerdoen and Bartels (1992) refer to the potential problems in deciding the range and sequential process of removing life-sustaining treatment in critically ill patients and implementing measures aimed at promoting comfort until a patient dies.

By examining these interpretations of technology and palliative care in the critical care environment, nursing has created a dichotomy between technology and the humanising aspects of palliative care. The technology is associated with the dominant perspective of medicine, and is promoted at the expense of the traditional, subjugated responses of palliative care. Juxtaposing technology and palliative care as polarised opposites is another effect of the tension between care and cure, rational and irrational, object and subject, nature and nurture. Nursing has attempted to exalt and privilege the virtues of the nurturing, subjective attributes of caring over the rational, dominant attributes of technology. For instance, Allan and Hall (1988) suggest that nursing should adopt a health model that incorporates the person-environment relationship rather than a biomedical model that advocates objective and dehumanising technology. In attempting to privilege the caring over technology, nursing has met with failure because such a measure only serves to perpetuate the dichotomy. The rationality of technology is still the standard by which the virtues of caring are judged. It seems more appropriate and beneficial, therefore, to critically examine the way knowledge is constituted through the power of discourses of technology and palliative care in the critical care environment.

The effects of power relationships through the discourses of technology and palliative care will now be considered from two perspectives: the nurse's role in technological competence and palliative care; and the expression of the patient's and family's vulnerability through communication.

## Technological competence and palliative holistic care

The subject positions of the critical care nurse are structured by technological competence and palliative holistic care. Ray (1987) explains that the association between technological competence and caring results from a maturation process. She suggests that when a nurse's needs are met from mastering the machinery, the nurse can then meet others' needs. Hence once a nurse is comfortable with the technology, then greater efforts can be placed on the patient and family (Benner, Tanner, & Chesla, 1992). Unfortunately, nurses' ability to speak about their knowledge of the patient's palliative care needs is constrained by dominant practices such as regular documentation of observations, communication of patient findings through handover and progress, and the silencing of nursing knowledge (Parker & Gardner, 1992).

An exploration of the assessment procedures undertaken by nurses in critical care environments helps to identify the subject positions they appropriate. The 24-hour observation chart or bedside computer database, where regular nursing observations are performed on the patient, provides insight into the nature of care surrounding the patient. The chart shows, through use of space and position, the relative importance of particular sections of information. This chart documents assessment of blood pressure, central venous pressure, respiratory rate, urinary output, wound drainage, and other physiological parameters. A small amount of space is made available on the chart for other aspects of care (which may include a palliative focus). Often, however, these data are objectified by the use of scales and are not descriptive in nature. Effectively, the nurse functions as a data collector for medical decision-makers and as an operator of medical decisions (Bruni, 1990, as cited in Goltz & Bruni, 1995; Liaschenko, 1994). As this information is accessed and updated at least on an hourly basis, it carries the power to regulate and control nursing practice. Documentation relevant to palliative care is lacking. This may include indications of suffering and sadness, grief and dying, trust and decisions about treatment options. Information relating to a patient's feelings is not used to understand the patient's emotional status concerning vulnerability, suffering or grief, but rather to assess pain levels, the need to alter sedation levels, or changes in conscious state. Thus, not only does this documentation practice categorises the patient according to discrete physiological parameters aimed at bodily conformity and stabilisation, but it also regularly and coercively prioritises for the bedside nurse the knowledges that are valued and take precedence over more subjugated forms.

The nature of nursing tradition is marked by an oral culture, and in contrast to the recording of observations, it is communicated in private (Parker & Gardner, 1992). Information conveyed among nurses in an oral manner occurs at the nursing handover at the start and at the end of a shift. In the critical care area, handover can take effect in many forms. Most commonly, a global handover is initially given where information is provided on all patients to all oncoming nurses before a nurse is assigned to a particular patient or group of patients. Once at the bedside, nurses then receive a more detailed handover of those placed in their care. Much of the talk that occurs among nurses during nursing handover remains private, behind closed doors, and excludes other health professionals. The nursing handover serves many purposes for nurses, and acts as a template from which nurses can demonstrate different subject positions in relaying information concerning their patients. Part of the handover alerts oncoming nurses to the technological domain of the environment and provides a sense of familiarity of the unexplored terrain of the patient. Some of this knowledge tends to be decontextualised, impersonal and medicalised, an empty repetition of unreflected, abstract facts (Parker & Wiltshire, 1995).

Nurses also communicate in a language that constructs and reconstructs the world of the critically ill patient. This occurs through nurses' attitude of the 'ordinariness' of the world surrounding the critically ill and dying patient. That is to say, nurses take for granted the environment in which they work and therefore re-present information relating to patients as everyday and ordinary (Parker & Gardner, 1992). Alternatively, the language used to express the suffering, pain, grief and anxiety of the patient and family, registers the messiness of human communication, an inherent aspect of palliative care. But for this very reason, critical nurses often dismiss this form of communication as being 'subjective' (Parker & Wiltshire, 1995). Instead, greater value is bestowed upon the abstract, medicalised knowledge associated with technology.

Nursing discussions at handover about the patient's and family's suffering and conflicts with the technology of treatment tend to occur behind closed doors. It is useful to understand the influence of spatial arrangements on critical care nurses' practice, and the effect these arrangements have on the patient's and family's palliative care needs. The global nursing handover environment is characteristically an isolated enclosure, a place separate from all others and closed in on itself. It therefore has the effect of controlling nurses from external influences. The spatial arrangement of the bedside handover involves partitioning. All nurses have their own space, and each space has its specific patient. The main aim in this instance is to know where and how to locate a specific patient, to set up useful communications with the oncoming nurse and to assess, judge and analyse the patient's response. This selective use of space that excludes other health professionals such as doctors, partially explains the invisibility of this rich communication to the 'educated eye of medical staff' (Street, 1995, p. 51) and also accounts for the 'silence of nurses' (Parker & Gardner, 1992, p. 8). Critical care nurses may sense a fear of embarrassment as the expression of subjugated knowledges may be perceived as unprofessional, non-medical and common. It also raises sensitivities about the mortality and precariousness of human life. Rather than viewing these knowledges in dichotomous ways, critical care nurses will benefit from addressing these subjugated knowledges as fields of resistance where nurses are prompted to examine the diverse relationships these occupy in reference to the technology. By directing attention to the intersecting views of the patient, family and health care professional, nurses will be in a better position to identify the contradictory meanings of technology and the way these meanings intersect with palliative care concerns.

## Identifying patient and family vulnerability through communication

One of the greatest challenges for the nurse caring for critically ill patients is effective communication about treatment when care moves from a curative to a palliative nature. Communication can be adversely affected by the nurse's identification with the powerful and invincible nature of technology as opposed to the powerless and vulnerable patient and family (Cooper, 1993). An unequal relationship develops between the nurse and patient.

Ethical and legal principles have been developed with the intention of shifting the responsibility of life and death decisions from health professionals to patients and their families, and therefore, creating a more balanced relationship between these parties. An examination of these ethical and legal principles will demonstrate that they share the tenets of liberal humanism. That is, these principles are based on the assumption that all individuals share rational consciousness, which allows for the opportunity and right to self-determination.

Ethically, the principles of autonomy, privacy and pluralism apply to issues of dignity and quality of life of a critically ill and dying patient (Van Eys, 1991). Privacy is generally considered as the right to master a person's environment and to have this environment protected from any unwanted intrusion. Pluralism enhances and strengthens the right for autonomy, suggesting the freedom for patients to follow whatever path they choose in the dying phase of their life. Autonomy may be regarded as the overriding principle whereby care should be solely determined by the patient once complete information is supplied by the healthcare team (Van Eys, 1991).

This focus for patient self-determination is also highlighted in Australian common law and legislation relating to dying with dignity. In common law, if competent patients who are aware of their condition refuse further life-saving treatment, that decision must be respected even if refusal means that death will result or if healthcare professionals regard that decision as ill conceived (Eburn, 1994; Otlowski, 1995). Alongside the common law, Australian legislation allows patients to express refusal for certain treatments at some future time when they lack decision-making competence. Such legislation enables patients to establish advance declarations where, in the event of their suffering from a terminal illness, they may request not to be subjected to life-saving treatment. Legislation has been enacted in the Northern Territory, South Australia and Victoria that permits patients to refuse certain treatment and requires their doctor to honour that decision (Otlowski, 1995). The Victorian legislation also allows patients to appoint an agent who makes decisions on their behalf if they become incompetent. In parts of Australia where legislation relating to dying with dignity does not exist, the patient's rights are reserved under common law.

Unfortunately, despite the humanistic intentions of ethical principles, dying with dignity legislation, and common law, the shift in responsibility of life and death decisions from health professionals to patients or appointed agents remains slight. Using these intentions, the construction of the relationship between the health professional and patient implies a redistribution in the exercise of patients' rights. It attempts to replace a discourse of medical paternalism with a discourse of egalitarianism, where the patient and family are equal partners with the critical care team. Such a construction fails to take account of the operation of the power relations and their impact on decision-making abilities of patients and families to issues of technology and palliative care. The legislation may not have the anticipated impact in upholding a patient's or family's decision, as they may defer to the expertise of health professionals (Henderson, 1994).

In an attempt to reverse this trend and emphasise the patient's and family's contribution in decision-making, critical care nurses need to embrace a responsive approach to patient care. This approach has the effect of blurring the distinction between the patient's public and private character (May, 1992). As a public character, the patient is reduced to the categories specified by the pathology of the body. The patient's visible and public character presents as a body to be disassembled, manipulated and modified. To expose the patient's private character requires nurses to extend their gaze beyond the material condition of the body. This effort enables nurses to gain intimate knowledge of the patient. However, as nurses attempt to reconstitute the public and private characters of the patient to make a whole person, there is the possibility that aspects of the patient's private character may be interpreted as being fixed in time and space. Instead, nurses need to develop an acute awareness of the frailties of the human condition and the possibilities for conflicting and changing positions of the patient in addressing a patient's needs. Using stereoscopic vision of their language and practice, nurses can establish a therapeutic gaze (May, 1992). In contrast to the medical gaze associated with monoscopic vision, this therapeutic gaze opens up the possibility of reassembling the patient as a person with anxieties, uncertainties and suspicions. The exchanges between nurses and a critically ill patient demand more than the nurses' rigorous assessment of their material practice. Rather, an understanding of the patient's and family's social history and intimate disposition is built up through communication. No doubt, however, a rhetoric of patient individualisation and self-determination exists in critical care nursing practice. Cooper (1993) points to the way in which nurses are able to demonstrate care in concert with technological competence but identify with the values imposed by technology at the expense of acknowledging their own and the patient's vulnerability. Similarly, Hockley (1989) showed that while nurses were aware of the emotional needs of terminally ill patients, they felt cheated if the patient did not allow them to carry out physical care.

The possibility for critical care nurses demonstrating this therapeutic gaze by communication often remains just that—a possibility. The adoption of a responsive discourse is impeded by the way these nurse–patient relationships take place. Power relations continue to place limits on the nurses' ability to have sensitive relationships with their patients in the dying phase of their life. Major structural inhibitions to these relationships concern the institutional code. Examples include the use of standardised and universal procedural regimens. Critical care environments often have intricately constructed policies and protocols relating to the use of curative and palliative treatments. These structural inhibitions limit the nurses' discretion in successfully developing conducive relationships with patients and families.

Resistance to the creation of effective interpersonal relationships also arises from the private qualities of patients, their families and nurses. The routinised, task-orientated work that characterises critical care nursing has relied on nurses having a moral dedication and sense of personal worth in the delivery of an ideology based on selfless devotion to duty (Wilkinson, 1992). Trying to incorporate relevant issues of palliative care into a system of structured rigidity and formality merely maintains a professional distance between the nurse and patient. Palliative care initiatives in critical care, therefore, tend to rely on the management of the patient's symptoms, including pain, anorexia, constipation, nausea, stomatitis and weakness (Heslin, 1989). With the ready availability of medication therapy and other complex forms of management, palliative care in the critical care environment could easily concentrate on the provision of symptomatic management with little emphasis on providing psychological, spiritual and compassionate support for the patient and family.

Nursing practice directed at penetrating and guiding the interpersonal relationship along a specific track can paradoxically make the patient more malleable (May, 1992). As such, this focus does not concentrate on the generation of humane and sensitive approaches of palliative care, but rather on 'ways of defining and mobilising the most technically efficient ways of penetrating the patient's intimate disposition' (May, 1992, p. 600). In mapping a predetermined journey along this track, we are forced to question the influence of the power–knowledge nexus. While the power to define and respond to the patient as being more than a malleable object rests with the critical care nurse, the type of knowledge espoused by the nurse sometimes is not powerful enough to foster meaningful interpersonal relationships as required for effective palliative care. Nursing must begin to focus on the importance of the unique person, in the production of knowledge that is organised around 'the constitution of the patient as a "real" or "authentic" subject' (May, 1992, p. 599).

The private quality of critically ill patients also limits the extent of palliative, responsive care. While it may appear legitimate to expect the critical care nurse to care for the patient, practice directed at exposing, examining and interpreting the patient's and family's private disposition and frailties demands voluntary admission from them that this is indeed legitimate. An interpretation of the private dispositions of the patient and family is an important component of palliative care. Some patients and families may resist attempts to become 'exposed' and therefore elect to remain silent. Unequal power between the nurse, patient and family relating to the vulnerability, health status, familiarity with the technological environment, and superhuman attributes associated with the healthcare team, contributes to this silence. Furthermore, the patient may become involuntarily silent through the implementation of paralysing and sedating medications, mechanical ventilation, and the metabolic effects of organ failure. Communication is further hindered by excessive noise levels, meaningless sensory stimuli, pain, fear and disrupted sleeping patterns. A decision to remove curative forms of treatment in preference to palliative care initiatives does not necessarily involve removal of all forms of technology. Indeed, the patient may continue to be tethered up to ventilation devices and other modes of complex technology, even though palliative measures have been instigated. This pervasiveness of technology in a patient receiving palliative measures may further exacerbate feelings of alienation between the nurse, patient and family, and hinder the nurse's sensitivity to unique palliative care requirements.

Structural and interpersonal aspects affect the extent to which the patient and family expose their own truth, in their constitution as unique people. Not only do these aspects constrain but they also produce particular modes of knowledge which modify the way the patient and family interpret and understand the critical care experience. Unlike the truth associated with the objectified body of the patient, visible by the Foucauldian concept of surveillance and the monitoring for specific effects, the truth relating to the therapeutic gaze can only function with permission from the patient and family. To achieve this level of acknowledgment, the nurse needs to gain the trust and acceptance of the patient and family before they can be expected to give voice to their own private and authentic concerns.

# Conclusion

Using Foucauldian notions of power, knowledge, discourse and subjectivity, this chapter has attempted to elucidate the conflicts between the discourses of palliative care and technology.

The silencing of the subjugated knowledges associated with palliative care in the critical care environment is examined at two levels of communication. At the first level, nurses communicate their technological competence with each other through oral and written modes of delivery. Although these modes of communication are constrained by technological dogma, there are opportunities for resistance where nurses do communicate the ordinary, messy world surrounding the patient and family. These opportunities are, however, limited by power relations concerning self and peer surveillance among nurses and the spatial arrangements of the different modes of nursing communication. Communication between the nurse, patient and family also affects the extent of the contribution of palliative care discourse in critical care. Currently, although a rhetoric of patient autonomy and self-determination exists, technological competence continues to overshadow the influence of palliation in critical care. Structural concerns and interpersonal, private qualities of patients, families and nurses constrain and produce the interpretation and understanding of the critical care experience.

The exposition of the power relations and their interrelationships with the knowledges informing the discourses of technology and palliative care is constructive in revealing new possibilities for critical care nursing practice. The critical care nurse will need to lay claims on knowledges relating to shared meanings and understandings of palliative care requirements, an appreciation of shared human frailties, the affirmation of human conditions of vulnerability and unpredictability, and concern for the intimate, unique disposition of the patient and family.

# References

Allan, J.D. & Hall, B.A. (1988). Challenging the focus on technology: A critique of the medical model in a changing health care system. *Advances in Nursing Science, 10* (3), 22–34.

Ashworth, P. (1990). High technology and humanity for intensive care. *Intensive Care Nursing, 6*, 150–160.

Benner, P., Tanner, C., & Chesla, C. (1992). From beginner to expert: Gaining a differentiated clinical world in critical care nursing. *Advances in Nursing Science, 14* (3), 13–28.

Blues, A.G. (1984). Hospice philosophy of appropriate care. In Blues, A.G. & Zerwekh, J.V. (Eds.), *Hospice and palliative nursing care* (pp. 1–9). Orlando: Grune & Stratton.

Buchanan, J. (1989). Psychological aspects of palliative care. *Cancer Forum, 13* (1), 17–21.

Coates, G. (1982). Palliative care: The modern concept. *Medical Journal of Australia, 2*, 503–504.

Cooper, M.C. (1993). The intersection of technology and care in the ICU. *Advances in Nursing Science, 15* (3), 23–32.

Diamond, I. & Quinby, L. (1988). Introduction. In Diamond, I. & Quinby, L. (Eds.), *Feminism and Foucault: Reflections on resistance* (pp. ix–xx). Boston: Northeastern University Press.

Eburn, M. (1994). Withdrawing, withholding and refusing emergency resuscitation. *Journal of Law and Medicine, 2*, 131–146.

Faber-Langerdoen, K. & Bartels, D.M. (1992). Process of forgoing life-sustaining treatment in a university hospital: An empirical study. *Critical Care Medicine, 20* (5), 570–577.

Foucault, M. (1980). *Power/Knowledge: Selected interviews and other writings, 1972–1977.* New York: Pantheon Books.

Foucault, M. (1990). *The history of sexuality. An introduction*, vol. 1. London: Penguin Books.

Goltz, K. & Bruni, N. (1995). Health promotion discourse: Language of change? In Gardner, H. (Ed.), *The politics of health: The Australian experience*, 2nd edn (pp. 510–549). Melbourne: Churchill Livingstone.

Henderson, A. (1994). The significance for critical care nurses of the 'Dying With Dignity' legislation. *Australian Critical Care, 7* (2), 23–26.

Heslin, K. (1989). The supportive role of the staff nurse in the hospital palliative care situation. *Journal of Palliative Care, 5* (3), 20–26.

Hockley, J. (1989). Caring for the dying in acute hospitals. *Nursing Times, 85* (39), 47–50.

James, M.L., Gebski, V.J., & Gunz, F.W. (1985). The need for palliative care services in a general hospital. *Medical Journal of Australia, 142*, 448–449.

Keenan, T. (1987). I. The 'paradox' of knowledge and power: Reading Foucault on a bias. *Political Theory, 15* (1), 5–37.

Liaschenko, J. (1994). The moral geography of home care. *Advances in Nursing Science, 17* (2), 16–26.

Marck, P. (1990). Therapeutic reciprocity: A caring phenomenon. *Advances in Nursing Science, 13* (1), 49–59.

May, C. (1992). Individual care? Power and subjectivity in therapeutic relationships. *Sociology, 26* (4), 589–602.

McGilly, H. & Haines, F. (1995). Care in a hospice. In Robbins, J. & Moscrop, J. (Eds.), *Caring for the dying patient and the family*, 3rd edn (pp. 243–250). London: Chapman & Hall.

Olsen, D.P. (1991). Empathy as an ethical and philosophical basis for nursing. *Advances in Nursing Science, 14* (1), 62–75.

Otlowski, M.F.A. (1995). Legal and ethical issues in palliative care. *Monash Bioethics Review, 14* (1), 33–47.

Parker, J. & Gardner, G. (1992). The silence and the silencing of the nurse's voice: A reading of patient progress notes. *Australian Journal of Advanced Nursing, 9* (2), 3–9.

Parker, J. & Wiltshire, J. (1995). The handover: Three modes of nursing practice knowledge. In Gray, G. & Pratt, R. (Eds.), *Scholarship in the discipline of nursing* (pp. 151–168). Melbourne: Churchill Livingstone.

Pearson, A. (1993). Guest editorial: Nursing, technology and the human condition. *Journal of Advanced Nursing, 18*, 165–167.

Ray, M.A. (1987). Technological caring: A new model in critical care. *Dimensions of Critical Care Nursing, 6* (3), 166–173.

Sandelowski, M. (1988). A case of conflicting paradigms: Nursing and reproductive technology. *Advances in Nursing Science, 10* (3), 35–45.

Street, A. (1995). *Nursing replay: Researching nursing culture together.* Melbourne: Churchill Livingstone.

Van Eys, J. (1991). The ethics of palliative care. *Journal of Palliative Care, 7* (3), 27–32.

Weedon, C. (1992). *Feminist practice and poststructuralist theory.* Oxford: Blackwell.

Wilkinson, P. (1992). The influence of high technology care on patients, their relatives and nurses. *Intensive and Critical Care Nursing, 8*, 194–198.

# 21

# From Cure to Palliation in a Bone Marrow Transplant Unit

## Yvonne Panek-Hudson

*This chapter is dedicated to Steven Ryle*
*who died on 25 May 1996, aged 30*
*a patient*
*a friend*
*an inspiration*

Since the 1960s, bone marrow transplantation has developed from a highly experimental to a first-line treatment modality (Szer, 1994). An enormous number of malignant and benign disorders are being treated with bone marrow transplants including leukaemia, lymphoma, breast cancer, multiple myeloma and aplastic anaemia. Many people who would previously have died from these diseases or treatment-related toxicities now experience long-term survival with bone marrow transplantation.

The advent and progress of this intensive form of treatment has seen an increase in curative potential but, simultaneously, a higher incidence of treatment-related morbidity and mortality. This knowledge leads to the understanding that there will be a percentage of bone marrow transplant (BMT) patients who will not survive. It is essential to highlight the importance of providing a suitable environment and resources for those patients for whom BMT has not been successful.

This chapter will briefly outline the historical background of BMT before moving to a discussion of the provision of palliative care within the BMT environment. The specific focus of the chapter is on the dilemmas faced by nurses in their attempt to provide optimal levels of care when they recognise the futility of treatment, often in advance of the patient, family or medical practitioner. The transition from cure to palliation is highlighted in the BMT context because the patient undertakes a potentially curative procedure associated with significant potential for treatment-related mortality.

# Background

BMT as a treatment modality has developed in Australia over the past 20 years. Worldwide it is estimated that 10 000 bone marrow transplants are conducted per year (Whedon, Stearns & Mills, 1995). The types of transplants performed include allogeneic, autologous, syngeneic, matched unrelated, mismatched, peripheral stem cell and, more recently, umbilical cord blood transplants.

Bone marrow transplants are performed for two major purposes. The first is to 'rescue' patients from the myelosuppressive effects of high dose chemotherapy (Crouch & Ross, 1994), and the second is to replace diseased marrow with healthy, functioning marrow, the main indication for allogeneic transplants. In both situations the ultimate purpose of BMT is to alter the course of an aggressive and fatal disease and achieve a cure. Most of the patients are young (less than 50 years of age) and are prepared to accept the multiple, disabling and potentially fatal side-effects as offsets against this chance at a cure of their disease. The increasing use of matched, unrelated (MUD) and mismatched familial transplantation is associated with a greater risk of severe and potentially fatal side-effects.

BMT is a relatively simple procedure where bone marrow is infused following a course of treatment aimed at destroying the patient's existing bone marrow. The usual in-patient admission is approximately six weeks, depending on the transplant type and the associated toxicities of treatment which may develop. Upon discharge, close outpatient follow-up care is necessary for at least three months post-BMT.

The growth and development of BMT has resulted in the discovery of treatment modalities and medications with a greater curative potential. Incidence of relapse post-BMT is significantly lower due to the utilisation of higher doses of chemotherapy and radiotherapy in conditioning therapy; however, treatment-related morbidity and mortality rates continue to be high as a result of the serious side-effects of many of these agents.

# Nursing implications

The knowledge that some patients will die receiving acute, potentially curative treatment has serious implications for nursing practice. Death may be due to a variety of factors such as multiple organ failure secondary to septicaemia, acute severe graft versus host disease, haemorrhagic cystitis and its associated complications, and relapse of disease.

Nurses often confront dilemmas in practice during the transition from curative to palliative care. While nurses are saddened by the impending death of the patient, the dilemmas that arise are likely to be related to issues of determining when further treatment is futile and palliative care should be implemented. Daily contact with the patient often means that nurses are the first professionals to recognise the potential futility of treatment. However, the contract between the BMT doctor and the patient to attempt a cure, the potential of some serious complications to be reversible, and the frequent difficulty in distinguishing between treatment toxicity and disease progression make the determination of a BMT patient's palliative care needs highly complex. Additionally, many people are involved in coming to a decision to abandon active treatment of both disease and toxicities, not least of whom are the young patient and family, the BMT doctors and the nurses providing daily care.

While it is possible to deliver palliative care in a curative environment, the tension between cure and palliation is an important barrier in the provision of palliative care in the BMT unit. The separate agendas of palliative and acute care environments are difficult to reconcile in practice, with one focused on pain and symptom relief and the transition to death, while the other is concerned with active and curative intent treatment (Samarel, 1989).

## Transitions

Transitions take place regularly throughout life and can be favourable or disruptive. Tyhurst (1957 cited in Murphy, 1990) defined transition as 'a passage or change from one place or state or act or set of circumstances to another'. People with cancer experience a range of transitions within their disease trajectory. The nursing role is actively involved in preparing patients for these transitions and in attempting to make them as smooth as possible. Assisting patients with disease- and illness-associated transitions often involves helping them to alter the views they have of their situation and incorporating their changed circumstances into a new reality. Schumacher and Meleis (1994) acknowledge that successful transitions allow for a sense of well-being. This is important, particularly in the transition of patient care from an acute curative focus to one of palliation.

The role of the nurse in any patient care situation is enormous; however, in the case of a patient for whom death is imminent, the input required by nursing staff is multi-factorial. The transition from being actively treated for their disease to being managed palliatively can take time for patients and their carers to understand and/or accept, especially when this transition is not clearly marked, with little difference in symptoms from the point when cure was still being attempted. Many patients and family members find this lack of clarity difficult to comprehend and need time and support to accept and plan for the impending death of the patient. The road between acute care and palliation can be convoluted and meandering; however, the nurse has an important role in this transitional period. Difficulties in distinguishing toxicity from disease and determining whether treatment is futile can lead to a trying time for all concerned.

Communication and the provision of accurate information is vital and it is often the nurse who is required to facilitate the opportunities for open discussion between the BMT doctor and the family and within the BMT team. Additionally, the nurse is often called on to clarify what has been said and to help the patient and family first deal with the uncertainties and then confront the knowledge that the BMT has not been successful and that the patient will die. However, many healthcare providers have difficulty discussing issues that contain uncertainty and ambiguity (Chekryn-Reimer & Davis, 1991). The nurse must be skilled in dealing with feelings of anger and uncertainty and in providing emotional support to the patient and family and to members of the healthcare team who will also have invested significant energy into the cure of a patient and also may find it difficult to acknowledge the patient's impending death. The nurse's efforts will also include ensuring symptom control for the patient.

# Two case histories

The following case histories illustrate the transition in care focus from cure to palliation in BMT and highlight the dilemmas and issues raised.

## Case 1: Simon and Sophie

Simon was a 25-year-old man with acute lymphoblastic leukaemia who underwent a mismatch transplant with bone marrow donated from his cousin. Simon was engaged to Sophie and they planned to marry as soon as Simon had recovered from the effects of the BMT. They both had a strong Catholic faith and believed that their strength and dedication would get them through.

Simon experienced the usual transplant-related toxicities such as infection, nausea, vomiting and mucositis; however, he recovered very well from his bone marrow suppression and was able to be discharged less than 30 days after his transplant. Sophie was the major support person for Simon during his transplant and was present in the BMT unit each day and many nights assisting with his care. Sophie was more outspoken than Simon and often answered questions and made decisions for him.

Several months following discharge, it became apparent that Simon's leukaemia had returned and that the focus of care would now be on symptom control and preparing Simon for his impending death. A course of oral chemotherapy was commenced as a symptom control measure only, and Simon and Sophie sought advice from alternative practitioners in the hope that a cure was still possible. During this time Simon and Sophie were married and moved into a flat that they had bought together.

Simon continued to become increasingly unwell and required admission to hospital for pain relief secondary to leukaemic infiltrates in his facial region. Gross periorbital oedema, which was unresponsive to treatment, meant that Simon had limited sight in both eyes with consequent impaired mobility. It was decided that Simon's optimum comfort was achieved through analgesia and relaxation methods.

Throughout the BMT and subsequent relapse, Simon never engaged in lengthy conversations with staff and appeared quite content for Sophie to ask the questions and be in control of decisions that needed to be made. Sophie made it quite clear that, regardless of nursing and medical staff believing Simon to be dying, she believed that he would live and be free of his leukaemia. Sophie insisted that treatment was to continue in an attempt to control his leukaemia and if necessary, Simon was to be resuscitated and transferred to the intensive care unit.

During this time Sophie maintained a vigil at Simon's bedside, rarely leaving his side and therefore making it extremely difficult for staff to enter into discussions specifically with Simon regarding his disease, prognosis and personal wishes. In view of Sophie's demands, medical staff were reluctant to commit to firm decisions relating to Simon's resuscitation status, leaving nurses in a dilemma over what action to take should Simon die in their care.

Simon died mid-morning, a number of weeks after his admission. No one was present at the time as Sophie had left his room briefly to make a phone call.

## Case 2: Jim

Jim was in his forties with refractory acute lymphoblastic leukaemia and underwent an allogeneic BMT using his brother's marrow. As Jim's disease had previously been unresponsive to conventional chemotherapy, a BMT was acknowledged as being his final opportunity for cure. Jim came from interstate and during most of his hospital stay had no support people with him and very few visitors. Jim was divorced but had a friendly relationship with his ex-wife, Maria. They had two adult sons, George and Paul. Jim was a placid and quiet man who attended to his daily care as independently as possible. He rarely made requests or voiced concerns, even when encouraged.

Early in Jim's BMT he began experiencing complications of impaired liver function, increasingly abnormal renal performance and persistent febrile episodes indicating overwhelming infection. Nursing and medical management focused on rectifying the toxicities Jim was developing secondary to his disease and BMT. As it became evident that Jim's condition was continuing to deteriorate despite intervention, Jim agreed that his family should be contacted and informed of his unstable condition. The family arrived promptly and, after discussion with Jim, medical and nursing staff, decided to stay in Melbourne to provide care and support to Jim.

Jim became increasingly unstable physically and was showing signs of confusion. Nursing staff were keen to make some realistic decisions regarding his plan of care, incorporating Jim's wishes, the needs of his family and advice from the nursing and medical staff. Staff felt some reluctance to discuss these issues with Jim's family, given their minimal involvement until this point, and Jim's deteriorating mental function made it difficult to discuss them with him. In view of this, active treatment continued for a further short period of time.

Nursing staff needed to encourage the medical staff to raise issues of resuscitation and intensive care admission with Jim's family. Nursing staff demanded that decisions be made regarding these issues so care could be focused on symptom relief and preparing Jim's family for the likelihood of his death.

Jim died peacefully with his sons and primary nurse present. All invasive treatment had been withdrawn following discussions with Jim's family. Palliative care measures had been commenced which allowed for fewer physical barriers between Jim and his family and improved comfort for Jim in an environment supportive of everyone involved.

## Discussion

These case histories reflect the very real practice dilemmas facing nurses during the transition to palliative care in the BMT Unit. In Simon's case, nurses' recognition of the need to implement palliative care was hampered by Sophie's understandable difficulty in accepting that her partner was dying. The differing timing of acceptance of the inevitability of death between the patient, family members and different staff requires careful negotiation of communication and sensitivity to each person's perspective. The nursing dilemmas associated with Simon's care revolved around not being able to gain Simon's perspective, not wanting Simon to die while hooked to a ventilator in the intensive care unit, and difficulties associated with implementing palliative care measures in the face of continuing belief in the possibility of cure. Nurses are required to work daily with the competing interests and perspectives of all involved and it can be enormously frustrating when attempts to meet the comfort and care needs of the patient are thwarted by a continued focus on cure.

Jim's story highlights the need for early discussion of the patient's wishes in regard to active treatment. His deteriorating mental condition precluded his involvement in decisions about his care, and the lack of an established relationship between the medical and nursing staff and Jim's family made the transition decisions all the more difficult to make.

The decision of whether to implement life-support in a patient following BMT is always difficult. Severe renal, liver and lung toxicity is common and at times intubation is indicated; however, few patients survive. The decision—between an attempt at a last effort at cure and an acceptance of death—is in no way as clear-cut as it might be in advanced solid tumours or other terminal illnesses.

The contract that is established between the BMT doctor and the patient in deciding to undergo BMT is one of attempted cure. Severe toxicity is expected and patients are prepared for this and accept it as inevitable that they will be very sick before they are better. The decision to end attempts to reverse toxicities is not easy and marks the breaking of this contract. Many doctors find this difficult to do, and there are examples of patients who did pull through despite the odds and many patients want to continue with treatment at any cost, including dying on a ventilator in intensive care.

The interface between curative and palliative care is complex and uncertain, making it difficut to anticipate precisely when treatment is futile. Nurses have a major role to play in helping bring into the open the uncertainties and dilemmas such decision-making raises. Input from all members of the team, the patient and the family early in the course of deterioration helps to reduce the isolation of all those involved, and to negotiate the transition.

## Conclusion

BMT staff are enthusiastic in their endeavours to cure patients who face the prospect of no further treatment and death. Nurses working within this specialist field of oncology are dedicated to the goals of care for BMT patients and make a significant contribution to the success of BMT procedures. However, they concurrently recognise the potentially life-threatening nature of this treatment and wish to ensure appropriate care of the person who will die during or following their BMT.

Dilemmas arising from the transition of care from curative to palliative are abundant and are directly related to the success of transition and role adaptation. A nurse's inability to meet the needs of the dying as a result of situations in their workplace can lead to role insufficiency (Williams, 1982, cited in Samarel, 1989). Many nurses believe that these dilemmas also result in suboptimal standards of palliative care being offered to BMT patients.

Future directions that may assist to develop an enhanced environment for the provision of palliative care for the BMT patient should include:

- nursing research into this issue;
- further improvements in multidisciplinary approaches to patient plans of care;
- initial and ongoing discussion with patients regarding their personal wishes relating to their treatment paths in the event of serious morbidity;
- work toward improving patient and family education;
- education of healthcare providers;
- a mutual understanding of the roles and benefits of each person involved in the care of patients, including the patient.

There are many survivors of BMT who experienced severe toxicities and have recovered from them. There are those who have survived and live with chronic conditions secondary to their BMT. There are those who did not survive but gave all their strength to fighting their illness. It is from all of these patients that we must learn about the importance of early and continual involvement in care decisions, of creating the opportunity to make choices and being hopeful in the face of cure no longer being possible. The nurse's challenge is to find ways to facilitate discussion of the transition to palliative care and to reduce the separation of curative and palliative care in the BMT unit.

# References

Carney, B. (1987). Bone marrow transplantation—Nurses' and physicians' perceptions of informed consent. *Cancer Nursing, 10* (5), 252–259.

Chekryn-Reimer, J. & Davies, B. (1991). Palliative care—The nurse's role in helping families through the transition of 'fading away'. *Cancer Nursing, 14* (6), 321–327.

Crouch, M.A. & Ross, J.A. (1994). Current concepts in autologous bone marrow transplantation. *Seminars in Oncology Nursing, 10* (1), 12–19.

Redler, N. (1994). A triumphant survival, but at what cost? Meeting the long term needs of cancer survivors. *Professional Nurse, 10* (3), 166–170.

Samarel, N. (1989). Caring for the living and dying: a study of role transition. *International Journal of Nursing Studies, 26* (4), 313–326.

Scumacher, K.L. & Meleis, A.I. (1994). Transitions: A central concept in nursing. *IMAGE: Journal of Nursing Scholarship, 26* (2), 119–127.

Szer, J. (1994). Bone marrow transplantation in 1994. *Modern Medicine of Australia,* March, 74–83.

Tyhurst, J. (1957). The role of transition states—including disasters—in mental illness. In Murphy, S.A. (1990) Human responses to transitions: A holistic nursing perspective. *Holistic Nursing Practice, 4* (3), 2.

Whedon, M., Stearns, D., & Mills, L.E. (1995). Quality of life of long term adult survivors of autologous bone marrow transplantation. *Oncology Nursing Forum, 22* (10), 1527–1537.

Williams, G.A. (1982). Role considerations in care of the dying patient. In Samarel, N. (1989) Caring for the living and dying: a study of role transition. *International Journal of Nursing Studies, 26* (4), 314.

Winters, G., Miller, C., Maracich, L., Compton, K., & Haberman, M.R. (1994). Provisional practice: The nature of psychosocial bone marrow transplant nursing. *Oncology Nursing Forum, 21* (7), 1147–1154.

# 22

# Dying of AIDS in Australia*

## Claire Parsons

This chapter addresses approaches to acquired immune-deficiency syndrome (AIDS) palliative care, mindful of how the sociopolitical context of AIDS permeates care even to the moment of death. In doing this, it highlights critical clinical and social issues associated with contemporary HIV (human immuno-deficiency virus) palliative care within Australia and in relation to Australian healthcare policy.

## History of the clinical management of people dying with AIDS

When AIDS was first being treated, there was little that could be identified as 'planned palliation' as most people died in hospital, often amidst confusion, fear and irrational testing of 'patients' for the blood-borne virus. Until the late 1980s, people dying with AIDS were often pressured to endure the experimental testing of drugs to the moment of their death. By the early 1990s, this approach to those dying of AIDS had largely ceased. With improvements in drug effectiveness, currently, it is often the person with AIDS (PWA) who pressures the clinician to allow access to experimental drugs as the only hope of recovery.

This is a disease of a mercurial nature, with multiple manifestations. People do not die of HIV or AIDS; they die from the array of opportunistic diseases that intrude upon a body where immune defences are severely compromised. The multifaceted, capricious nature of the disease often includes episodes of rapid deterioration and rapid recovery. Not surprisingly, people with HIV/AIDS often experience multiple signs and symp-

*I am most graftful for comments on earlier drafts of this paper from Dr Brian MacDonald, Palliative Care, Fairfield Hospital, and Mr Nigel Arberdour, Clinical Specialist, Royal District Nursing Service, which I took into consideration as I prepared the final draft. Any interpretations or errors of fact are, in the final analysis, entirely mine.

toms, such as pain, confusion, dementia, depression and anxiety, fatigue, fever, dyspnoea, headache (for several reasons, including cryptococcal meningitis), deteriorating vision or blindness, nausea and vomiting, diarrhoea, dehydration, wasting, ataxia, peripheral neuropathy, myopathy, Kaposi's sarcoma, skin diseases (such as psoriasis, folliculitis, seborrhoeic dermatitis, herpes zoster, molluscum contagiosum) and fungal infections (such as candidiasis). Many of these are common to the clinical manifestations of dying with AIDS and cause high levels of distress for the PWA and carers (Kermode, Emery, Parsons, & Edwards, 1994).

Pain management emerged early in the epidemic as a major issue as, initially, health providers struggled with ad hoc arrangements, without realising that this new disease required management of complex pain syndromes such as may occur with peripheral neuropathy. While some health providers endeavoured to provide adequate symptom control, others were sometimes unable or unwilling to appreciate the need for preventive pain management. Some took a punitive approach to people living with HIV/AIDS (PLWHA), embracing the multiple stigmas and social retributions meted out to homosexuals, injecting drug users (IDU), sex workers and others. Injecting drug users suffered the most, given that their desperate requests for relief of pain were often interpreted as a political calculation for drug attainment, not pain containment. Some professional carers believed IDU deserved to suffer for their reprehensible lifestyles (Parsons & Spicer, 1992; Jones & Molaghan, 1995; Flaskerud & Ungvarski, 1995).

Increasingly, biomedical knowledge has demonstrated the benefits of prophylaxis for opportunistic diseases such as pneumocystis carinii pneumonia (PCP), and has facilitated some improvement in symptom control of cytomegalovirus (CMV, with its associated blindness) as well as cryptosporidial diarrhoea.

While some opportunistic conditions could be treated, the antiretroviral AZT (azido-thymidine, Retrovir, Zidovudine) was the first drug licensed in Australia (1987) with proven benefits in stalling the virus (albeit over a limited period as the Anglo-French AZT trial, known as the Concorde study (1993–94), was to show). Drugs such as DDI (Didanosine, Videx) and DDC (Zalcitabine, Hivid) were to follow and, in 1995–96, 3TC (Crixivan) was to further the recognition of HIV disease as one of potential chronicity, rather than one leading to an inevitable and rapid death. In 1995, clinical trials of protease inhibitors began to show some success in inhibiting viral reproduction. In addition, the finding in 1995 that combination therapy constituted 'best practice' in medical treatment endorsed the view that HIV disease was shifting in profile from a necessarily fatal, to a chronic disease trajectory.

While HIV disease is becoming less a mandatory death sentence, AIDS is generally fatal and there is a greater realisation that people with HIV disease need to plan for their living and dying early in their disease, in case an opportunistic disease should cause a rapid decline in physical capacity, or induce mental changes that diminish the capacity to prepare for death.

## Contemporary management of palliation

Some insight can be gained of changes that have taken place over the past decade in palliative care management for people with AIDS. This section reports on such a comparison and then develops a broader understanding of the physical, mental, social and spiritual dimensions of the experience of dying with AIDS.

### A clinical profile of a death from AIDS

#### The male PWA

In 1995, at a seminar held in Victoria, 1986 and 1995 profiles of Victorian PWA were compared. It was reported that in 1986, 80 per cent of those presenting with pneumocystis carinii pneumonia (PCP) also received their HIV positive diagnosis for the first time. Ten per cent of PWA did not leave hospital following their first AIDS-defining illness. The mean survival rate following AIDS diagnosis was seven months. By 1995, the profile had changed markedly. Usually, an HIV positive man would have known about his serostatus for around a decade, would still be employed, and would be on combinations of drugs, taking around 25 tablets (including PCP prophylaxis) per week. The mean survival rate following AIDS diagnosis was reported as 42 months (within the range 0.4–67 months) in 1995. Cytomegalovirus (CMV) has now replaced PCP as the most common opportunistic disease (as most PWAs have been prescribed preventative medication for PCP). The PWA will have regular ophthalmology screening following HIV diagnosis—recommended 6-monthly when CD4 count is below 50 (Jennens, 1995). He will receive treatment at home, administered by a registered nurse and will only be admitted to hospital if there are complications (Mijch, 1995). A recent survey of drug therapies given in the last year of life showed that in the terminal stage of HIV disease, PWAs are being treated with an average of five medications, usually in multiple doses per day, and this raises an issue regarding the difficulties of late stage polypharmacy to be managed by palliative care teams (MacDonald, 1995).

This profile will vary little across Australia today. Unlike those dying of any other disease, the male PWA also commonly has a history of multiple grief due to loss of partners, friends and associates who have already died of this disease and possibly a partner who is also dying of the same condition. This gives him an intimate second-hand experience of the conditions and outcomes that lovers and friends have endured and that he may now experience personally.

## The female PWA

The issues for women differ, as does the clinical trajectory. HIV positive women often subordinate their own health and well-being for the sake of partners and children (Moore, 1993; Patton, 1994; Jones & Molaghan, 1995; Lawless, Kippax, & Crawford, 1996). Women tend to be diagnosed late because they do not regard themselves as being 'at risk' when within what they see as a stable relationship, and because of persistent failure on the part of the health professions and society to overcome the stereotype that women who are HIV positive must be deviant ('prostitutes' or IDU) (Stuntzner-Gibson, 1991). Therefore, the married woman, the upper middle-class schoolgirl, the lesbian, is often not perceived as needing investigation. Late diagnosis also occurs because doctors often fail to recognise that some gynaecological conditions, such as persistent or recurrent unexplained vaginal candidiasis, cervical dysplasia, and pelvic inflammatory disease, might be a manifestation of HIV disease (Mijch, Clezy, & Furner, 1996). Indeed, since 1993, the Centres for Disease Control classification has identified invasive cervical cancer as a major indicator of AIDS in women.

While in Australia there appears to have been no study comparing gender life expectancy differences for PWA, in the USA, a woman's life span from HIV diagnosis to AIDS diagnosis to death has been reported as being shorter than that for men (Patton, 1995), although this has been disputed as reflecting late diagnosis (Stuntzner-Gibson, 1991; Melnick, Sherer, & Louis, 1994). However, internationally, HIV-infected women are a third more likely to die without an AIDS-defining diagnosis.

Most positive women have lower self-esteem than do most positive men, often have young children (some of whom are HIV positive [Mijch et al., 1996]) and are slow to disclose their HIV status in order to protect others in the family from stigma, especially children from violence and discrimination at school (Moore, 1993; Patton, 1994; Lobb, 1995). However, a child's diagnosis of HIV will often disclose the mother's HIV status.

Women will frequently receive less than optimal medical care, will often cease taking medications where allergies, drug interactions and side-effects affect their ability to care safely and effectively for their children. Community-based organisations working with positive women report that these women frequently do not have the finances to access alternate treatments, and are sometimes unable to pay for recommended treatments under orthodox medicine, with Medicare covering a minimum of the expensive AIDS medications; this latter problem is common to many with a life-threatening illness. Nor are they likely to be in a situation where they can leave work and retire on a substantial superannuation payout as can a proportion of the positive men, factors that have yet to be investigated systematically in Australia. Indeed, as Patton (1993) points out, the poverty and isolation in which HIV positive men may suddenly find themselves following diagnosis is often the ongoing lived experience of women. These are women who may have HIV positive partners, or have been rejected by partners, may face isolation and poverty and have few (if any) support and care providers in the community. They may also be women grieving for the loss of future involvement in their children's development, having to make custodial arrangements for their children when the children's fathers and their own biological family may have deserted them but want control of their children (Patton, 1994; Lobb, 1995). Carers from community-based organisations working with positive women report that this is true in Australia. However, again, this requires detailed research.

During the terminal stage of HIV disease, the women with children often have great difficulty finding ongoing child-care support, especially when they are obliged to disclose their HIV status, and occasionally the HIV positive status of their children. Given that 'quality of care' for PWA is supposed to include stress reduction (to limit the impact of stress on immune function) and hence promote life quality and duration, this can compound the other major contributor (late diagnosis and treatment) to shorten the life of the female PWA (further social and clinical issues are discussed in Duckett, 1994; Lucke & Raphael, 1994; Mijch et al., 1996). The issues pertaining to the care of HIV-positive women, a minority group within a marginal group of people with terminal illness, have yet to be appropriately addressed by the majority of health providers. Palliative care teams, even in AIDS-dedicated units, seldom have specialist training in the special needs of male PWA, let alone female PWA. Nor do they understand PWA in a cross-cultural context despite planning to redress this issue (cf. Palliative Care Advisory Council, 1991). As Horton (1995) concluded in his paper on women and HIV, 'without an appreciation of the context of HIV infection, much effort will be squandered on overly simplistic and impracticable programmes' (p. 530).

## Physical dimensions

During episodes of acute care, a PWA may be hospitalised. However, the remainder of the process of living and dying with HIV disease is spent in ambulatory care, sometimes managing treatments in a day unit, or in the home. Indeed, home-care or community-care nurses have altered the face of healthcare delivery, setting new standards of care and community management including the effective use of technologies, such as nutrition via a gastrostomy (PEG) or the administration of parenteral medications including pain relief. The alimentary tract is highly susceptible to the opportunistic infections associated with HIV disease, from oral hairy leucoplakia and disseminated candidiasis, to profound malabsorption syndrome, secondary to a wide range of gastroenteric pathogens, to intestinal and rectal infections. Clinical management of AIDS, no matter where it is delivered, involves adequate nutrition, often being administered by non-oral means.

CMV retinitis is a late stage condition associated with HIV disease, occurring in around 20 per cent of PWA and can be asymptomatic until the pathology is advanced whereby the PWA may begin by reporting flashes of light, floaters in the visual field, or optic pain and later, blurred vision or partial visual field loss (Jones & Molaghan, 1995, p. 687). While gancyclovir (DHPG) or foscarnet may be administered as a therapy, close monitoring (on a monthly basis) of changes in the PWA vision is important to health management.

The greatest barrier to the delivery of quality care to HIV positive women is the remnant myth of women as vectors of disease (Report of the 'HIV infection in women' conference, 1995; Lawless et al., 1996) as are the effects of the association between sexism, poverty and drug use. As the gynaecological manifestations of HIV disease are usually severe, persistent, recurring and debilitating, the doctor and nurse need to employ all their knowledge from gynaecological training to recognise and assist with early treatment of conditions that may manifest in various ways, including menstrual irregularities, vaginal infections (candida, herpes), cervical dysplasia, pelvic inflammatory disease, and genital ulcers. As palliative care may be provided over a prolonged period, the health provider becomes clinician, educator and counsellor, taking seriously and sensitively issues around sexuality, STD management, and even contraception as essential to quality care.

Home palliation or hospice care has been considerably restructured to allow many PWA to die in the comfort and privacy of their own home and in the presence of loved ones. Home management is complex, requiring the PWA to have no impairment to mental faculties (or have full-time supervision and home support), as well as to manage equipment, including safe disposal of needles and (where applicable) cytotoxic waste; and for those who are IDU, to have a clear understanding of possible outcomes if an intravenous line is used to inject non-prescribed drugs (Jones & Molaghan, 1995).

Pain is often managed by nurses and the PWA in the home facilitated by technologies such as syringe drivers and intravenous lines. Adjuvant medications may be used to boost the effectiveness of pain medications. Here the health provider as observer, practitioner and advocate must differentiate between acute and chronic pain, pain associated with drug withdrawal, and pain related to the disease manifestations. Establishing trust, valuing the PWA's account of a pain experience, and understanding the PWA's cultural and personal mode of pain expression, are crucial to the assessment and management of the pain experience to maximise quality of life. Tolerance to pain medications can occur quickly and needs to be taken into account when assessing the PWA's pain experience. Lack of adequate sleep and rest, nausea, depression, anxiety, anger, or fear will amplify the pain experience.

Symptom management is paramount in palliative care, as is knowledgeable and sensitive communication, including the early preparation and provision of support for the dying process. The primary caregiver as patient advocate may challenge medical orders, or family decision-making, if the PWA does not believe it is in his or her best interests.

## Mental dimensions

By the late 1980s, as medications began to stall the progression and incidence of opportunistic diseases, increasing observations were being made about mental changes concomitant with HIV disease. Several years passed before such changes were clinically distinguished from the array that concatenated the symptoms of depression and anxiety as anticipated psychological responses to what was effectively 'a death sentence', and those that indicated neuropsychiatric pathologies. Some PWA with such mental changes were being diagnosed for the first time as having both HIV and their first AIDS-defining illness. The major neuropsychiatric diagnosis was labelled AIDS Dementia Complex (more recently redefined as AIDS-related dementia). The realisation that psychological and psychiatric changes manifested in several ways further complicated the more typical case scenario of palliation where a gradual deterioration occurs until, finally, palliative care management is required in the last few days or weeks of life. In contrast, AIDS-related palliation and control of multiple and diverse symptoms might be required intermittently over a period of months to more than a year.

Along with severe pain, it is AIDS-related dementia that PWA fear most although the incidence has not increased markedly among PWA over time, this being largely attributed to the beneficial effects of AZT (Brew, 1995).

Parsons and Spicer's (1992) study in Australia showed that general trained nurses lacked the skills of psychiatric nursing to undertake appropriate diagnosis and management of the psychological and neuropsychiatric changes among PWA. The distinction between the two not only requires some knowledge of psychiatric nursing, but also an understanding of the socio-political context of this disease. Understanding the psycho-emotional pain of rejection, blame, fear of contagion and disassociation guides the health provider in interpreting the silence, depression and anxiety, withdrawal, anger, aggression, or suicidal thoughts that the PWA may express or exhibit. Learning effective assessment techniques assists the health provider to advocate for early psychological or psychiatric assessment for the treatment, support and protection of those with AIDS. The diagnosis of neuropsychiatric symptoms of HIV disease remains problematic, usually being made through methods of exclusion rather than through each having its own discrete nosology.

## Social and spiritual dimensions

There are a number of social issues to be dealt with in HIV palliative care. In addition to the usual ethical concerns over confidentiality, informed consent and 'best practice' are other ethical and practical issues of patient advocacy and appropriate communication regarding the PWA as his or her condition deteriorates. The politicising of HIV disease has impressed on health providers the need to remember, daily, 'who' knows 'which' aspects of the individual's diagnosis, as with this disease perhaps above all others, confidentiality of diagnosis may vary even between family members. For example, a mother may know her son's diagnosis while a father may not even know his son is gay, let alone that he is dying of AIDS. Rhetoric masks HIV/AIDS under the more socially acceptable constructs: 'your son has cancer', 'your daughter has pneumonia', 'your son has tuberculosis'. Thus an issue to be confronted by both patient and health provider is 'who to disclose to'. Having AIDS raises multiple issues: dying, dying of a stigmatised disease, 'coming out', loss of employment with ensuing impoverishment and isolation, challenges over who claims the body (partner, family or friends), who claims the assets, who claims custody of children, who is willing to handle the body (funerary practices) and so on. Health providers can be involved in all these potentially contentious issues, which adds to the complexity of patient advocacy.

Health providers in the community must also recognise the support needs of the PWA, the time when carers need respite, especially as partners and family who provide the most support may still do so in a climate of ignorance and disapproval. They must also be responsive to the PWA need for spiritual, philosophical, or religious support and know when and how to summon such support.

Lego-ethical issues surrounding euthanasia, power of attorney, health insurance, pauperisation, viatification, funeral preparation are currency in planning for disease management in HIV disease and alleviating the psychoemotional stresses associated with terminal illness.

# Euthanasia and dying of AIDS

Suicide, assisted-suicide, self-delivery and euthanasia are concepts implicit in the debate about PWA's palliative care options in terminal illness. Suicide is usually a concept associated with a lonely death, chosen individually and without support. Assisted suicide implies that someone who is supportive and has some expertise in the management of a quick and painless death is involved in assisting the individual to make a reasoned choice between living and dying. In this situation, there are more factors involved than a single means–end choice influencing the decision. These factors may include those pertaining to personal, family and social values, quality of life and life meaning.

Self-delivery refers to the fact that the individual who wishes to end his or her life in this sphere of existence is capable (both mentally and physically) of choosing to press a button, or drink a solution (or the like), but requires expert assistance to prepare the apparatus, or cocktail, to terminate life. Euthanasia draws on the latter concepts. It is the termination of life at the behest of the individual who has a terminal condition. This is usually undertaken in a supportive environment with chosen loved ones and friends in full knowledge that the action is to be taken and often with them in attendance.

In Australia, the debate has been clouded by Judeo-Christian values that impede both reasoned debate and a recognition that all concepts and realities are socially constructed. Listening to the voices of medicine, nursing, people living and dying with AIDS, and other community sectors, the debate conflates the legitimised and powerful discourses of culture, religion and science.

While this is not the place to debate the pros and cons of euthanasia, in some instances political and medical opinion has become coterminous with the emotive lay discourses on 'murderers' and 'killers' (cf. Pollard, 1990). These do little to enlighten the issues involved. Euthanasia as a 'desire' is grounded on multidimensional experience and decision-making. It is linked to values, life philosophies, social relationships, a sense of autobiography and identity, as well as a belief about whether anyone should own or control the life and death decisions of another.

As nurses and doctors listen to these debates and ponder their personal accountability as professionals, they are caught between the people they have come to know as patients with a terminal illness who wish relief from their existence and the professional narratives legitimising the speaking of the 'experts' over that of the individual. While they may have some empathy with the patient's plight, they also see the issue as one of real life legal and professional consequences in terms of self.

In 1995, seven doctors in the fields of HIV medicine and oncology in

Australia declared publicly that they had supported 'patients' with 'assisted suicide'. This opened a public debate on an issue that had been in the shadows for some years. Indeed, the ingredients of a 'cocktail' to be used for an effective and painless suicide had been released in the gay press prior to the doctors' declaration. Researchers began surveying medical attitudes toward euthanasia and assisted suicide and found that a majority among doctors treating HIV disease supported the measure as a choice negotiated between the patient and doctor (Fagan, Smith, McMurchie, Byliss, & Magnussen, 1995). The medical survey responses were given in the recognition that although many PWAs discuss or report considering these options as they face their first AIDS-defining diagnosis, few plan to undertake such action once they are able to access effective care, including specialist palliative care.

In 1995, Marshall Perron, chief minister of the Northern Territory of Australia, undertook a referendum on the issue of euthanasia. The referendum returned a 'yes' vote and the first measures for assisted suicide to be passed into law were implemented in 1996 to take effect 1 July. Crucial amendments were passed in February of 1996 (Leach & McLean, 1995; Voluntary euthanasia, 1996). The other states in Australia have yet to hold such a referendum. While the bill passed into law in the Northern Territory, and a few people with terminal illnesses took advantage of it, federal legislation overturned it.

For health providers, there remains the dilemma of awaiting professional policies on the issue of their role in euthanasia while continuing to be privy to confidences of patients wishing to discuss euthanasia as an option and the occasional voicing of the desire to 'end it all'. In the face of a lack of guidelines on how to process requests for euthanasia, palliative care professionals seem the best suited to make sensitive and detailed non-judgmental assessments of such requests.

## Policy and the politics of dying with AIDS

In the socio-political management of the dying process, discrimination in service provision, the partial and partisan availability of particular human and technological services, limited out-of-hours backup for services, the restricted availability of new drugs for survival or palliative management, delayed approval of newly trialled HIV drugs, limited Medicare provisions for the expensive and multiple medications required by PWA even during palliative care stages are only some of the more visible manifestations of the politics of care of those dying with AIDS, although each is not necessarily unique to AIDS. As Watney (1988) and Small (1993) have argued, the politics of the discourses on AIDS has presented people living with HIV disease as largely invisible and passive receptacles of the virus and its consequences. Yet, in Australia, PWA are often well educated and politically astute, and have been proactive in driving aspects of the quality and priority issues of AIDS research, treatment and care (including palliative/hospice care) to the best of their ability.

This chapter has raised issues pertaining to the impact of AIDS in the context of the political, social, and experiencing (phenomenological) body (Turner, 1984; Scheper-Hughes & Lock, 1987), including dimensions of the mind, identity and experience of dying, and has raised palliative care policy implications of such discursive discourses at the level of education, clinical management and health service delivery. The issue of quality of care available to PWA in Australia is currently focused on the availability of specialist palliative care services, although mainstreaming of such service provision is planned but has yet to be supported by widespread health provider training. While health provider training, counselling and debriefing also remain inadequate, successful strategies for achieving this have been demonstrated by non-government and community-based organisations who offer education, counselling and support for their care teams. Issues remain as to how to institutionalise and/or deinstitutionalise dying with dignity and the resources, services, quality of care and continuity of care required by individual PWA.

## What makes AIDS different

Some health providers, such as Woodruff (1993) have argued that AIDS-related palliation is little different (if at all) from that required for people dying of cancer. However, others argue that HIV disease is different from beginning to end (Palliative Care Advisory Council, 1991; Jones & Molaghan, 1995; George, 1995). The multifaceted, capricious nature of this disease attests to its clinical difference. Few, if any, diseases manifest the range of opportunistic illnesses and multi-systemic effects that arise in HIV disease. There are also therapeutic differences including the fact that most PWA have embraced alternative or complementary therapies, and the management of the high level of polypharmacy and the balancing of allopathic and naturopathic medicinal properties become very complex.

At the psycho-emotional level, the impact of this disease has a profound effect on the PWA, not only because he or she is young and facing death. To the PWA, physical appearance, such as that associated with wasting, Kaposi's sarcoma, or PEG tubes, central venous access devices (such as PICC lines), or the occasional indwelling urinary catheter, can be devastating, especially in a gay lifestyle where the body is often one's major currency of 'selfhood', identity and social companionship. Issues around intimacy and sexuality are intrinsic to relationships and ongoing normalcy in everyday life, and may remain important even into the palliation stage. Fear of dementia is ever present. Furthermore, grieving for the multiple loss of partners, friends and associates who have already died of this disease takes a toll greater than any other disease this century. Each of these distinguish this disease from all others, even in the palliation stage.

Although all diseases have their elements of unpredictability and uncertainty, these features are amplified in HIV disease. For example, while pain relief and other symptom relief are central to the final stage of management, preventative and curative therapies may be aggressively pursued, such as when active treatment is continued in order to prevent blindness from CMV, the severe manifestations of disseminated candidiasis, or raised intracranial pressure.

The historical and political context of AIDS has profoundly influenced the human (individual and collective) experience of this disease to ensure it is different from all others. As Patton (1994) has pointed out, if it were not for the fact that gay communities mobilised to put 'gay rights' on the political agenda in America the decade prior to the epidemic being recognised, HIV probably would not have become labelled first as GRID (gay-related immune deficiency disease) or regarded as a gay disease and would never have been politicised and stigmatised in the way it has. Rather, it would have been seen as a disease which appeared to indiscriminately afflict men, women and children across social classes and continents, a pandemic about which everyone became concerned and to which the various sectors of all societies would have demanded the equitable mobilisation of resources and care.

Stigma and discrimination has held sway over reason among lay and professional alike. Irrational 'fear of AIDS' among health professionals has been documented in many countries (Ross & Hunter, 1991; Cydulka, Mathews, Born, Moy, & Parker, 1991; Sergeant, 1992; Parsons, 1995; Hunt, 1996). To ascertain the real meaning of 'care' that a society is prepared to provide for those living and dying with a particular disease, we must take account of these contexts of the social construction of diagnostic labelling as well as of what are deemed appropriate therapeutic and palliative care options.

# References

Brew, B. (1995). Dementia: There's hope. *Talkabout*, Sept., 20–21.

Cydulka, R., Mathews, J., Born, M., Moy, A., & Parker, M. (1991). Paramedical: Knowledge base and attitudes toward AIDS and hepatitis. *Journal of Emergency Medicine*, 9 (1–2), 37–43.

Duckett, M. (1994). Women, children and AIDS. Paper presented in HIV Studies, Western Sydney University.

Fagan, D., Smith, D., McMurchie, M., Byliss, H., & Magnussen, R. (1995, Nov.). Euthanasia, assisted suicide and other medical decisions concerning the ending of life: A quantitative survey of attitudes and practices among doctors who are members of the Australasian Society for HIV Medicine Inc. Paper presented at the ASHM conference, Coolum.

Flaskerud, J. & Ungvarski, P. (1995). *HIV/AIDS: A guide to nursing care*, 3rd edn. Philadelphia: W.B. Saunders Company.

George, R. (1995, 2 Dec.). Symptom control in advanced AIDS. Paper presented at the seminar on 'HIV palliative care', Fairfield Hospital, Melbourne.

Horton, R. (1995). Women as women with HIV. *Lancet, 345*, 531–532.

Hunt, R. (1996). The hospice movement matures. *Medical Journal of Australia, 164*, 452–453.

Jennens, I. (1995). Cytomegalovirus retinitis. In Bowden, F., Hoy, J., Mijch, A., & Robinson, J. (Eds.). *HIV medicine handbook: A manual for clinicians working with HIV infection.* Melbourne: Melbourne University Press.

Jones, D. & Molaghan, J. (1995). HIV nursing care. In Sande, M. & Volberding, P. (Eds.), *The medical management of AIDS.* Philadelphia: W.B. Saunders Company.

Kermode, M., Emery, K., Parsons, C., & Edwards, H. (1994). *Orientation to infection control including HIV/AIDS.* Melbourne: La Trobe University.

Lawless, S., Kippax, S., & Crawford, J. (1996). Dirty, diseased and undeserving: The position of HIV positive women. *Social Science & Medicine, 9* (43), 1371–1378.

Leach, T. & McLean, S. (1995). Euthanasia law passed in the Northern Territory. *HIV/AIDS Legal Link, 6* (2), 1, 6.

Lobb, D. (1995). Palliative care for women with AIDS: Identifying the issues. *Journal of Palliative Care, 11* (2), 45–47.

Lucke, J. & Raphael, B. (1994). HIV and AIDS: Issues for women in Australia. *Health Care for Women International, 16*, 221–228.

MacDonald, B. (1995, 2 Dec.). Drugs used in final stages of AIDS. Paper presented at the seminar on 'HIV palliative care', Fairfield Hospital, Melbourne.

Melnick, S., Sherer, R., & Louis, T. (1994). Survivial and disease progression according to gender of patients with HIV infection. *JAMA, 272*, 1915–1921.

Mijch, A. (1995, 2 Dec.). Medical aspects of AIDS: The challenge of change. Paper presented at the seminar on 'HIV palliative care', Fairfield Hospital, Melbourne.

Mijch, A., Clezy, K., & Furner, V. (1996). Women with HIV. *Medical Journal of Australia, 164*, 669–671.

Moore, R. (1993). Support for women with HIV/AIDS: An interview with Bev Greet of Positive Women, the support group for women with HIV/AIDS. *Health Sharing Women, 4* (1), 1.

Palliative Care Advisory Council (1991). *Caring for people with terminal illness: A manual outlining the palliative care standards and guidelines.* Melbourne: Health Department Victoria.

Parsons, C. (1995). Infection control and HIV/AIDS. In Bennett, L., Miller, D., & Ross, M. (Eds.), *Health workers and AIDS: Research, intervention and current issues in burnout and response.* London: Harwood Press.

Parsons, C. & Spicer, M. (1992). *HIV/AIDS nursing: Changing minds.* Melbourne: La Trobe University.

Patton, C. (1993). With champagne and roses: Women at risk from/in AIDS discourse. In Squire, C. (Ed.), *Women and AIDS: Psychological perspectives.* London: Sage.

Patton, C. (1994). *Last served? Gendering the HIV pandemic.* London: Taylor & Francis.

Pollard, B. (1990). Some medical aspects of euthanasia. *Pallicom, 9* (4), 3–6.

Report on the 'HIV infection in women' conference, Washington (1995). *AIDS Alert*, p. 55.

Ross, J. & Hunter, C. (1991). Dimensions, content and validation of the fear of AIDS schedule in health professionals. *AIDS Care, 3* (2), 175–180.

Scheper-Hughes, N. & Lock, M. (1987). The mindful body: A prolegamenon to future work in medical anthropology. *Medical Anthopology Quarterly, 1* (1), 6–41.

Sergeant, J. (1992). Not only a room with a view. *Pallicom, 11* (1), 19–20.

Small, N. (1993). Dying in public places. In Clark, D. (Ed.), *The sociology of death: Theory, culture, practice.* Oxford: Blackwell Publishers.

Stuntzner-Gibson, D. (1991). Women and HIV disease: An emerging social crisis. *Social Work, 36* (1), 22–27.

Turner, B. (1984). *The body and society.* Oxford: Basil Blackwell.

Voluntary euthanasia Northern Territory (1996). *Monash Bioethics Review, 15* (2), 7–8.

Watney, S. (1988). AIDS, moral panic theory and homophobia. In Aggleton, P. & Homans, H. (Eds.), *Social aspects of AIDS.* Lewes: The Falmer Press.

Woodruff, R. (1993). *Palliative medicine.* Melbourne: Asperula.

# 23

# Motor Neurone Disease

## Helen Austin

Motor neurone disease (MND) is an uncommon degenerative disease that affects men and women of all ages but more commonly older people in the 60–80 year age group. In Victoria with a population of four and a half million, 90 people die of MND each year, some living with the disease for less than 12 months, others for 20 years or more. The majority of people have symptoms for between two and five years (Kurtzke, 1982).

While no treatment is available yet for MND, a great deal of research is being carried out around the world and some therapeutic trials are underway in Australia and overseas (Orrell & Lane, 1994). However, much can be done to deal with the symptoms produced by the disease. The focus must always be on improving the quality of life, providing comfort for the person with MND and support for the family and carers.

The care these people require will depend on the symptoms the disease produces (Sedal, 1987). As many people will lose the ability to speak, but not to communicate, it is best that the palliative care team be introduced earlier rather than later so that a relationship can be established while oral communication is still possible. The length of contact the MND patient will have with the palliative care team is not unlike that of the AIDS patient and, increasingly, of patients with other life-threatening diseases (Oxtoby, 1993).

Traditionally, the palliative care team has been involved with cancer patients for the last three to six months of life, but with motor neurone patients that period may well be one to two years. It is relatively easy to determine when the person with cancer requires palliative care: they have often reached the end of treatment that was directed against the disease itself, the disease is continuing to progress and the patient's general condition is deteriorating. The situation is different for the person with MND: no treatment significantly alters the course of the disease and the period of the illness that is relatively symptom free is short once the diagnosis has been made. The emphasis from the moment of diagnosis is on anticipation of the symptoms and the development of means to overcome them. The symptoms are often in the form of a disability such as weakness or dysarthria rather than pain or nausea, which are more typically seen in palliative care. Patients with MND have been heard to say that they don't feel ill, but rather disabled. Perhaps the rapidly progressing disability rather than a rapidly progressing illness makes these people seem different in a palliative care setting. Whether it is disability or illness that we are dealing with, the same principles apply—what is it that is distressing the patient or their carer and what can we do to alleviate that distress?

## The clinical team

Because symptoms vary from patient to patient and result in a mixture of disability and illness, they require the skills of a palliative care team supported by a specialist rehabilitation team (Oliver, 1989). It may be a large team, with the core members being medical, nursing, speech pathology, pastoral care and social workers, but a physiotherapist, occupational therapist and on occasions a neuropsychologist will also be required. Because this is a large team it is critical that members work well together. The important feature of such a team is that every member understands and respects the skills and knowledge of every other member. To spare a patient being inundated by well-meaning health professionals, the team members are introduced as they are needed. It is important to identify key members of the team who are usually those with skills that are particularly relevant to the problems the patient is experiencing or who develop a good relationship with the patient or carer. They provide the bulk of care and use the other team members as consultants. When team members know that their skills are recognised and valued by other team members and the goals of treatment are clear, the team will work well together for the benefit of the patient.

## *Team members*

The *doctor* needs to have access to detailed information about the disease so that questions can be answered honestly and the patient, carer and other team members have time to plan for the care needs. As the progression of the disease is often rapid, anticipation of care needs is vital. Most patients have seen at least one neurologist, usually two and on occasions many more, as they seek information and honest answers to their questions. With only 80–100 new cases of MND each year in Victoria, many neurologists will only see a few people each year and the patient's general practitioner may see only one person with MND in 20–30 years of general practice. Thus, the general practitioner may know much about the patient and their family but very little about the disease itself. Access to specialist medical advice is therefore essential. Continuity of medical care must be maintained and communication between the specialist and the general practitioner must be regular and open.

The *nurse's role* obviously depends on where the patient is being cared for. In the community, the nurse often acts as the case manager, co-ordinating all aspects of the care the patient is receiving from a variety of health professionals. Nurses need to be attentive to changes in symptoms and to understand the roles of other health professionals who may be able to offer expert advice. They offer support to the families and carers as well as providing hands-on care when necessary.

The role of the *speech pathologist* can be critical in good management, as this disease affects the patient's ability to speak and to swallow. Many people have heard frightening stories of 'choking' to death, but our experience of caring for over 400 people indicates that 'choking' does not occur. The speech pathologist's role is twofold: to ensure that adequate communication skills are maintained and developed, and to enable the patient to swallow and receive food and fluids in the most suitable form.

Access to a skilled *physiotherapist* is important as mobility is often a concern. The shoulders may become painful as the muscles supporting the joint become weaker; the chest muscles weaken and respiratory function is compromised and the ability to deal with secretions is reduced. The physiotherapist also has a role in general comfort and positioning.

MND can result in fairly rapid loss of independence for many people and the early introduction of an *occupational therapist* can facilitate access to aids necessary for personal independence and the alterations that may be needed in the home.

MND is a chronic condition and the patient and carers require support and practical help from *pastoral carers* and *social workers* as they come to terms with the diagnosis and the consequences of the illness and its progression.

In a small proportion of cases, dementia may be a feature. It may occur as part of the disease or, on occasions, alongside the disease (Muller et al., 1993). A *neuropsychologist* can provide assessment and ongoing advice.

# Specific symptoms

## Dysarthria

Oral communication is the most effective form of communication, with most people speaking up to 200 words/minute. With MND, the speed of communication is reduced and the intelligibility is severely compromised. If the speed of communication is reduced to 50 per cent (i.e. to 100 words/minute), conversation is prolonged. If intelligibility is also reduced, oral communication is extremely difficult.

Communication is a two-way interaction: we have a responsibility to make ourselves understood and to understand. There is no need to apologise for not understanding if some basic steps have been taken. These involve closing the door and windows to external, extraneous noise, turning a television set or radio off, positioning oneself to watch the patient's face and get as many non-verbal clues as possible and then to focus on the conversation. If speech is still unintelligible, it is time for an alternative method of communication to be used. The patient needs to accept responsibility for communication. What method they will choose and be able to use depends on a number of variables. If they have adequate hand function they may be able to write, either on paper or on a 'Magna Doodle'. The latter has the advantage of the communication being transitory—nothing is left for others to read. The Magna Doodle is not just a toy; it is in fact a quite sophisticated communication tool.

If hand function is adequate, the use of an electronic communicator may be appropriate and referral to a speech pathologist to determine which type is most appropriate is vital—the range is now considerable and professional assessment of the patient followed by introduction to, and instruction in, the use of the aid is essential. These aids will range from the simple, with a visual display or tickertape print out, to the complex, with voice output. It is vital to remember that once an aid is required, the speed of communication will fall dramatically and this has implications for everyone providing care—patient and carers will need time.

Even if hand communication is lost completely, there are still means of communicating. Eye movement is only very rarely affected in MND, so people who loose speech and hand movement can still be provided with an effective means of communication. The E tran board allows for sophisticated communication provided the carer is adequately trained in its use. The patient will usually adapt quickly to its use, spelling out their message by looking at the letters on the board and the person to whom they are communicating will be able to record the letters and the message.

It should be possible to ensure that every person with MND is able to communicate in a meaningful way with their carers and family. It is important to remember that alternative means of communication can be very slow.

## Dysphagia

Fear of choking is common in this condition. People with bulbar involvement may have significant swallowing problems and referral to a speech pathologist with skills in this area is essential.

We eat for reasons other than simply to provide nutrition for our bodies. Eating is usually a pleasurable activity and attention should be paid to the colour, taste and texture of the meal, its nutrient content and the effect various foods have on saliva composition. The social aspects of eating, such as the companionship of a shared meal also need to be considered, as do the volume of the meal and the amount of fluid required to feel comfortable.

Swallowing is an enormously complex function, involving the psyche as well as the lips, tongue, teeth, oropharynx, naso-pharynx, larynx and oesophagus. In the early stages of MND, decisions may need to be made about the avoidance of certain foods that affect the volume and consistency of saliva—milky products in particular will cause a thickening of the saliva by increasing mucous production and this alteration may be just sufficient to cause difficulties with swallowing. Grape and papaya juice, on the other hand, may thin the saliva. For some patients the volume of saliva may appear excessive and they may have trouble swallowing it, especially at certain times of the day. Sometimes a patient may take an agent to thin their saliva and another to help dry it up. This may seem inconsistent but it works for some people. The thickening of fluids may help, but again the aesthetics need to be considered—thickened water is like mucous, thickened beer has no fizz but slightly thickened orange juice may be quite acceptable. Commonsense and the patient's preferences need to be taken into account.

As swallowing deteriorates, assessment via video fluoroscopy can be very helpful. It can assist in determining the best position in which to feed the patient, the most appropriate volumes to feed (teaspoonful rather than tablespoon), and the texture most safely dealt with by the patient.

It is not common for devices and procedures to be considered to ease the dysphagia. Cricopharyngeal myotomy is of no value and the use of a nasogastric tube or gastrostomy needs to be considered in the light of the patient's overall condition. It has been shown that the use of a nasogastric tube neither improves the quality of a patient's life nor extends the length of their life (Scott & Austin, 1994). The effectiveness of gastrostomy feeding in people with MND is yet to be evaluated. It is important to ask why a gastrostomy is being performed. Is it for symptom relief? Is the patient hungry or thirsty? It is important to keep in mind that MND is a wasting disease and the weight loss and weakness are due primarily to the disease rather than a lack of food intake. The caloric needs of people with severe neuro-muscular disorders are very limited (Gaden et al., 1987).

The ethical dilemmas of ceasing parenteral feeding are complex and the right questions need to be asked—and answered—before these methods are implemented.

## Pain

Motor neurone disease affects the motor neurones and spares the sensory neurones. This means that patients are often very sensitive to pressure and require frequent repositioning to be comfortable. This can be very time consuming for staff and carers, and much patience and understanding is required. Opioid analgesics may be necessary and can usually be given orally. A night-time dose may be helpful to enable the patient to settle and sleep.

The loss of movement and changes in muscle tone can lead to stiffness and pain around certain joints. The shoulder joints being supported by muscles are commonly affected and care must be taken when handling a patient with painful shoulders. Anti-inflammatory agents, especially in the evening, can be helpful. Diazepam may be helpful in relieving muscle cramps which are also relatively common.

## Dyspnoea

The respiratory muscles of the chest and the diaphragm are commonly affected by motor neurone disease. Dyspnoea is a frightening symptom. An open window or a fan may produce a gentle movement of air, bringing comfort. On occasions, small doses of opioids are needed and, if anxiety is significant, diazepam may be helpful. Monitoring oxygenation of the blood is not helpful as it can engender significant anxiety for the patient and their carers.

Ventilatory support is considered by some patients. Occasionally acute respiratory failure is the first presentation and ventilatory support is initiated before the diagnosis is clear. Once ventilatory support has been commenced, decisions to cease it can be very difficult (Goldblatt & Greenlaw, 1989).

## Anxiety and depression

Not unexpectedly in a condition which produces dyspnoea, dysarthria and dysphagia, anxiety is common. It is important that carers are calm, confident and well trained. Anxiety may become more marked in the late afternoon and evening, and a small dose of diazepam in the late afternoon, followed by a larger one on settling, may be helpful.

## Where is care to be provided?

Most people can be cared for in their own homes provided they have carers who are well informed and supported. As the person with MND is often elderly, the carer may also be elderly and possibly in poor health.

Respite care is available in some centres and home-based respite care may be provided by local councils and other organisations. 'Respite care' may be a misnomer as admission to hospital can be a time for the clinical team to reassess symptoms and the need for new appliances. Respite care is often sought when the carer is feeling stressed or a new problem has arisen in the care of the patient. Carers may be reluctant to accept respite admissions, and describing them as periods of reassessment may offer a different perspective.

Patient support organisations exist in all states and can provide support and information for the patient and their carers. They can often assist with the provision of aids and appliances for which there may be a lengthy delay from other sources, such as the government-funded PADP scheme. It is important that the needs of these people are anticipated as the disease progresses rapidly and any delay in the provision of aids may mean they will no longer be appropriate when they become available.

## End stage care

People with MND may access palliative care services at an earlier stage than patients with other terminal conditions and may require services for a longer period. The mode of death varies enormously. Some patients die relatively unexpectedly from respiratory failure—evidence of aspiration or pneumonia is not always apparent and it is postulated that the process is due to the involvement of the respiratory centre itself. With others, aspiration and pneumonia may be clinically evident. Prevention of aspiration is important, as is symptomatic management of infection. The use of antibiotics is appropriate for some people, but needs to be carefully considered for those whose respiratory function is already severely compromised and who are unable to cough or tolerate physiotherapy. Benzodiazepines and morphine may be more appropriate in such cases.

Agents that dry secretions can be helpful but they may produce constipation in some patients, particularly those with diminished food and fluid intake, frailty, and immobility and poor abdominal muscles to help with elimination. Drugs which alter bowel function such as hyoscine and morphine may be the final straw, yet they may also relieve symptoms which are producing greater distress and their use requires good clinical judgment.

It is important to remember at all times that the person with MND has an incurable and progressive disease and all treatment must be directed at symptom relief and comfort. Each person, with their own symptom complex and psychosocial situation, is unique and decisions regarding treatment must involve the clinical team, the patient and their carers. It is of overriding importance that those who are managing the patient's care ask the right questions: what are we trying to achieve? and what will be the consequences of intervening or not intervening? Only when these questions are answered honestly with the involvement of the treating team, the patient and family, will the most appropriate care be delivered (Oliver, 1993).

# References

Gaden, L. & Groom, H.E., et al. (1987). Energy balance, body weight and composition in hospitalized multiple sclerosis patients. *Proceedings* of the 1st Deakin/Sydney University Nutrition Symposium.

Goldblatt, D. & Greenlaw, J. (1989). Starting and stopping the ventilator for patients with amyotrophic lateral sclerosis. *Neurological Clinics, 7*, 798–805.

Kurtzke, J.F. (1982). Epidemiology of amyotrophic lateral sclerosis. *Advances in Neurology, 36*, 281–302.

Muller, M. & Vierregge, P., et al. (1993). Amyotrophic lateral sclerosis and frontal lobe dementia in Alzheimer's disease. *European Neurology, 33*, 320–324.

Oliver, D.J. (1993). Ethical issues in palliative care—An overview. *Palliative Medicine, 7* (supp. 2), 11–13.

Oliver, D.J. (1989). *Motor neurone disease.* Exeter: Royal College of General Practitioners.

Orrell, R. & Lane, R.J.M. (1994). Recent developments in the drug treatment of motor neurone disease. *British Medical Journal, 309*, 140–141.

Oxtoby, M. (1993). *Multidisciplinary management from day one: The neuro-care approach to motor neurone disease.* Romford, Essex: Harold Wood Hospital

Scott, A.G. & Austin, H.E. (1994). Nasogastric feeding in the management of severe dysphagia in motor neurone disease. *Palliative Medicine, 8*, 45–49.

Sedal, L. (1987). The management of motor neurone disease. *Patient Management*, Feb., 85–110.

# 24

# In the Twilight: Alzheimer's Disease and Palliative Care

## Katrina Breaden

She lay curled up like a fetus, showed no reactions, had epileptic spasms, and was given antiepileptic agents. She was spoon-fed with great difficulty. The food had to be inserted deep into her throat in order to elicit her swallowing reflexes. She regurgitated after feeding, and often had to be suctioned. Primitive reflexes had reappeared. She was as powerless as a human being can be and still be alive. (Akerlund & Norberg 1990, p. 16)

Alzheimer's disease (AD) is a devastating condition as the above quote attests. It is a degenerative disorder of the brain that insidiously and progressively affects memory, learning and judgment (Nuland, 1993). While it initially affects recent memory, language and functional abilities gradually deteriorate, until the performance of such tasks as eating, toileting and walking become impossible (Enck, 1992). The cause of Alzheimer's disease is subject to much speculation, and the theories of causation range from environmental toxins to genetic factors. As yet there is no known cure, although several drugs aimed at partially reversing the progression of the disease are presently being trialled (Shapira, 1994).

While AD is primarily a disease of the aged, it is not the natural result of ageing (Mace & Rabins, 1981). Nonetheless, the '85 years and over' group contains the highest incidence of AD (Douglas, 1994). According to recent predictions, the prevalence of those with AD is going to increase, posing challenges for long-term care facilities and for healthcare providers (Breaden & Coulson, 1994).

The terms 'dementia' and 'AD' have been used interchangeably in this chapter for ease of discussion. While there are many causes of dementia, AD does account for the highest proportion of cases (Dept of Community Services & Health, 1990). AD is also sometimes referred to as 'Progressive Dementia of the Alzheimer Type' (Enck, 1992) in recognition that dementia has under its umbrella a number of diseases and conditions.

Dementia has been defined as 'a syndrome due to disease of the brain, usually of a chronic or progressive nature, in which there is a disturbance of multiple higher cortical function' (World Health Organization, 1992, p. 312). This definition, while technically correct, does not reveal the enormous suffering and human cost involved in a disease such as AD, nor does it reveal the mistrust and fear the term evokes in our imaginations.

This chapter is primarily concerned with those nurses and other health care providers who care for people with AD. The discussion is centred around the time in the disease process when the sufferer is as powerless as a human being can be and yet still be alive—that is, its end stage. It starts by outlining the chronic nature of AD and its relationship to palliative care philosophy and then discusses the challenges nurses face when looking after people in the end stage. This discussion is insufficient, however, without offering some solutions to the challenges nurses face. The final section deals with a number of strategies that may enable nurses to continue working in this very demanding area.

## The chronicity of AD

In the end stage, the client no longer ambulates . . . skin breakdown, contractures, urinary tract infections, and pneumonia are common. (Hall & Buckwalter 1991, p. 40)

From the first symptoms of memory loss and mood swings, to the eventual death of the sufferer, the average survival period for a person with AD is eight years. The majority of patients die from its complications, such as pneumonia, rather than from the disease itself (Volicer, Volicer & Hurley, 1993).

Hall and Buckwalter (1991) have assigned descriptive terms to the particular phases of AD in order to outline the management of the disease as it progresses. The terms that they have used are 'forgetfulness', 'confused', 'ambulatory demented', and 'terminal'. Although there is a predictable course to the disease, the phases do not always occur in a linear fashion, nor are there defined boundaries between them. In the 'terminal' or end phase, the sufferer often lies suspended in time and confined to a space which lies at the very edge of existence as we understand it. It is a world that Breaden and Coulson (1994) have termed the 'twilight zone'. Although there are some studies that explore the care of a patient in this terminal phase (Volicer et al., 1989; Fabiszewski, Volicer & Volicer, 1990), little has been written about the issues those nurses and other health care providers who care for these people must deal with.

## AD as a terminal disease

Palliative care is concerned with conditions where cure is no longer possible. Its aim is to 'provide the best quality of life for patients by the control of symptoms and the emotional, psychological and spiritual support of the patient, family and staff' (Gibbons, 1993, p. 127). While cancer is usually the focus of concern, AD as an incurable disease also falls within the scope of palliative care practice. Although the principles of palliative care apply to both AD and cancer, AD differs significantly from the disease process of cancer in a number of important areas. First, families of those with AD have usually dealt with the burden of caring for someone at home for a great deal longer, given that AD may last from between two and sixteen years after the onset of symptoms (Enck, 1992). Second, the sufferers themselves, at the end stage, are seldom able to make decisions regarding their care, which poses with it certain ethical dilemmas. Third, although people in the end stage of AD are considered to be 'terminally ill', it is difficult to predict just how long they will survive (Volicer et al., 1993). Finally, approximately half of the people with mild to severe AD end up in long-term care facilities such as nursing homes (Sax, 1993), and not in family homes, hospices or acute care institutions.

An approach to care that centres around a palliative care philosophy has been shown to be appropriate for a person in the terminal phase of AD. Mortality rates do not significantly increase (Volicer et al., 1989), and a hospice or palliative care approach provides a supportive environment that maximises quality of life for both patient and family (Volicer, 1986; Luchins & Hanrahan, 1993).

## The challenges

> They lie wherever we put them. Awake or asleep, silent or noisy, immobile and seemingly purposeless, the patients with dementia in the terminal stage challenge our clinical skills most acutely. (Hall, 1991, p. 3)

AD has unique care requirements in the terminal stage, which pose certain challenges for all who enter into the circle of care. Breaden and Coulson (1994), in their conversations with the nurses, identified a number of challenges that exist for nurses during this final phase of AD process. These are: the challenges of pain management, caring for a lived body in illness, coping with ethical dilemmas, and the issue of facing loss after loss as each person dies.

## Pain and its management

> Pain is as elemental as fire or ice. Like love, it belongs to the most basic human experiences that make us who we are. (Morris, 1991, p. 1)

Pain is a universal human experience and the management of pain in terminal illness is a cornerstone of palliative care practice. During the end stage of AD, when the individual lays mute and immobile, assessing the prevalence of pain can be especially difficult. The contracted way a person lies in bed must at times involve the experience of pain, as he or she is repositioned, washed and cared for on a daily basis. In addition, the elderly experience other chronic conditions concomitantly with AD, many of which can cause pain (Eland, 1988, cited in Marzinski, 1991). Breaden and Coulson (1994) suggest that nurses who care for people in this terminal phase need to remain vigilant to the possibility of pain, reading the body as text and interpreting facial cues and other non-verbal behaviour. They need to recognise that pain and the possibility of pain forms part of the day-to-day management in this end stage. Therefore, appropriate and reliable pain assessment tools are required for this patient population.

A number of studies have looked at the difficulty of pain assessment in AD patients. Marzinski (1991), in her study of 26 patients with AD who had potentially painful conditions, found that the staff of the unit knew the patients well—that is, they knew what was normal for each patient and took appropriate action when the behaviour deviated from this pattern. As one nurse said, '[w]hen she hurts, she gets very quiet, and doesn't eat. Then I know something's wrong with her' (Marzinski, 1991, p. 27). Jansson et al. (1993) highlighted the importance of reading patients' facial expressions in order to try to understand how they were feeling. The researchers videotaped a number of interactions between two caregivers and four patients in the end stage of AD. They found that 'it was possible to see the patients as capable of having experiences and of communicating them to their caregivers although their ordinary caregivers reported that they were more or less unable to communicate' (Jansson et al., 1993, p. 320). Therefore, nurses caring for people in the end stage need to act as though the person is still able to experience the world around them and can communicate this understanding to others. It is easy to believe that the ability to communicate is lost; however, 'the person will have some remaining abilities, even if they may be inconsistent, fragmented and even momentary' (Douglas, 1994, p. 98).

Pain is obviously not the only symptom requiring attention that emerges in the terminal phase. As Hall and Buckwalter state '[a]t a minimum, these clients should be observed for pain, discomfort, infections, fear, and loneliness' (1991, p. 41).

Some researchers refer to 'knowing a patient' as the basis for nursing interventions (Breaden & Coulson, 1994; Tanner et al., 1993). But how do nurses gain this knowledge? Tanner et al. (1993) suggest that knowing the patient is accomplished first by knowing the patient as a person, and second by knowing the habitual patterns of responses of the patient in certain situations. For the nurses who care for people in the terminal stages of AD, this knowledge is crucial. Knowing the patient as a person is accomplished through the shared interactions nurses have with the families of the person concerned. Through shared stories, nurses are able to find out a patient's likes and dislikes, fill in some of the contextual knowledge that is missing in the end stage when the sufferer can no longer communicate verbally. By observing the patient's non-verbal communication in day-to-day interactions, nurses become able to identify patterns of responses. It is because of 'knowing the patient' that nurses can act as an advocate: 'They talk about their commitment to be vigilant in ensuring that adequate care is given, that early warnings of patient change are attended to, that medical therapies are given with an understanding of the particular patient's responses' (Tanner et al., 1993, p. 278).

There are a number of barriers to nurses getting to 'know' the patient. Organisational structures that move nurses regularly can mitigate against this process. As nurses move from ward to ward, contextual knowledge is lost unless passed on from carer to carer. Economic restrictions on staffing levels in long-term care institutions can also prevent nurses from getting to know the individuals well. Time is inadequate to get to know a patient's likes and dislikes, and habitual patterns of responding, and this knowledge therefore does not form the basis of nursing interventions.

## A lived body in illness

A long term care institution can be a haven, with living, humane, and personalised care. It can also become a snakepit, turning living beings into dehumanised, neglected bodies. (Bergman, 1986, p. 363)

Another challenge in the end stage of AD is to humanise the care of these 'bodies' that lie mute in bed. This care is given by the nurses and the families who surround the patient at this time. It involves a perspective that moves beyond seeing the body as an object, to seeing and remembering the body in which and through which the world is experienced—the lived body (Emden, 1991). This perspective can be difficult for nurses who do not always carry with them the historical knowledge of the person with AD. Nurses face the challenge of delivering care 'somologically' (Lawler, 1991), taking into account both the body as an object and the body as it is lived, and integrating these two aspects in their day-to-day care. Some nurses are able to do this. As one nurse explained it, mind and body are involved in a connected way and so 'how do you separate the person from the body? ... for me the person remains until the end' (Breaden & Coulson, 1994, p. 20). For other nurses, all that remains is the object body, a vacant container; 'the person dies first, the body lingers on' (Breaden & Coulson, 1994, p. 20). The body, however it is perceived, is central to the care nurses give in the end stage.

People in the terminal phase of AD are at a 'nothing more to do' phase, as Glaser and Strauss (1965) have described it, meaning that quality of life becomes the aim rather than interventionist treatments. Lawler refers to the demanding work of this end stage as 'typically women's work' (1991, p. 187). The work is physically tiring—turning and lifting, and dirty, dealing with excretion and decaying flesh. It is work that generally is not valued and is of low status.

As nurses are the keepers of the body in this 'nothing more to do' phase, they face the challenge of providing care for the patient without taking over control of the body, nor of the space that surrounds the body. Strongly connected to the challenge of looking after the person somologically is the challenge of entering into the lived space of another. Bodily boundaries do not end at the skin's surface, they extend into the spaces that surround them. The body becomes the space in which it finds itself (van Manen, 1990). The person who is confined to bed as a result of the disease process is a prisoner in this space:

> The bed ridden demented patient in the final stage of the disease has a very small territory of his own—his bed. He will not even be able to reach his bedside-table and his bed will often be invaded by the caregivers for cleaning, dressing, feeding and so on . . . (Norberg, Melin & Asplund 1986, p. 316)

The challenge for nurses is to be mindful of this unconscious invasion while still keeping the patient's physical environment aesthetically pleasing. As the disease process progresses, the greater the impact the external environment has on the person who 'is a prisoner of the environment, (Douglas, 1994, p. 112). Maintaining pleasant aromas, appropriate temperatures, and familiar objects are some of the ways of providing support and reassurance for the person with AD (Douglas, 1994).

## To feed or not to feed: An ethical dilemma

> During the terminal stage, the nurse and family grapple with difficult ethical issues . . . (Hall & Buckwalter, 1991, p. 41)

In the terminal stages of AD, a patient will often refuse food and fluids. As one nurse said: 'what is left for these people other than to refuse food? No longer can they mobilise . . . no longer can they put a hand up, but they can shut their mouth' (Breaden & Coulson 1994, p. 21). This action by the patient heralds an ethical dilemma—to feed or not to feed.

Nurses who care for severely demented patients often show ambivalent feelings towards the instigation of nasogastric tube feeding when patients are no longer able to take food voluntarily (Akerlund & Norberg, 1990).

Nurses face the choice of inserting a nasogastric tube or continuing to encourage the person to eat. As the main goal of palliative care is to provide comfort, the nurses wonder how that goal can be achieved in this situation. The person in the end stage is unable to communicate his or her wishes, and so the nurse must interpret the person's wishes based on non-verbal communication (Jansson, Norberg, Sandman, & Astrom, 1995). Yet the nurses can never be absolutely certain of the patient's wishes. These decisions are not made in a vacuum—they are always made in consultation with the family and on the basis of the contextual knowledge the nurse has in relation to the patient. It is not an easy decision nonetheless, and nurses require support from each other and from the organisation in which they work, in order to bring to the foreground stories of ethical conflict that Parker (1990) argues have been silenced and devalued: 'Stories once spoken of with passion have been silenced, rendered unspeakable by the threat of being ignored, intimidated, or judged morally inept. Consequently many of these stories stay within the confines of nurses' private dreams' (Parker, 1990, p. 39).

## *Loss on loss: Confronting death, again and again*

> The process of dying and the eventuality of death affects individuals personally, socially and psychologically . . . It is thus difficult for the health care professional to relinquish his/her innate feelings, fears and personal attitudes towards death when caring for the dying and confronting death, in the course of work. (Copp, 1994, p. 552)

Generally death and dying are not discussed openly in our society, and, to use the words of Clark (1991, p. 253), 'we usually know death from a distance'. Nurses are no exception. The progressive nature of AD slowly robs the sufferer of abilities that previously enabled them to interact with the world in a meaningful way. The nurses who enter into a relationship of care with this person cannot help but be affected. They become attached as they follow the sufferer over time, interacting with the family, sharing the vigil and often the pain. Coping with death and dying has traditionally involved denial of feelings of loss, and stoicism (Robbins, Lloyd, Capenter & Bender, 1992).

It has been argued by a number of authors (Kingma, 1994; Copp, 1994; Degner & Gow, 1988) that educational institutions need to better prepare health professionals to care for the dying person and the grieving families. Repeatedly watching and caring for a person who eventually dies can be stressful for the nurses concerned, leading to feelings of helplessness and depression (Kingma, 1994). How do nurses cope with these feelings? They often cope by distancing and suppressing feelings and by concentrating on routines and tasks, rather than on personal interactions (Quint, 1966).

The challenge is for nurses not to suffer from burnout and leave the profession, but to remain in nursing and to develop a positive attitude towards death and dying.

# Strategies to support staff

## Education

Nurses working in the area of palliative care, wherever this care is situated, require education. The International Society for Nurses in Cancer Care (ISNCC) has published a core curriculum in palliative nursing that services the needs of nurses who deliver palliative care (ISNCC, 1991). The ISNCC stresses that education in the areas of palliative care philosophy, communication and counselling skills, pain management, and the control of symptoms other than pain, are core elements in the framework of palliative care delivery. Education in these areas is essential for nurses caring for patients in the terminal phase of AD. This view is supported by nurses who work in the area (Breaden & Coulson, 1994).

## Support

> Social support from fellow nurses is the most effective way to reduce stress and burnout. (Norbeck, 1985, p. 373)

Nurses working in this demanding area require support, not just from the organisation in which they work, but from their peers as well. This support can be accomplished in a number of ways, but the most effective is probably the formation of support groups.

Support groups can provide a forum for both ongoing education and acknowledgment of the shared emotional burden of care. Caring for someone in the terminal phase of a disease process requires an awareness of one's own fears and anxieties in relation to death, and also of the fears and anxieties that the patient's family and friends may hold. Such an awareness is facilitated by a process that looks at motivations, attitudes, coping strategies and the personal limits of the nurse (Hines, 1989).

It has been suggested that nurses who work in long-term care institutions do so because they like working with people (Robertson, Herth & Cummings, 1994). However, nurses may have a more specific reason—the notion of reparation where, because of some previous experience with a death that was poorly handled, they want to atone for this 'failure' in some way (Hines, 1989). Therefore, what motivates someone to care for the dying is an important area that needs to be covered in support groups. In addition, nurses also go through the grieving process with the death of each resident. How this process is handled will often depend on the nurse's own values and beliefs in relation to death and dying. Nurses are not always comfortable with the thought of their own death, let alone the death of each patient they look after. Values, beliefs and the possibility of death anxiety can be explored through death education courses.

Regardless of how it is accomplished, either through group or one-to-one interaction, support is vital if nurses are to stay working in the area of aged care and/or to resist hiding behind a professional mask: 'If they [the nurses] do not have the opportunity of sharing their strain and questions, they are likely to leave this field [terminal care] or find a method of hiding behind a professional mask' (Saunders, 1984, p. 240).

## Rituals of remembering

Ritual behaviour softens the phases of life when we are reminded how hard it is to be human. (Fulghum, 1995, p.113)

Rituals perform important functions in our lives. From birth to death, the procession of time is marked by ritual acts that provide meaning and structure to our everyday existence (Fulghum, 1995).

Rituals form an important part of the behaviour that surrounds the care of a person in the terminal phase of AD. There is a ritual of 'hello' as the nurse enters the room, the ritual of 'goodbye' that accompanies the last breath as it leaves the body. There is the ritual of attending the funeral service to bring to an end one part of a shared journey. One method of support for the nurses who carry out this demanding work is to engage in the ritual of remembering (Fulghum, 1995). Once the person has died, the nurses can join with the family, remembering and sharing, telling stories about the crossing over of the threshold from life to death. The ritual of retelling is one way of 'sanctifying the memory' (Fulghum, 1995, p. 41). The retelling of personal moments, good days and bad, shared with family members and other nurses, provides a conversational space from which to consider and celebrate the life of the person who has died.

## In conclusion

Living with AD brings with it many challenges, for the nurses who care for the sufferer, and for the families. This chapter has explored some of the challenges that exist for nurses working with people suspended in the 'twilight zone'. It began by placing the chronicity of AD within the framework of palliative care, and suggested that as an approach, palliative care was as suitable for the diseases of dementia as it was for other life-shortening conditions. The difficult issues of pain management, caring for a lived body, the dilemma of ethical decision-making and the stress involved in repeatedly caring for the dying was discussed. Strategies for dealing with these issues, including education, support, and the ritual of remembering, have been suggested as ways to assist nurses to continue working in the complex area of end stage dementia care.

This chapter is just a beginning. It can only ever hint at the complexity of what nurses and other health care professionals have to face in the course of their day-to-day work. The work is demanding, but humane nursing care can lessen the anguish of living and dying with AD:

There are no consolations in the diagnosis of Alzheimer's disease. The anguish may be mitigated by good nursing care, support groups, and the closeness of friends and family, but in the end . . . [t]here is no dignity in this kind of death. It is an arbitrary act of nature and an affront to the humanity of its victims. If there is wisdom to be found, it must be in the knowledge that human beings are capable of the kind of love and loyalty that transcends not only the physical debasement but even the spiritual weariness of the years of sorrow. (Nuland, 1993, p.117)

# References

Akerlund, B. & Norberg, A. (1990). Powerlessness in terminal care of demented patients: An exploratory study. *Omega, 21* (1), 15–19.

Bergman, R. (1986). Nursing the aged with brain failure. *Journal of Advanced Nursing, 11,* 361–367.

Breaden, K. & Coulson, I. (1994). Images in the twilight: Alzheimer's disease and palliative care. *The American Journal of Alzheimer's Care and Related Disorders & Research, 9* (5), 15–23.

Clark, G. (1991). To the edge of existence: Living through grief. *Phenomenology and Pedagogy, 9,* 253.

Copp, G. (1994). Palliative care nursing education: A review of research findings. *Journal of Advanced Nursing, 19,* 552–557.

Degner, L. & Gow, C. (1988). Evaluations of death education in nursing: A critical review. *Cancer Nursing, 11* (3), 151–159.

Department of Community Services and Health (DCSH) (1990). *The problem of dementia in Australia.* Canberra: AGPS.

Douglas, E. (1994). Care of people with dementia. In Davis, J., *Older Australians: A positive view of aging.* Marrickville: Harcourt Brace & Co.

Emden, C. (1991). Ways of knowing in nursing. In Gray, G. & Pratt, R. (Eds.), *Towards a discipline of nursing.* Melbourne: Churchill Livingstone.

Enck, R. (1992). Alzheimer's disease. *The American Journal of Hospice and Palliative Care,* September/October, 12–13.

Fabiszewski, J., Volicer, B., & Volicer, L. (1990). Effect of antibiotic treatment on outcome of institutionalised Alzheimer patients. *JAMA, 263,* 168–172.

Fulghum, R. (1995). *From beginning to end: The rituals of our lives.* Moorebank: Bantam Books.

Gibbons, N. (1993). Palliative care provided to patients within an extended care institution. In *Proceedings of the Australian Nursing Federation Gerontology Special Interest Group: First National Conference.* Perth: Promoco Conventions.

Glaser, B. & Strauss, A. (1965). In Lawler, J. (Ed.) (1991), *Behind the screens: Nursing, somology, and the problem of the body.* Melbourne: Churchill Livingstone.

Hall, G. (1991). Examining the end stage: What can we do when we can't do any more?. *Journal of Gerontological Nursing, 17* (5), 3–4.

Hall, G. & Buckwalter, K. (1991). Whole disease care planning: Fitting the program to the client with Alzheimer's disease. *Journal of Gerontological Nursing, 17* (3), 38–41.

Hines, N. (1989). Caring for the carers. In Sherr, L. (Ed.), *Death, dying and bereavement*. Oxford: Blackwell Scientific Publications.

International Society for Nurses in Cancer Care (1991). *A core curriculum for a post-basic course in palliative nursing*. England: Haigh & Hochland Ltd.

Jansson, A., Norberg, A., Sandman, P., & Astrom, G. (1995). When the severely ill elderly patient refused food: Ethical reasoning among nurses. *International Journal of Nursing Studies, 32* (1), 68–78.

Jansson, L., Norberg, A., Sandman, O., Athlin, E., & Asplund, K. (1993). Interpreting facial expressions in patients in the terminal stage of the Alzheimer disease. *Omega, 26 (4)*, 309–325.

Kingma, R. (1994). Revising death education. *Nurse Educator, 19* (5), 15–16.

Lawler, J. (1991). *Behind the screens: Nursing, somology, and the problem of the body*. Melbourne: Churchill Livingstone.

Luchins, D. & Hanrahan, P. (1993). What is appropriate health care for end-stage dementia? *Journal of the American Geriatrics Society, 41*, 25–30.

Mace, N. & Rabins, P. (1981). *The 36 hour day: A family guide to caring for persons with Alzheimer's disease, related dementing illnesses, and memory loss in later life*. Baltimore: Johns Hopkins University Press.

Marzinski, L. (1991). The tragedy of dementia: Clinically assessing pain in the confused, nonverbal elderly. *Journal of Gerontological Nursing, 17* (6), 25–28.

Morris, D. (1991). *The culture of pain*. Berkeley: University of California Press.

Norbeck, J. (1985). Cited in P. Benner & J. Wrubel (1989). *The primacy of caring: Stress and coping in health and illness*. Menlo Park: Addison-Wesley.

Norberg, A., Melin, E., & Asplund, K. (1986). Reactions to music, touch and object presentation in the final stage of dementia. An exploratory study. *International Journal of Nursing Studies, 23* (4), 315–323.

Nuland, S. (1993). *How we die*. London: Chatto & Windus.

Parker, R. (1990). Nurses' stories: The search for a relational ethic of care. *Advances in Nursing Science, 13* (1), 31–40.

Quint, J. (1966). Awareness of death and the nurse composure. *Nursing Research, 15*, 449–455.

Robbins, I., Lloyd, C., Carpenter, S., & Bender, M. (1992). Staff anxieties about death in residential settings for elderly people. *Journal of Advanced Nursing, 17*, 548–553.

Robertson, J., Herth, K., & Cummings, C. (1994). Long-term care: Retention of nurses. *Journal of Gerontological Nursing*, November, 4–10.

Saunders, C. (1984). *The management of terminal disease*. London: Edward Arnold.

Sax, S. (1993). *Aging and public policy in Australia*. Sydney: Allen & Unwin.

Shapira, J. (1994). Research trends in Alzheimer's disease. *Journal of Gerontological Nursing*, April, 4–9, 47.

Tanner, C., Benner, P., Chesla, C., & Gordon, D. (1993). The phenomenology of knowing the patient. *IMAGE: Journal of Nursing Scholarship, 25* (4), 273–280.

van Manen, M., (1990). *Researching lived experience*. New York: State University of New York Press.

Volicer, L. (1986). Need for hospice approach to treatment of patients with advanced progressive dementia. *Journal of the American Geriatric Society, 34* (9), 655–658.

Volicer, L., Seltzer, B., Rheaume, Y., Glennon, M., Riley, M. et al. (1989). Eating difficulties in patients with probable dementia of the Alzheimer type. *Journal of Geriatric Psychology Neurology, 2*, 188–195.

Volicer, L., Volicer, B., & Hurley, A. (1993). Is hospice care appropriate for Alzheimer patients? *Caring*, 50–55.

World Health Organization (1992). *International statistical classification of diseases*, (10th rev.). Geneva: WHO.

# 25

# The Meaning of Death in Residential Aged Care

## Rosalie Hudson and Jennifer Richmond

Demographic data showing the increasing incidence of terminal illness in nursing homes alert gerontic nurses to the option of providing palliative care services in residential settings. While the average length of stay for a nursing home resident is one to two years, a significant number of deaths occur within the first three months and most discharges are due to death (Dept of Health, Housing, Local Government and Community Services, 1993). In the absence of specific, funded specialist services, gerontic nurses have much to offer residents in their care. When the last years of life are recognised as the final stage of growth, residents may be encouraged to move beyond being mere passive recipients of care to offer insights into the meaning of death and dying. While the nurse's rational, problem-solving expertise provides a basis for comfort, security and dignity, intuition and imagination allow the nurse to enter the resident's story so that caring becomes a shared experience.

This chapter focuses on the arena of meaningful care in a residential setting at the end of life, an arena within which the principles of palliative care take their place.

'For the older person, it is not death that is feared as much as the events that surround the experience of dying' (Health Department Victoria, 1991, p. 50). The accuracy of this statement may be attested to by all those who have managed nursing home waiting lists, for issues of death and dying are often apparent in initial conversations surrounding such a significant event as entering institutional care. From the first contact, relationships are established with the resident and family that set the scene for good palliative care. When trust is established, opportunities abound for this stage in the resident's life to be filled with meaning. When the resident enters a community of care, potential for personal growth is acknowledged, a safe passage through the last chapter of life is assured and fears of an undignified death are allayed.

While palliative care principles emphasise the importance of accommodating the dying person's expressed wishes and choices, many of the frail aged in nursing homes lack the cognitive ability to enter such discussions. Such factors do add to the complexity of the care, but opportunity also arises for the gerontic nurse to utilise creative skills to ensure that the care is responsive to each dying resident's needs. Directive care gives way to an exploration of the meaning inherent in each person's experience.

Despite such difficulties as the lack of funding, ageist attitudes and the impaired cognitive function of many residents, it is the role of the gerontic nurse to respond to the needs of the dying resident. In offering palliative care, the nurse discerns what is of significance and value to each resident within the network of their relationships.

# When does palliative care begin?

When an older person enters a nursing home thoughts of dying are often evident.

> 'This is probably my last move.'
> 'I suppose this is where I'll die.'
> 'I wonder what it will be like here, I'd rather die in my own home.'
> 'Will they move me out if I get really sick?'
> 'Will they know to call the priest?'

Families will also have questions, even if they are not articulated.

> 'Will they know how to treat Mum's pain?'
> 'What will happen if Doreen dies in the night? Will I hear the phone?'
> 'How will they possibly have the time to care for Eric the way I've done for the past fourteen years?'

If palliative care is to be family centred and holistic, these questions, concerns and anxieties need to be addressed soon after the resident is admitted. Prompt reassurance invites a positive response. 'Yes, this seems a caring place. I'll be all right here.' The promise of expert palliative care is conveyed not only in the personal and professional encounter with staff, but also in the written information supplied by the nursing home. In listing the services provided, the advertising brochure may include a statement such as:

> This nursing home approaches issues surrounding death and dying with open communication. Regular review is encouraged between resident, family, doctor and staff to formulate an agreed plan of care. Principles of palliative care (where treatment is aimed at providing maximum comfort rather than attaining a cure) are practised so that a resident who is approaching death is cared for with dignity and the best skills available. Wherever possible the resident's and family's wishes are given every consideration. Pastoral care and chaplaincy services are available as required.

# How does palliative care continue?

Although the importance of first impressions is undeniable, it is also important that the many residents who live for years after admission to a nursing home are given every opportunity for personal development in their last stage of life. Through meaningful relationships, the residents may discover what are the important elements in the closing chapter of their lives. Nurses and their allied health colleagues foster self-development by identifying any impediment to growth which may occur through stereotyping the dying person as 'hopeless', 'difficult', 'stubborn', 'confused' or 'demanding'. Carers may conclude the dying resident is 'non-communicative', 'withdrawn', 'depressed', when issues of perception and meaning may hold the key. Through professional observation and enhanced perception, the nurse may uncover factors that influence the dying resident's attitudes to life and death. Personal meaning and growth may be acknowledged through positive influences such as increased self-esteem, dignity and comfort.

Humour plays an important part in self-understanding, both for the nurse and for the dying resident. To recognise a dying resident's humour and wit, to acknowledge the ludicrous and the absurd is to go beyond logic and rationality and to enter with the resident into those precious moments which transcend the immediate tasks and functions and foster self-development even in the last stages of life (Ebersole & Hess, 1994, pp. 717–18). Research has shown that terminally ill patients welcome nurses' humour rather than an undue seriousness at all times (Arblaster, Brooks, Hudson & Petty, 1990, p. 39). The use of creative arts, such as music or story-telling, may also offer a powerful medium for expression of inner feelings, uncovering further meaning hidden within the experience of dying.

Good preparation for palliation is based on thorough knowledge of each resident and family. Careful admission assessment is reinforced by regular reviews when basic data are checked and amended, when changes in family processes are noted and where spiritual, psychological, emotional, and physical needs are explored. Time set aside for regular review is time well spent and may facilitate palliative care at a stage when critical issues emerge. Assessment in an informal atmosphere may elicit important details, as in the following example.

> Mary and Frank, a professional couple, appeared to have a thorough understanding of all the issues of death and dying. At the end of the meeting to review Frank's father's care, they were asked if there were any other issues they wished to raise. Mary, embarrassed and reluctant at first, admitted she often wondered how long the body would remain in the bed after death. Her concern was that sufficient time would be

given for other family members to be contacted. She had heard of other places where the body seemed to be removed with undue haste.*

When an attitude of trust develops between staff, residents and families, the opportunity also arises for fears and anxieties to be explored. However, Mary's final question came as a surprise, prompting the nurse to explore the meaning behind the question. Was there a fear based on past experiences? Was the underlying concern really: how can we be sure he is really dead? Uncovering such anxieties may take time, signifying the need for continuous re-evaluation of each set of circumstances.

Regular review of care arises from the nursing home's policy, a framework which provides a reassuring reference point for residents, families, doctors and staff. Such a policy includes the aim of offering palliative care to every resident. For example, at the review meeting to discuss the care of Frank's father, the breadth of his needs were fully analysed with specific focus on palliative care issues. Among matters discussed were symptom management, dignity factors, preferred site of care (including the option of returning home), resuscitation, nutrition and hydration, medications, use of allied therapies such as aroma, music and massage. Spiritual issues were extremely important to this family and continued liaison with the chaplain was essential. In discussing the context of care, it was apparent that home care was not an appropriate option. It was important, therefore, to ascertain the family's needs in relation to visiting and to reassure that 'out of hours' visiting was appropriate and acceptable.

Mary and Frank were encouraged to participate in the resident's care. They thought this would not be allowed, so the offer was accepted tentatively, their confidence increasing with staff support and encouragement. The family appreciated being consulted prior to each change of treatment, such as the introduction of narcotics. They were given an article to read on the issue of dehydration and were greatly reassured that their father would not be experiencing discomfort when he no longer accepted food and fluids. (Another family, however, may not appreciate such a formal explanation.) Referral to a palliative care specialist was discussed. Mary and Frank appreciated the offer but were content with the local doctor's supervision at that time.

Some of the meaning of Frank's father's death was conveyed in the closing pages of the clinical record. 'Mary and Frank described the grief attached to their loss of community, relationships developed through daily visits over a period of seven years. Frank commented:

---

*Unless noted otherwise, the examples presented in this chapter are composite illustrations drawn from actual events and experiences of various people.

"What will I do without this regular routine in my life?" Mary summed up her feelings: "I will miss coming here. This has been like a second home to me."' '

## New learning opportunities

Each resident's death provides learning opportunities for nursing home staff, signifying the need for responsive education programs. Issues such as multidisciplinary team building, sharing professional expertise and skills, utilising family resources and disease-specific education all become matters of significance when exploring the meaning of death.

Cultural issues require specific understanding based on careful assessment of each resident's and family's needs and the nurse's knowledge of available resources. To explore the meaning of death, in some instances, may involve creative partnership between the resident, family, nurse and culturally appropriate consultant. Being open to learning opportunities in each situation, the gerontic nurse ensures that the care matches the individual's changing circumstances.

Within the broad principles of palliative care, there is an emphasis on 'the notion of continuity of care underpinned by effective communication' (Health and Community Services, 1995, p. 50). Constant reflection on practice may highlight areas for new learning which focus on these issues of continuity and communication. When such a co-ordinated approach is streamlined, doctors, staff, residents and families are given a reliable reference point, minimising elements of confusion and misunderstanding.

## When does palliative care end?

The holistic nature of palliative care indicates that concern for the resident does not end at the moment of death. What does this person's death mean to this particular family, nurse, doctor, other staff, other residents? How does this death affect the whole nursing home community? Inherent in the concept of 'a good death' are such elements as guardianship of the body, completion and closure of the clinical record, emotional care of other residents and staff, and a commitment to bereavement follow-up, formal or informal.

In response to each unique death, the nursing home may interpret and broaden the principles of palliative care in a variety of practical ways:

- announcing the death in an appropriate manner (to other residents, for example);
- the facilitation and management of family viewing at the bedside if this is desired;

- ensuring specific personal, religious or cultural preferences are observed;
- supervision of the transfer of the body, ensuring dignity is maintained;
- notification of funeral times, encouraging attendance from other residents and their relatives, staff and volunteers, where appropriate;
- ensuring family's wishes are respected;
- due care of the deceased resident's belongings.

## De-briefing

Implicit in the concept of continuity of care is the obligation to acknowledge the staff and residents who were significant others, particularly of long-term residents. After the death it may be appropriate to offer some form of staff de-briefing. This may include funeral attendance, a memorial gathering to share memories, or a forum where issues of death's meaning may be uncovered, as illustrated in the following reflection.

> After the death, staff were invited to an informal meeting 'to remember Joe'. Although this is not the practice after every death, it seemed appropriate considering the unusual events surrounding Joe's death and the impact he had on many staff. The meeting was intended as a de-briefing, without the formal title, an opportunity to complete unfinished business with respect to a man whose influence in the nursing home was widespread. Staff from many departments attended, one of the rare times so many of the part-time health professionals met together. All brought their own agendas and needs, from the ego-boosting to the confessional. Many different views of death emerged, staff learned from each other. Why had they never talked like this before?
>
> There were those who said very little, disclosed little, who just seemed to come and observe, to vicariously de-brief, perhaps because this way of communicating in a group was so new. There were others who didn't come, and one boasted, 'I'm no good at group things like that', but then de-briefed informally and expertly in a group of staff talking at the desk just before lunch!
>
> In the end, the experience was esteem enhancing, each person's contribution to Joe's care was recognised. Predominantly, positive events and feelings were emphasised, which left some feeling emotionally warm but carrying unexpressed negative memories to deal with alone.

## Closure of the record

Clear documentation comprises a lasting and tangible record of good palliative care, not only of specific symptom control but of conversations and situations where the meaning of this unique death has been explored.

> Recording practice over time enables nurses to chart the movement in understanding and subsequent actions. This can be the source of encouragement for nurses engaging in critical reflective processes as they identify the impact of new understanding of their existing knowledge, along with the development and instigation of more empowering practices. (Street, 1991, p. 26)

In the clinical record, a description is made of the setting and achievement of goals, providing a valuable source for follow-up reflection and education, and a wealth of material for research. Care at this point centres on clarity in recording what actually happened, not only in the clinical area but also as 'a narrative account of a significant life experience . . . not only the dominant voices, but also the shadows and the silences' (Parker & Gardner, 1992, p. 4).

> 'Edward may have achieved a more peaceful death had the priest been notified earlier. The apparent failure of pain management may have been due to lack of recognition of his spiritual pain.'
>
> 'Amy died as she wished, "alone and with no fuss"'
>
> 'George had expressed fear about dying alone. Staff expressed immense satisfaction that in his last hours a vigil was maintained by his bedside.'
>
> 'Colin had expressed his fear of dying. We listened to one of his favourite Irish tapes. As I sat beside him he even let me stroke his hand, and we shared a joke about his long lost Irish relatives 'hoping to get their hands on my money'. We sat together for two hours until his death at 4 am. All fear had gone from his eyes.'

These extracts from nurses' final entries depict the true meaning of 'progress notes'. They show the nurse's response unfolding in direct relationship to the dying resident's needs, demonstrating the dynamic flow of each interaction. While such responses may be spontaneous, they are often the result of the nurse's intimate knowledge of what is important to the particular resident, in life and in death.

And after the death, where is the informal bereavement visit recorded?

> Agnes visited this morning to speak with some of the residents who shared a room with her sister. Nursing staff welcomed Agnes warmly. Agnes said she had passed by several times and only today felt brave enough to come in. Staff expressed their appreciation of Agnes' courage and admiration of her strength in maintaining such a constant vigil during her sister's last days. Agnes expressed appreciation for the care of her sister and for the promise of a continued welcome by the staff.

The charge nurse's final entry constituted her own de-briefing: 'Agnes and her sister will always have a place in our hearts.'

The neat ordering of all the deceased resident's files provides a source of satisfaction for the nurse responsible for 'tying up the loose ends'. Here is the opportunity to include a photo of the resident, a copy of a letter of thanks forwarded to the doctor, a comment from the music therapist or physiotherapist about their involvement, and relevant comments conveyed by the volunteer. These final touches give meaning to this particular resident's life and death, testifying to this person's significance within the whole nursing home community. With pages neatly ordered, this file becomes a repository of good palliative care practice. Used for formal research or for informal staff discussion, further meaning may be extrapolated to benefit both the carers and future recipients of care.

Staff's efforts to ensure a resident's smooth transition from life to death should not go unacknowledged. Palliative care skills may be advanced and enhanced by a note of praise and encouragement from the director of nursing, congratulating staff on the use of specific innovative strategies, sound clinical management and sensitive communication.

## *Bereavement*

In the absence of formal, funded bereavement follow-up (Hudson & Richmond, 1994, pp. 63, 115–17), staff's attendance at the funeral may have positive implications, not only for staff members, but also for the bereaved family (Hodder & Turley, p. 101). Here, meaning is shared when staff may learn from the eulogy facets of the deceased resident's life which were not formerly known. Staff may gain greater understanding of the significance of this person's life and death, bringing deeper meaning to the nurses' relationship with the family and greater sensitivity towards other dying residents.

Ongoing informal relationships with the family may require flexibility and goodwill from staff who may be required to pause during a busy day and spend a moment with the deceased resident's daughter who 'just popped in while I was passing', or greet the deceased resident's wife who is making an unannounced anniversary visit. While the close relationship established between staff, dying resident and family does not necessarily cease when the resident dies, it may be difficult to manage follow-up visits. A distraught family member may need to be referred to a counsellor when needs and demands outstrip available resources and when staff's attention is, of necessity, focused on the particular needs of those living residents still in their care.

Regardless of intentions, nurses cannot make every death a 'good death'. Neither is the outcome of a resident's death always positive for the family. Depending on the circumstances, family grief may be expressed in negative, critical or recriminative ways, as Irma's story conveys.

> Her husband died in hospital after a fall in the nursing home. She had always been an anxious woman, reluctant to accept that staff would

ever care for him adequately. Staff responded to her vulnerability, tried to understand, listened to her anxieties endlessly, but she never noticed she was being cared for too. The fall seemed to confirm her worst fears and she cursed the day she ever allowed herself to be convinced he should leave home.

It was six months later when a nurse met her in the street. Walking home after a busy day, her mind on what to cook for dinner, the nurse did not notice Irma approaching. Before she knew what was happening Irma was clutching at her, face contorted with emotional pain, words spilling out all around. For ten minutes she harangued the nurse on the street corner, going over and over her husband's care, biting back angry words, talking fast, bitter, bitter. The nurse thought Irma might strike her, but instead she used her words to batter. It was as if the nurse did not exist, the only reality was Irma's anguish.

People waiting for the tram stared at the furious little woman in black. More and more words poured out. She said she could never, never come back, could not even walk past the street of the nursing home. She was not able to recall how fondly her husband had been regarded, nor how much time, care and support the staff had given her. She did not hear the nurse say staff had been thinking of her and that her husband would always be remembered. Suddenly she scurried off, driven by her despair, shopping bags crashing around her, bent low with guilt and deep, deep grief—but trailing anger.

When does palliative care end? Holistic care encompasses all the strategies, efforts and gestures that convey respect for the deceased person and their family. Good palliative care finds its tangible expression in the proper, seemly and dignified closure of one unique life—and its relationships with others. Good palliative care involves exploring new meanings and building on new learning experiences.

## Conclusion

Aged care institutions have the potential to provide for the dying person a sense of community rather than the isolation so often feared. This community of family, residents, nursing and non-nursing staff, volunteers and visitors provide a tangible witness to death as a shared experience where one person's death affects the whole. When a resident's length of stay may be months or years, the nursing home community has time to develop relationships, time to plan carefully each resident's care and to build a climate of trust. Nurses who are attuned to the deeper meaning in a resident's life may then explore, with the resident and family, some of the pertinent issues in relation to death and dying. However, when death occurs soon after admission, little time is available to develop a meaningful relationship. Working against an excellent outcome in each situation is the inadequately structured and funded time for family counselling, staff de-briefing, bereavement visits, staff education, reflection on practice and the research necessary to build on practice.

More research is needed into clinical experience in aged care facilities in order to increase awareness of the broad opportunities for gerontic nurses to practise palliative care. With well-educated gerontic nurses as their role models, students may respond positively to increased opportunities in this area. Gerontic nurses are learning to provide expert physical, spiritual, emotional and social care underpinned by a continuous exploration of the unique meaning attached to each resident's dying.

However, in order to close the gap between the ideal (Health Department Victoria, 1991) and reality, the funding issue needs to be addressed in such a way that older persons in residential care have access to all necessary resources (Hudson & Richmond, 1994, pp. 5–13). As Jecker (1991, p. v) states:

> The aging of society casts into vivid relief a number of deep and troubling questions. On the one hand, as individuals, we grapple with the immediate experience of aging and mortality and seek to find in it philosophical or ethical significance. We also wonder what responsibilities we bear toward aging family members and what expectations of others our plans for old age can reasonably include. On the other hand, as a community, we must decide: What special role, if any, do older persons occupy in our society? What constitutes a just distribution of medical resources between generations? And, how can institutions that serve the old foster imperilled values, such as autonomy, self-respect, and dignity?

In this chapter we have outlined a range of opportunities that exist for gerontic nurses to practise palliative care in the residential aged care setting. In doing so, we invite nurses to enter into creative partnership with dying residents and families, and so bring meaning to each unique life.

# References

Arblaster, G., Brooks, D., Hudson, R., & Petty, M. (1993). Terminally ill patients' expectations of nurses. *The Australian Journal of Avanced Nursing, 7* (3), 34–43.

Department of Health, Housing, Local Government and Community Services. (1993, July). *Nursing homes for the aged: A statistical overview 1991–1992.* Melbourne: Aged and Community Care Planning Section, Residential Program Management Branch.

Ebersole, P. & Hess, P. (1994). *Toward healthy ageing: Human needs and nursing response.* Chicago: Mosby.

Health and Community Services Promotions Unit. (1995, June). *Palliative care in Victoria: A vision: report of the palliative care task force to the Minister for Aged Care.* Melbourne: Department of Health and Community Services.

Health Department, Victoria. (1991). *Caring for people with terminal illness: A manual outlining Victorian palliative care standards and guidelines.* Melbourne: Health Department Victoria.

Hodder, P. & Turley, A. (Eds.) (1989). *The creative option of palliative care.* Melbourne: Melbourne Citymission.

Hudson, R. & Richmond, J. (1994). *Unique and ordinary: Reflections on living and dying in a nursing home.* Melbourne: Ausmed Publications.

Jecker, N. (Ed.) (1991). *Aging and ethics: Philosophical problems in gerontology*. Totowa, NJ: Humana Press.

Parker, J. & Gardner, G. (1992). The silence and the silencing of the nurse's voice: a reading of patient progress notes. *Australian Journal of Advanced Nursing, 9* (2), 3–9.

Street, A. (1991). *From image to action: Reflection on nursing practice*. Warrnambool, Victoria: Deakin University.

# Index

residential care 59–61, 301
*see also* healthcare, influence of
management on
Foucault, Michel 238–9, 247

## G

Gawler, 146
general practitioner 51–2, 76–7, 78, 194, 196, 205, 222
Gleitzman, Morris 98
'good death' *see* death and dying
grief xxxii, 77, 131–2, 136–7, 232, 234–7, 261–2, 263, 269–70, 287–8, 295, 299–300
*see also* bereavement
Grollman, Earl 234

## H

health care, influence of management
on xxviii, 8, 11–12, 14, 16, 57, 72, 74, 79, 80, 110, 112, 136, 178, 188, 198, 246
healthcare providers 107–8, 165
as advocates 266
and decision-making 70–1
doctors 77–8, 143–4, 167, 189–90, 192, 194, 229, 201, 274–5, 299
nurses 167, 275
occupational therapist 275
pastoral carers 78, 167, 275, 293
physiotherapist 275, 299
psychologists 78
social workers 167, 275
speech pathologist/therapist 181, 275, 276
volunteers 77, 78, 299
*see also* nurse, palliative care; team, multidisciplinary; territorialism
Helen House 233
HIV/AIDS 215, 259, 260–1, 262–3
children with 263
females with 262–3
gynaecological symptoms 262, 264
males with 261–2
*see also* AIDS
Hodgins, Philip 98
holistic care ix, xxvii, 5–6, 15, 16, 17, 27, 28, 72, 77, 80, 127, 167, 209, 230–1, 240, 279, 296, 300
home
care xxviii, 37, 62, 71, 73, 158, 166, 195, 199, 219, 222, 263–4, 278–9, 295
as place of death 5, 26–7, 37, 64, 116, 141–2, 155, 163, 195
Home and Community Care (HACC) 58–9, 61
hope xxxi, 91–2, 108–9, 110, 123, 229, 240
*see also* despair
hospice xxi, 218
development xxvii–xxviii, 3, 4–5, 48, 49, 56, 149, 208–9

evaluation 3–4, 7–8
mainstreaming xxi, xxviii, 3–17
models 6, 201–2
movement 3, 4–7
values xxi, xxvii–xxviii, 4–5, 6, 13, 14, 15, 16, 30, 150, 151, 173
hospitals
and palliative care xxxii–xxxiii, 167–8, 173, 191, 193, 195, 199, 206, 218–27, 241–3
as place of death 64, 71, 128, 130–1, 141, 142–4,149, 218, 259
for respite care/reassessment 278–9

## I

ideology 21–2, 30–1
Illich, Ivan xxv–xxvi
immigrants 34–6
intercultural dynamics 35–6
improvement on practice
environment to encourage 169, 214–16
through education and training 43, 112, 130, 169, 212–13
through reflection 111–12, 132–5, 212
*see also* research
integrated care *see* co-ordinated care; continutity of care

## K

Kübler-Ross, Elisabeth xxiv, 103–4, 234

## L

Lawson, Henry 92
legal issues
for doctors 176
for nurses 179–81, 181, 182
*see also* euthanasia
locations of death *see* home; hospital; residential care

## M

mainstreaming of palliative care xxi, xxiii, xxviii, xxix, 11, 13–14, 15–16, 71–2, 73, 79
funding 12–14, 62–6
medicalisation xxi, xxviii, xxix, xxxi, 12–14, 15–16, 73, 79
*see also* palliative medicine
medical dominance xxvi, 15, 58, 77–8, 238
Medicare Incentive Packages (MIP) 48, 62, 64
mental function difficulties 255, 256, 265–6, 282
*see also* AIDS; dementia
multi-infarct dementia *see* dementia
motor neurone disease (MND) 273–9
symptoms 275–8
treatment 273, 276, 277, 278, 279
Murray, Les 92